DESIGNING
ARCHIVAL PROGRAMS
TO ADVANCE KNOWLEDGE
IN THE HEALTH FIELDS

DESIGNING
ARCHIVAL PROGRAMS
TO ADVANCE KNOWLEDGE
IN THE HEALTH FIELDS

Edited by

Nancy McCall

and

Lisa A. Mix

The Alan Mason Chesney Medical Archives
The Johns Hopkins Medical Institutions
Baltimore, Maryland

The Johns Hopkins University Press
Baltimore and London

The Johns Hopkins University Press
2715 North Charles Street, Baltimore, Maryland 21218-4319
The Johns Hopkins Press Ltd., London

A catalog record for this book is available from the British Library.

Library of Congress Cataloging-in-Publication Data

Designing archival programs to advance knowledge in the health fields
  /   edited by Nancy McCall and Lisa A. Mix.
      p.   cm.
    Includes index.
    ISBN 0-8018-4761-3 (hc.   :   alk. paper)
    1. Medical records.   2. Medicine—Archival resources—Management.
I. McCall, Nancy.
    [DNLM: 1. Archives.   2. Information Systems—organization &
administration.   3. Medical Records.   WX 173 D457 1995]
R864.D47   1995
651.5′02461—dc20
DNLM/DLC
for Library of Congress   93-40454

To the memory of Richard H. Shepard, M.D.
1922–1991

Our mentor and our muse

Contents

Figures

Foreword

IN THE HEALTH SCIENCES, archivists, like their cousins, librarians, are faced with both an increasing volume of materials and a proliferation of the formats in which these materials are recorded. The documentation of science, and especially the medical sciences, has increased dramatically in the last half century. Today's medical librarian, for example, must be familiar with not only the traditional paper forms—books and journals—but also online reference databases, full-text electronic knowledge sources, information on compact disks, interactive educational software, and the Internet and the many tools, services, and information resources growing up about it.

The challenges that face the medical librarian also face the archivist who works in the health sciences. For that person, this book is ideal. The contributors rightly emphasize the diversity of archival forms and the essential role of computational techniques in managing records. Because of the immensity and complexity of modern medical documentation, the cost of preserving it, and the built-in redundancy of the data, archives must become more selective about what they decide to acquire and preserve. In many cases, the focus must be on preserving "intellectual integrity" rather than original formats. These points are well made by the authors.

It is reassuring to note that there is an emphasis on the many users (individual, institutional, multi-institutional) and the manifold uses to which archival material is put. This emphasis is apparent in the cogent discussions of such issues as privacy, for example, in the context of student records and patient records. These contemporary considerations are blended with sound advice concerning traditional collection-handling practices.

Compartmentalization in how we produce, handle, and preserve information is no longer acceptable. I believe that the key to success in archival endeavors is close collaboration between scientists, scholars, clinicians, librarians, and archivists. Only by working together to develop new approaches to selecting, organizing, and preserving useful information will today's documents be of maximum use to future generations.

Donald A. B. Lindberg, M.D.
Director
National Library of Medicine

Preface

THIS BOOK EVOLVED largely as an outgrowth of the archival program at the Johns Hopkins Medical Institutions. The archives was founded in 1978 under the direction of Thomas B. Turner, dean emeritus of the School of Medicine; it is dedicated to the memory of Alan Mason Chesney. A former dean of the School of Medicine and a chronicler of its early history and that of the Hospital, Alan Chesney had years before initiated plans to establish an institutional archives.

Whereas the Alan Mason Chesney Medical Archives devoted its first years of existence to locating and processing the late nineteenth- and early twentieth-century records of the Medical Institutions, it soon became clear that the main challenge facing the archival program was how to deal with the uncontrolled proliferation and destruction of contemporary documentation. Because a mechanism was urgently needed to protect critical administrative documentation from loss, the Medical Institutions established a records management program. Operated under the aegis of the archives, the records management unit began on a small scale, concentrating primarily upon central administrative records. As the program expanded to the departmental level, many other types of records, including clinical and research documentation, were deposited in the records management unit. However, precedents could not be found for archival management of the broadening range of clinical and research documentation.

A. McGehee Harvey, who was then archivist, urged that the archives staff undertake a comprehensive study of contemporary documentation at academic health centers. A physician-historian and former director of the department of medicine, Harvey had become concerned about the fate of contemporary documentation while researching the recent clinical and scientific contributions of the staff of the Medical Institutions. Recognizing the value of clinical and scientific documentation for the study and teaching of history, he was alarmed by the large-scale loss and destruction of critical contemporary documentation at Johns Hopkins and at other institutions in the health fields.

Richard H. Shepard, as associate archivist, played a major role in the early stages of the study of contemporary documentation. A physiologist, biomedical engineer, and pulmonary specialist, Shepard guided the staff in the study of scientific and clinical documentation. As a pioneer in computation in the health fields, he encouraged us to explore the technology and use of computers.

Victor A. McKusick, as Chairman of the Archives Advisory Committee, has provided staunch support for the development of both the archival program and this book.

Gert H. Brieger, as director of the Institute of the History of Medicine, has encouraged the archival program and also research for the book to focus on the study of the health fields in the twentieth century. In 1987, the Medical

Archives became part of the Institute of the History of Medicine.

The quality of the archival program has been augmented by the research for and the writing of this book. While the daily work of the archives has provided an opportunity to study contemporary documentation in the health fields on a firsthand basis, research for the book in turn contributed new ideas to the archival program. The confluence of expertise from professionals in many different fields has enriched our research and has also helped to focus the development of the archival program. Collaboration with archivists, librarians, records managers, physicians, scientists, and historians has been crucial to both the management of the archival program and the creation of the book.

Notice: Because practices in the archival, legal, scientific, clinical, and technological fields are constantly changing, the editors and publisher of this volume advise the reader to monitor the most current literature for new developments in these respective fields.

Acknowledgments

A COMBINATION of fortuitous circumstances has fostered the development of this volume. We are particularly grateful for the willingness of colleagues to collaborate with us in this publishing venture and for the availability of financial resources. The National Historical Publications and Records Commission (NHPRC) supported the basic research for this work through a grant for the Johns Hopkins Medical Institutions Records Project and made the book's publication possible through a subvention grant. At the same time, we extend appreciation to the Johns Hopkins Medical Institutions for contributing matching funds for these grants and for supporting the additional research and editing efforts that were needed.

Strategic planning for the archival program afforded a timely opportunity to utilize findings from the NHPRC-supported records project. Ultimately the synthesis of ideas from the records project and strategic planning helped to focus our research. Because of the collaborative nature of the records project, strategic planning, and processes of writing and editing, many individuals have been involved in the evolution of the book. Confronting the archival issues of contemporary documentation in the health fields demanded the expertise of specialists from a wide range of disciplines. Altogether the research, writing, and editing benefited greatly from their involvement. Work with these colleagues from the archival, library, and health fields yielded important insights that helped to shape our ideas.

Our personal thanks go to all those people who provided us with wise counsel and enduring support. First and foremost, we want to recognize our families and friends for their patience and kindness. We are particularly thankful to Charles Mann and Moira Egan for keeping our spirits elevated and our humor intact and to Phoebe B. Stanton for strengthening our resolve.

Past and present staff members of the Medical Archives—William R. Day, Jr., Frances Dukissis, Mary Garofalo, Agota Gold, Nancy Heaton, Catherine Hidalgo-Nuñez-Wohlleben, Marjorie Kehoe, Arian Ravanbakhsh, Gerard Shorb, and Anne Slakey—deserve recognition for their creative ideas and their hard work. Also we thank our student assistants from Johns Hopkins for their contributions: Jeffrey Charles, Alvin Egerer, Daryll Hart, M. Crawford Keenan, Minda Mella, Alison Mneek, John Park, and Mark Stewart. They have helped to pave the way for new concepts and practices in both the archival program and the book. Frances Dukissis has been a mainstay, providing loyal support. She has overseen the administrative details of the grants and has extended herself in numerous other ways to keep the projects on course. We owe her a tribute for her dedication and her attention to everyone's morale.

The Archives Advisory Committee and the archival policy committees in the various divisions of the Medical Institutions have helped to guide our research as well as our planning endeavors. The members of these committees made contributions both collectively and individually. Whenever we have needed their assistance, they have been unfailingly accessible and receptive.

In general, the community of the Medical Institutions—the Johns Hopkins Hospital, the School of Hygiene and Public Health, the School of Medicine, and the School of Nursing—provided an intellectually stimulating ambience for our work. The opportunity for discourse with faculty members, students, and staff members enabled us to hone thoughts and at the same time broaden perspectives. Colleagues from Johns Hopkins to whom we are particularly grateful include Susan Abrams, S. William Appelbaum, Dorothy Brilliantes, Gert Brieger, Louise Cavagnaro, Frederick DeKuyper, Elizabeth Fee, Patricia FitzGerald, Patricia Friend, Sukon Kanchanaraksa, Raymond Lenhard, Nina Matheson, Victor A. McKusick, Robert E. Miller, Julia B. Morgan, Edward Morman, Kathleen Mulford, Lori Ocvirk, Phoebe Sharkey, Earl Steinberg, and James Wirth.

We extend special appreciation to the following individuals for their participation as consultants to the Records Project: Haroutune K. Armenian, Queta Bond, Cecelia DiGiacomo, John Dojka, Clark A. Elliott, Richard Giordano, Victoria Harden, David Himmelstein, Peter Hirtle, Susan Horn, Ward Houston, Mary Littlemeyer, Kenneth Ludmerer, Harry M. Marks, Whitney Minkler, Charles Rosenberg, Kenneth Thibodeau, and Steffie Woolhandler.

Communication with colleagues from abroad has enriched both our research and writing: Ann M. Mitchell and Irene Kearsey (Australia); Barbara L. Craig and Heather MacNeil (Canada); and Richard Giordano, Julia Sheppard, and Jane Williams (England). In addition, colleagues from various parts of the United States have also been generous with their time and expertise: Patsy Gerstner, Sona Johnston, Richard Knapp, Joan Krizack, Adele Lerner, Edward Papenfuse, Helen Samuels, Nancy Seline, Robert Sink, Laura G. Thomforde, Joan Warnow-Blewett, and Marianne Zawitz. Frank Burke performed a

particularly valuable professional service by reading and critiquing the manuscript in its entirety. We hasten to add, however, that any errors in fact or judgment that may be found are our responsibility and not that of those many colleagues who have advised us.

A highly talented and dedicated team has enhanced the overall publication process: Deborah McClellan, Susan Shock, Patricia Stephens, Miriam Kleiger, and Linda Forlifer provided excellent copyediting assistance; their skills of composition and verbal precision have helped to articulate complex subject matter. Agota Gold and Marjorie Kehoe assisted in the research for illustrations and coordinated the reproduction of photographs. Barbara Lewis spearheaded concepts for graphics, design, and layout. Peter Smith served as an arbiter for visual refinements.

Wendy A. Harris, the medical editor for the Johns Hopkins University Press, deserves special recognition for her efforts in nurturing the development of the book and shepherding it into print. Laurie Baty, Richard Jacobs, and Nancy Sahli of the NHPRC staff smoothed the administration of grants for both the records project and the publishing subvention. We particularly appreciate the forbearance they showed in arranging extensions for the publishing grant when other commitments interfered with our original schedule.

In compiling this list of acknowledgments, we are reminded that a remarkable number of colleagues have collaborated with us at every major juncture—research, writing, editing, and production. Our sincere thanks go to one and all.

Introduction

THIS BOOK is intended to serve as a catalyst for change. We hope that it will stimulate archives in the health fields to reconceptualize their programs so that they can deal more soundly and effectively with the surfeit and the complexity of contemporary records. In essence the book is to be used by archival programs as a guide to chart a course of change. Because of the vast quantity of documentation being generated in the contemporary health fields, archival programs must resort to new strategies for acquisition. Rather than expand their acquisition activities to keep pace with the growing amount of records, they need to adopt strategies with stricter controls over content and quantity. They must begin to develop their holdings more selectively and on a smaller scale. However, if they are to accommodate a representative selection from the broadened base of documentation in the health fields, archives must also widen the scope of their holdings to include a range of different formats and media and new areas of scientific and clinical practice. We recommend that each archives design an acquisitions plan that is to be based upon the scope and scale of available resources. These resources include not only fiscal opportunities for program development but also the quality of the documentation itself and the presence of a vital user population.

In this era of diminishing resources in the health fields, approaches to the development and management of archival programs must become more practical and cost-effective.

Our objective is to help archives launch program change through concepts of rational planning based on available resources. To this end we introduce strategies for development and management of holdings as well as user services. We recommend that the focus of the various acquisition activities of an archival program be made more unified and that policies and procedures for the management of these activities be standardized and integrated.

Our ultimate goal is to introduce a program model that will function as a vehicle for advancing knowledge in the health fields. To accomplish this end, the model is fundamentally use-oriented. At the acquisitions level, this model advocates a highly selective approach. The selection of acquisitions is to be guided by a rational plan that will serve the mission of the parent institution. Criteria and standards for selection should be based on the intellectual scope and values of the institutional mission. The concept for the program should be rooted in the mandated functions of the institution. These may include teaching, research, and health care delivery. On a broader and more visionary level, the program should be designed to serve as a vital cultural force for education and research.

A five-year grant from the National Historical Publications and Records Commission (NHPRC) enabled the staff of the Alan Mason Chesney Medical Archives of the Johns Hopkins Medical Institutions to conduct studies of contemporary records not only at

Johns Hopkins but also at other academic health centers. The research activities supported by the NHPRC grant in turn contributed enormously to strategic planning efforts in the Chesney Archives. Through these two projects the staff has studied the changing documentation base of the health fields and has analyzed the implications of these changes for archival programs. A synthesis of the findings from these projects has formed the approach that we introduce.

Our work has also benefited greatly from several congruent studies conducted by archival colleagues working in related areas. Studies being conducted at the Center for the History of Physics, and the Beckman Center for the History of Chemistry, have enabled us to gain a better overview of the terrain of "big science"—the large-scale collaborative studies that span many fields and involve many institutions. In addition, documentation strategy studies of the broad-based and complex institutions in which "big science" is practiced have also contributed significantly to our approach. The opportunity to participate in Joan Krizack's documentation study of the U.S. health care system marked a major turning point in our work. Krizack's project enabled us to hone our focus on the study of documentation at academic health centers through analytic studies of the major functions of these institutions.

What emerges in the archival field is a need for both inter-institutional and intra-institutional collaboration in the selection and preservation of critical contemporary documentation, as well as a shift in archival theory to accommodate the vast size and the complexity of the contemporary documentation base. Archives must make adjustments in both theory and practice if they are to manage the documentation from large collaborative studies, as well as other documentation being generated within the specific context of their parent institutions.

Because the studies from the Beckman Center and the Center for the History of Physics describe the range of documentation in various scientific fields, these studies also serve as a guide to the types of documentation that are found in modern science. Moreover, Krizack's project demonstrates how archivists in the health fields may more effectively document the types of institutions that compose the U.S. health care system through functional analysis. In the intellectual progression of these projects, which go from fields of science to institutions in the health system, our work focuses largely on the repository level. At this focal point we suggest how archival programs may adapt both philosophically and pragmatically to accommodate the range of new documentation being generated at institutions in the health fields.

Although the tasks facing archivists in the health fields are daunting, they nevertheless present challenging opportunities for archivists to participate in the information revolution that is occurring in these fields. To deal with transformations in the use and communication of documentation, archivists are compelled to introduce new modes of archival practice. Managing the rapidly expanding documentation base requires the collaboration of many professionals from varied disciplines. Because of the complexities of format, content, media, and means of communication, the knowledge and the technical expertise of many individuals, ranging from clinicians and scientists to librarians and archivists, must be enlisted in the effort to develop new approaches to the selection and preservation of critical data and information that are needed for ongoing and future use.

Now more than ever, archivists have the opportunity to work directly with both the creators and the users of documentation. Archivists must gain a better understanding of content and of patterns of use to make more informed selections of acquisitions. The ephemeral and fragile media of contemporary documentation demands that archivists become more actively involved in the management of current records, in order to ensure that critical data and information in these media are targeted early and are either scheduled for regular refreshment or transferred to a more stable medium. To guarantee the survival of an archival base for future generations, it is the professional responsibility of archivists to recommend quality controls for the generation and maintenance of current documentation.

Contributors

PAUL G. ANDERSON, PH.D., Associate Director for Archives and the History of Medicine, Washington University School of Medicine, St. Louis, Missouri

JOHN DOJKA, M.A., M.L.S., Institute Archivist and Head of Collections Development, Rensselaer Polytechnic Institute, Troy, New York

NANCY A. HEATON, M.L.S., C.A., Former Processing Coordinator, Alan Mason Chesney Medical Archives, Johns Hopkins Medical Institutions, Baltimore, Maryland

JOEL D. HOWELL, M.D., PH.D., Associate Professor, Department of Internal Medicine, Department of History, Department of Health Services Management and Policy; Director, Program in Society and Medicine; University of Michigan Medical Center, Ann Arbor, Michigan

JOAN D. KRIZACK, M.A.T., M.S., Hospital Archivist, Children's Hospital, Boston, Massachusetts

NANCY MCCALL, M.L.A., Archivist, Alan Mason Chesney Medical Archives, Johns Hopkins Medical Institutions, Baltimore, Maryland

DEBORAH MCCLELLAN, PH.D., Research Associate, Department of Pharmacology and Molecular Sciences, Johns Hopkins Medical Institutions, Baltimore, Maryland

NINA W. MATHESON, M.L., Director Emeritus, William H. Welch Medical Library, Johns Hopkins Medical Institutions, Baltimore, Maryland

LISA A. MIX, M.L.A., Processing Coordinator, Alan Mason Chesney Medical Archives, Johns Hopkins Medical Institutions, Baltimore, Maryland

ARIAN D. RAVANBAKHSH, B.A., Former Archival Assistant, Alan Mason Chesney Medical Archives, Johns Hopkins Medical Institutions, Baltimore, Maryland

GERARD SHORB, M.L.A., Coordinator for Reference and Records Management, Alan Mason Chesney Medical Archives, Johns Hopkins Medical Institutions, Baltimore, Maryland

ANNE SLAKEY, B.A., Former Archival Assistant, Alan Mason Chesney Medical Archives, Johns Hopkins Medical Institutions, Baltimore, Maryland

PHILIP D. SPIESS II, M.A., M.PHIL., Museum Consultant, Associate Professorial Lecturer in Museum Studies, George Washington University, Washington, D.C.

JANE WILLIAMS, M.S., European Liaison Manager, University of Manchester, Manchester, United Kingdom

PART I

THE BROADENING BASE AND CHANGING MEDIA OF EVIDENCE IN THE HEALTH FIELDS

AN ARCHIVES IS defined primarily by the scope of its holdings and the type of institution in which it is based. To gain a better understanding of the role of archives at institutions in the health fields, it is first necessary to study the mandated functions of these institutions, their administrative structure, and the kinds of evidence that they generate and use in their corporate and functional activities. For appraisal purposes it is particularly important to consider how evidence is used within the context of the mandated functions of these institutions, such as teaching, research, and health care delivery. Patterns of current usage are usually reliable indicators of the ways evidence may be utilized in future archival reference and research.

The chapters that follow in Part I serve as an introduction to archival appraisal issues in the health fields. They provide an overview of the kinds of evidence that are produced at teaching, research, and health care delivery facilities in the health fields and discuss both current and potential uses of this broad spectrum of evidence. Particular attention is devoted to how these types of evidence may be employed to further studies in the social sciences as well as in the health, life, and biological sciences.

In general, the nature of how empirical evidence is generated and used in a particular field affects the terms of archival practice for that field. To assess the place of archival practice in the health fields, it is therefore logical to proceed by examining the range of evidence in these fields and analyzing how it is used in various key functions.

As a means of focusing the discussion of archival practice in the following chapters and throughout the other sections, this preamble to

Documentation—the manifestation of empirical evidence. *Documentation* includes both physical and intellectual manifestations of evidence. The term may refer either to a single item or to multiple items.

Format—the way by which evidence is articulated. The term *format* may refer either to an intellectual representation of evidence or to an actual material sample of evidence. In turn the two main categories for classifying the formats of evidence are recorded documentation and material evidence. Recorded documentation encompasses inscriptive, visual, and aural recordings of evidence. Material evidence includes a broad range of natural and chemical specimens and artifacts (materials made by human work).

Medium—the intrinsic composition of evidence. The term *medium* refers to the state (physical, chemical, electronic) in which the evidence exists.

Fig. I.1   **Constituent elements of empirical evidence.**

Part I defines general concepts of evidence in the health fields. These definitions in turn serve as a common vocabulary for the entire volume. See Figure I.1 for a definition of the constituent elements of evidence and Figure I.2 for the range of empirical evidence in the health fields.

Most theoretical and practical activity in the health, life, and biological sciences is grounded in the use of empirical evidence. Because of this innate empiricism, institutions in the health fields function mainly in an inductive mode, collecting large bodies of physical and intellectual evidence to analyze for purposes of research, teaching, policy making, administration, and clinical care. Maintaining such vast amounts of empirical evidence imposes severe strains on the institutions that have generated them. See Figures I.3 and I.4 for an overview of the uses of empirical evidence in the health fields.

In general, the dictates of professional ethics and regulatory bodies require that individual scientists and clinicians and their parent institutions preserve the evidence upon which their research findings, clinical decisions, and policy making are based; furthermore, this evidence must be retained for varied, and of-

ten unspecified, periods of time. As a result, large quantities of often redundant evidence accumulate at institutions in the health fields. The constantly mounting collection of evidence and the pressing need to manage it present special administrative and economic challenges at these institutions.

The sheer quantity and complexity of the accumulated evidence in the twentieth-century health fields also bring many new issues to archival theory and practice. Chief among these are the appearance of new forms of evidence and fundamental changes by which evidence is produced and communicated. These transformations in the scale and basic phenomena of evidence call for a reexamination of traditional archival concepts. New criteria and standards for archival practice must be adopted to accommodate the broadening base and changing media of evidence in the health fields.

To balance the evidential and informational needs of their institutions, archival programs in the health fields will have to function more in the mode of manuscript repositories. They will have to limit and refine their acquisition policies and base selections upon the criteria and standards of highly specific documentation plans, and thus leave inappropriate and out-of-scope materials behind for disposal or transferral to other types of repositories. The intellectual objectives of the acquisition policies should be to select a core of documentation that will advance the evolution of knowledge in the health fields (Fig. I.5).

In combining both archival and manuscript principles, these archival programs will have to develop acquisition plans that enable them to document the corporate structures as well as the mandated functions of their institutions. These plans should allow for a statistically representative selection of evidential and informational documentation in a wide variety of formats, including inscriptive, visual, and aural formats, as well as examples of material evidence when such evidence is necessary to augment recorded documentation. In the health fields the presence of new formats of evidence has commanded archival attention. The expanding functions of health care delivery, teaching, and research have contributed to the broadening scope of evidence in new formats and to the rapid profusion of such evidence. In addition, the rise of technology in the health fields has also had an impact on the ability of individuals and institutions to produce and disseminate evidence. Technological developments have not only contributed to the genesis of new formats for presenting evidence but also greatly accelerated the means by which that evidence is produced and communicated.

As archival programs acquire a wider range of documentation in new and varied formats, they will nevertheless have to concentrate on acquiring evidence that supports key institutional objectives and reflects the scope and scale of their parent institutions. To serve their institutions more appropriately, archival programs must also widen their pool of selection. In addition to administrative records, they will have to include a variety of other types of documentation from the full spectrum of the institution's mandated functions such as teaching, research, and health care delivery.

As archival programs are pressed to examine a wider range of institutional evidence, they must in turn broaden their criteria and standards for selection. Archival programs in the health fields are faced with a particularly pragmatic dilemma: while the overwhelming quantity of evidence compels them to collect more selectively and on a smaller scale, the greater variety of materials requires that they expand the scope of their acquisitions to include a more representative selection of documentation. However, with astute planning, intelligent compromises can be made between these competing demands.

In archival practice, the acquisition policies of repositories are usually focused around the missions of the parent institutions. The objectives of the institutional mission should ultimately set the agenda for the selection of acquisitions. For instance, if the parent institution specializes in health care delivery and research, the archival program bears an obli-

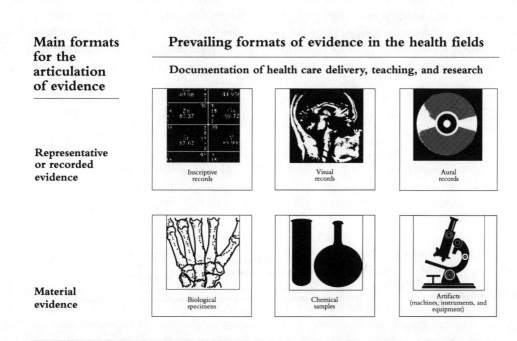

Fig. I.2   **The range of empirical evidence in the health fields.**

gation to make provisions in its acquisition policy for the institution's clinical and scientific documentation. In selecting clinical and research evidence to add to its holdings, an archival program must consider the multifaceted value of these materials. To assess the reference and research value of these materials, archival programs should weigh not only their administrative and historical significance but also their relevance for scientific and clinical research. The acquisition of materials for purposes other than administrative requirements and historical study marks a departure in traditional archival practice. At archives in the health fields one of the most compelling reasons for urging the acquisition of clinical and scientific evidence is to conserve untapped resources for new research applications. Some of these materials may still be viable for ongoing clinical and scientific study. See Figure I.6 for an overview of issues concerning the preservation of data, information, and knowledge in the health fields.

In the decades since World War II, more clinical and scientific evidence has been produced than at any other time in history. While government and private foundations financed expansion of research at institutions in the health fields, the payment plans of federal and private insurers enabled unprecedented growth in health care delivery services. The surge in research and health care delivery activities has been accompanied by a commensurate increase in the production of evidential and informational documentation.

Technological advances have also contributed to the proliferation of research and clinical documentation. Innovations in technology have expanded both the formats and media of documentation; in addition, they have accelerated both the production and the dissemination of documentation. Although these new technical applications have led to many refinements in the recording and communication of evidence, they have also contributed to redundancy.

An unfortunate result of the overproduction of evidence is that a large portion of it is underused. Because of the resources that have gone into the creation of research and clinical documentation, some pragmatic-minded legislators, policy analysts, and administrators of funding agencies, foundations, and institutions in the health fields are interested in finding ways to increase the yield of knowledge from the materials that have been amassed. They have recommended that the scientific and clinical documentation that is routinely amassed be put to more productive uses. In recent years officials from both the private and the public sector have urged that researchers expand their collaborative efforts and conserve basic resources by sharing the data and information that they have generated in ex-

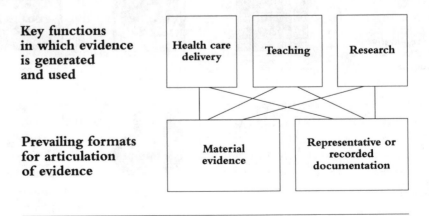

Fig. I.3 **The generation and use of empirical evidence in the health fields.**

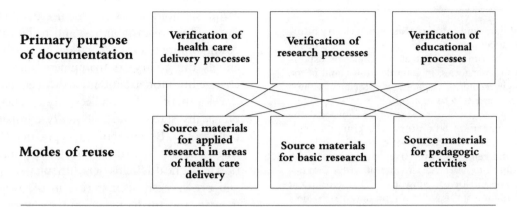

Fig. I.4 **Multiple uses of empirical evidence in the health fields.** Documentation that is generated to verify processes of health care delivery, teaching, and research is frequently reexamined and reutilized for purposes other than those for which it was originally intended.

perimental and observational studies.

Thus, a new role for archival programs in the health fields is emerging. They must begin to promote the recycling of research documentation at their institutions. Furthermore, they will have to expand the scope of their acquisition policies to acquire research and clinical documentation that may be viable for reuse in related or other forms of study. In view of the quantity of documentation being generated in the health fields, archival programs are, however, limited in what they may reasonably acquire. Yet, if they were to restrict their preservation activity to the boundaries of their repositories, they would not serve their institutions well. They will have to assume a broader share of the professional responsibility for recycling institutional documentation that has the potential for reuse by rescuing critical research and clinical documentation and, if their own programs are faced with collecting limitations, they must make a concentrated effort to transfer this documentation to other types of repositories where it may be put to effective intellectual use. In some cases it may be more appropriate to place certain materials in scientific or clinical data centers or to transfer them to other appropriate repositories where they will be made accessible for research.

As more archival programs in the health fields begin to focus on the clinical and re-

search activities of their institutions, they will find that they must accession a broader spectrum of formats and media, thus departing from the long-held archival concentration on textual materials in paper-based media. Repositories in the health fields now face new challenges as they attempt to accommodate the full range of formats that are used in the presentation of evidence at their institutions. Their acquisition policy must include provisions for both recorded documentation (inscriptive, visual, and aural formats) and actual samples of material evidence (biological, chemical, and artifactual).

During the twentieth century, recorded documentation in the health fields has become increasingly visual. Beginning with applications of still photography at the turn of the century, the use of visual formats for the presentation of scientific and clinical evidence has grown considerably. The advent of motion pictures, x rays, and radiological imaging has further altered research, clinical, and teaching practices. Likewise, but on a smaller scale, the use of sound recordings has transformed some common research, clinical, and teaching practices.

The expansion of formats and media presents vexing problems and at the same time new opportunities for archival practice. Whereas the passive and indiscriminate acquisition of these highly varied formats and media may

Production of raw data and information—the primary manifestation of recorded documentation. This stage of recorded documentation occurs at the time of direct observational or experimental intervention in laboratories, in clinical settings, and in the field. Examples include records of diagnostic and therapeutic procedures (e.g.,blood chemistries, fetal monitor charts, electrocardiograms, MRIs, x rays, photographs of gross specimens, dictated operative notes, etc.); charts of laboratory experiments (e.g., autoradiography, karyotypes, etc.); collections of statistical data and information (e.g., health census records, survey records, etc.). This documentation is utilized to chart the activities of health care delivery and research. The intellectual content of documentation at this stage is usually unique and is seldom reproduced or widely circulated at the time of origin. However, it may be recalled for future purposes of patient consultation, to be used as defense in legal and regulatory reviews, and to support clinical and scientific findings that are eventually published. Whereas many journals in the health fields now request that raw data be included with manuscripts at the time of submission, some even stipulate that raw data be issued in conjunction with the publication of articles.

Interpretation of data and information—the secondary manifestation of recorded documentation. At this stage raw data and information are assessed and classified. Examples of interpreted documentation range from diagnostic reports and results of experiments to survey and statistical summaries. These interpretations are used to evaluate the course of research and health care delivery. They serve as indicators of quality and monitors of progress. Clinicians, scientists, and students present analyses of new data and information for discussion with their peers. These analyses may consist of case presentations in medical grand rounds, seminar papers, poster presentations, papers at professional meetings, etc. Because such reports are intended to convey news of the most recent scientific and clinical findings, the professional community regards them as important sources of information about evolving knowledge. This stage of documentation is often an antecedent or precursor to publication.

Synthesis of knowledge—the tertiary manifestation of recorded documentation. At this stage the highly refined intellectual products of basic and applied research evolve. It includes studies that are synthesized from analysis of the primary and secondary stages of data and information. Most documentation at the tertiary stage is published or issued under the aegis of peer review, which bestows credibility and professional endorsement. Forms of this tertiary documentation appear in books, journals, video and audio tapes, and computerized data and information bases. These various vehicles of communication are mass-produced, intensely marketed, and widely disseminated throughout the health fields. Because new knowledge is postulated and verified at the stage of tertiary documentation, this form of documentation is classified as knowledge-based.

Fig. I.5 **Key stages in the evolution of knowledge in the health fields.**

result in holdings with intellectual limitations, physical instabilities, and technical incompatibilities, a more focused approach that entails the ability to manipulate and interchange both format and media will enable the development of intellectually coherent, physically stable, and technically compatible collections. Because of the ephemeral and fragile nature of many types of documentation in the health fields, it is difficult to acquire and preserve some materials in the original formats and media in which they were produced. Because some of the formats and media are easily transmutable, opportunities do, however, exist for the interchange of content. The same data and information may be transmuted from one format and medium to another, allowing archives an unprecedented choice in determining the composition of their holdings. For instance, digital computer processes allow the rapid transformation of certain data and information from inscriptive formats to digitized visual analogues that may be easily manipulated and rapidly communicated. Because errors may occur when information and data are transferred from one format and medium to another, standards and controls must be followed to protect the integrity of evidence when archival programs engage in the retrofitting of documentation for preservation purposes.

To guard against redundancy and duplication of basic evidence in their acquisition activities, archival programs will have to be especially discerning in their selection of formats. Their appraisal procedures must consider whether particular formats augment or overlap others. For instance, the numerical entries from an experiment that are recorded in a logbook may be sufficient to verify the researchers' findings and to recreate a visual analogue in the form of a graph or a chart. In such a case, it may not always be necessary for the archives to maintain the graphic holdings that accompany the logbooks. If, however, the graphs were heavily annotated with handwritten notes containing unique information, a greater argument would exist for maintaining them.

In some instances in which a particular body of evidence is difficult to articulate in any one format, different formats may have to be assembled, from recorded documentation to actual samples of specimens, chemicals, and artifacts. When certain evidence is articulated in one format more clearly than in others, the most definitive example should be considered for selection.

The introduction of new media for the production and communication of evidence presents especially compelling challenges to archival theory and practice. The fact that some new media are not only highly ephemeral but also largely machine-dependent raises many complex issues regarding their long-term preservation and use. Whereas archival philosophy has long been rooted in the preservation of the original physical manifestation of evidence, such an approach is no longer feasible in the case of many new media. Archival theory and practice must readapt concepts of preservation to fit the conditions that twentieth-century technologies have imposed; archivists are called upon to focus on preserving the intellectual integrity of evidence rather than its specific physical manifestations.

Data and information (raw and interpreted)—Much of this primary and secondary stage documentation is ephemeral in terms of both media and use. The media in which most primary stage documentation is manifested (electronic, chemically-coated strip charts, etc.) are often fragile, with short life spans. If special measures are not taken to provide long-term back-up for both electronically stored and hard-copy documentation, these materials will not survive for long periods of time. Generally documentation from these stages is most intensely used shortly after it is produced. Various laws and regulatory requirements stipulate that research and clinical data be maintained for designated periods of time by the institutions in which they were generated. After statutes of limitation expire, these materials may be destroyed. In some instances, selections of primary and secondary documentation that have long-term and ongoing use in clinical and research activities may be preserved and placed in repositories such as data centers and archives where they will be available for further study.

Knowledge-based documentation—The principal repositories for knowledge-based documentation are libraries. Because of the rapid production of new knowledge-based documentation, the management of these materials within libraries is constantly changing with older materials being supplanted by newer ones. As a result libraries in the health fields frequently readjust their collecting priorities and regularly weed their holdings. Even though these libraries focus on literature from the mainstream of modern medical knowledge, they also preserve examples of classical precedents. Libraries in the health fields as a rule place older tertiary materials in rare and historical book collections. Archives and manuscript repositories normally limit their holdings to unique forms of primary and secondary documentation; they do not acquire mass-produced tertiary documentation unless it is a rare example that augments their holdings. Libraries in the health fields have played an active role in establishing preservation programs for printed and computerized materials.

Fig. I.6 **Issues concerning the preservation of data, information, and knowledge in the health fields.**

BIBLIOGRAPHY

ATHEY, T., AND R. ZMUD. 1988. *Introduction to Computers and Information Systems*. Glenview, Ill.: Scott, Foresman and Co.

BADASCH, S.A., AND D.S. CHESEBRO. 1988. *The Health Care Worker: An Introduction to Health Occupations*. Englewood Cliffs, N.J.: Prentice-Hall.

BARZUN, J., AND H. GRAFF. 1977. *The Modern Researcher*. New York: Harcourt Brace Jovanovich.

BELL, D. 1976. *The Coming of Post-industrial Society: A Venture in Social Forecasting*. New York: Basic Books.

CLARKE, E., ED. 1971. *Modern Methods in the History of Medicine*. London: Athene Press.

COMMITTEE ON SCIENCE, ENGINEERING, AND PUBLIC POLICY. 1992. *Responsible Science: Ensuring the Integrity of the Research Process*. Washington, D.C.: National Academy Press.

HUFFMAN, E.K. 1972. *Medical Record Management*. 6th ed., ed. E. Price. Berwyn, Ill.: Physicians' Record Co.

KOHLSTAD, S.G., AND M. ROSSITER, EDS. 1986. *Historical Writings on American Science: Perspectives and Prospects*. Baltimore: Johns Hopkins University Press.

LEE, P.R., AND C.L. ESTES, EDS. 1990. *The Nation's Health*. Boston: Jones and Bartlett.

LIEBER, J.G. 1980. *Managing Health Records: Administrative Principles*. Germantown, Md.: Aspen Systems.

LILIENFELD, A.M. 1976. *Foundations of Epidemiology*. New York: Oxford University Press.

LOWENTHAL, D. 1985. *The Past Is a Foreign Country*. Cambridge: Cambridge University Press.

MCKUSICK, V.A., ED. 1978. *Medical Genetic Studies of the Amish*. Baltimore: Johns Hopkins University Press.

ROTHSTEIN, W.G. 1987. *American Medical Schools and the Practice of Medicine: A History*. New York: Oxford University Press.

TEMKIN, O. 1977. *The Double Face of Janus*. Baltimore: Johns Hopkins University Press.

TEMKIN, O., W.K. FRANKENA, AND S.H. KADISH. 1976. *Respect for Life in Medicine, Philosophy, and the Law*. Baltimore: Johns Hopkins University Press.

U.S. PUBLIC HEALTH SERVICE, DEPARTMENT OF HEALTH AND HUMAN SERVICES, OFFICE OF THE ASSISTANT SECRETARY FOR HEALTH, OFFICE OF HEALTH PLANNING AND EVALUATION, AND OFFICE OF SCIENTIFIC INTEGRITY REVIEW. 1990. *Data Management in Biomedical Research: Report of a Workshop*.

WILLS, C. 1991. *Exons, Introns, and Talking Genes: The Science Behind the Human Genome Project*. New York: Basic Books.

1

Assessing the Context for Archival Programs in the Health Fields

Joan D. Krizack

ACADEMIC HEALTH CENTERS are institutional complexes composed of multiple units and often affiliated with several outside institutions. An academic health center generally comprises an allopathic or an osteopathic school of medicine, one or more teaching hospitals, and at least one other school or program for educating health care professionals. Most academic health centers are administratively linked to a parent university, although a few are freestanding. Externally, they are often linked to affiliated health care delivery facilities, research institutions, licensing and accrediting associations, funding bodies (including governmental agencies, private corporations, voluntary associations, and foundations), and governmental regulatory agencies.

Selecting appropriate materials to document academic health centers has become an increasingly challenging task for archivists. Since the 1960s, academic health centers have become more highly regulated and have forged increasingly complex interconnections with other institutions both within and outside the health care system. In addition, reprographics and communications technologies have created new record formats and have increased the quantity of records produced and the amount of information stored at academic health centers. The once-reliable appraisal techniques and tools that archivists employed to decide which records should be accessioned into an institution's archives are no longer adequate to deal with the complexity of modern institutions. Responding to this problem, archivists have developed a proactive approach to selection, grounded in careful planning and based on an analysis of both the institution and its larger context. This approach is known as institutional documentation planning (Krizack 1993).

Institutional documentation planning as applied to academic health centers consists of two stages: analysis and selection. The first stage involves understanding the place of academic health centers within the larger U.S. health care system, analyzing the individual health center to be documented, and comparing it to other academic health centers. The second stage consists of formulating a documentation plan that identifies what functions and activities will be documented and for what purposes: institutional operations, historical research, and/or scientific research. Crucial to the plan is the identification of the institution's core records, which comprise the nucleus of materials that should be preserved to facilitate institutional operations and to provide a basic record for historical research. To document the institution more fully, the documentation plan is likely to identify for preservation in the institution's archives certain series of records that are not part of the core records.[1]

The significance of documentation planning is that its analysis of the academic health center's societal context provides archivists with an understanding of the entire range of functions and activities in which their institutions engage. Not only does this insight enable them actively to select the aspects they wish to document but it also provides them with a framework for reappraising materials already housed in their archives and for appraising unsolicited records that may be sent to the archives.[2] The analysis stage of documentation planning for academic health centers is critical because it enables archivists to devise rational documentation plans and assemble archival collections specifically tailored to the functions, goals, and resources of their respective institutions.

THE CONTEXT FOR DOCUMENTATION PLANNING IN ACADEMIC HEALTH CENTERS

The U.S. Health Care System: Functions and Institutions

The U.S. health care system is a vast, complex, and decentralized amalgamation of public and private institutions and organizations. Broadly viewed, the health care system has six major functions:

- The delivery of health care (diagnosis and treatment)
- Health promotion (activities aimed at fostering good health, e.g., fitness programs and informational campaigns)
- Research (basic and clinical)
- Education (of health care professionals)
- Formulating policies (coordinating health care services within a specified region or jurisdiction on a suprainstitutional level) and regulations (establishing standards for institutions and practitioners)
- The provision of goods and services (e.g., pharmaceuticals, wheelchairs, diagnostic and therapeutic equipment, and malpractice and health insurance)

These functions are carried out by diverse institutions and organizations that interact and overlap with one another. Each institution encompasses one or more functions in its mission, sometimes along with other functions that are not related to health care.

1. More detailed information on documentation planning, including a sample documentation plan for the anesthesia department of Children's Hospital (Boston), comprises chapter 8 of Krizack 1994.
2. For an informative discussion of the rationale and value of functional analysis, see Samuels 1992.

The institutions and organizations comprising the U.S. health care system may be classified as belonging to one of the following types:

- Health care delivery facilities (e.g., hospitals, nursing homes, and hospices)
- Health agencies and foundations (e.g., the U.S. Department of Health and Human Services, the National Health Council, and the Robert Wood Johnson Foundation)
- Biomedical research facilities (e.g., the Boston Biomedical Research Institute, the Center for Human Genetics, and the Cold Spring Harbor Laboratory)
- Educational facilities for health professionals (e.g., the Massachusetts College of Pharmacy and Allied Health Sciences, the Forsyth Dental Center School for Dental Hygienists, and the Harvard Medical School)
- Professional and voluntary associations (e.g., the American Nursing Association, the American Association of Health Care Administrators, and the American Cancer Society)
- Health industries (e.g., Merck; Codman and Shurtleff; Johnson and Johnson; and Blue Cross and Blue Shield)

These institutions are funded by governments, voluntary contributions, investors, philanthropic foundations (notably the W.K. Kellogg Foundation, the Robert Wood Johnson Foundation, and the Rockefeller Foundation), or consumers, or by a combination of these methods.[3]

Academic Health Centers

Academic health centers are the nucleus of the U.S. health care system. They are primarily engaged in health care delivery, education, and research, and comprise two main types of institution: health care delivery facilities and educational facilities (Fig. 1.1). Academic health centers control and deliver the most highly specialized patient care (tertiary care),[4]

educate health care professionals, and alter medical practice through biomedical research. In addition, they usually also provide primary care for members of their local communities, many of whom may be economically disadvantaged and uninsured.[5]

At the core of the academic health center is a medical school and one or more teaching hospitals, which may be owned by the university or may merely be affiliated with it. Academic health centers may also include other components—most often, schools of dentistry and schools of nursing. Other possible components are schools of pharmacy, schools of allied health professions (e.g., medical technology, occupational therapy, and physical therapy), schools of public health, schools of optometry, and schools of veterinary medicine. In addition, academic health centers often offer graduate programs in health-related scientific fields. Not all schools in academic health centers are equal in size, prestige, or power; usually the medical school has the largest budget and is the most influential.

The primary, if not the only, reason for the existence of academic health centers is the fact that the education of physicians, nurses, and other health care professionals requires clinical or practical experience in addition to classroom teaching. This fact was generally realized in the late nineteenth century, as diagnostic instruments were introduced and surgery became a prominent feature of medical practice. By the 1920s the integration of medical education with clinical training in a hospital setting was complete (Rosenberg 1987, 191–210). This was accomplished through a formal association of medical schools with local governmental or charitable hospitals

---

3. See also Krizack 1994.

4. It should be noted, however, that because of the rapidly changing environment of health care, university hospitals no longer have a virtual monopoly on providing tertiary care (Choi et al. 1986, 4).

5. Although hospitals affiliated with academic health centers regard health promotion as one of their primary functions, it is not a primary function of academic health centers per se.

rather than through direct ownership of the hospitals by the schools. In most cases, the medical school and the hospital were relocated to the same geographic site to form one health center (Stevens 1989, 61–62).

After World War II, academic health centers expanded as the federal government extended its funding of wartime scientific and technological projects to the funding of biomedical research in universities. By 1950 academic health centers had become a fixture in the U.S. health care system and had also become centers for tertiary care. In the 1960s they flourished, growing in size, number, and complexity because federal and state governments began funding the education of health care professionals and paying for health care for aged and poor people through the Medicare and Medicaid programs (Lewis and Sheps 1983, xiii). This trend changed in the 1980s as governmental funding for biomedical research and education decreased significantly and the cost of health care increased dramatically.

Most academic health centers are components of universities, public or private. As such, they must deal with the fact that although they are part of the academic "ivory tower," they also must function in the world at large. Specifically, university hospitals are less competitive in the commercial sector because the costs of teaching and research are factored into the cost of delivering health care, making treatment more expensive at these hospitals. Tensions also exist between academic health centers and other segments of their parent universities because of the health centers' quasi-independent status and their perceived wealth. The education and research functions of academic health centers, which are also functions of the university as a whole, are inextricably linked to their patient care function, which the university does not share. This distinction is especially evident in the current call for academic health centers' hospitals to pay more attention to providing primary care and other services to their surrounding communities, instead of focusing on tertiary care as they did in the 1950s.

Statistical Overview In 1992 the Council of Teaching Hospitals (COTH) recognized 123 academic medical centers in the United States (COTH 1992), and the Association of Academic Health Centers (AAHC) counted 97 members (AAHC 1992). According to the 1992 *Academic Health Centers Directory,* approximately 60 percent of academic health centers are publicly owned, and 40 percent are private institutions. Each AAHC member institution is composed of from one to seven schools or programs for educating health care professionals; more than 75 percent have three or more schools. Each member owns and/or is affiliated with between one and twenty-seven hospitals, with the majority (about 63%) linked to between two and five hospitals (AAHC 1992).

The American Hospital Association's annual statistical summary for 1990 (the 1991–92 edition) identified 1,238 teaching hospitals, which represented 19 percent of all U.S. hospitals. Of these, about one-third were owned by the government (18% state and local, 12% federal), and the remainder were privately owned (67% not for profit, 3% for profit).

Functions and Administrative Organization The primary functions of academic health centers are patient care (including services to the local community), education, and research. Administration, including financial management, human resource management, information management, and facilities management activities, is also a function, as it is a function of all institutions and organizations. The scope of an academic health center's administrative function varies according to the division of administrative activities between the university and the academic health center.

The primary functions (patient care, education, and research) are not separable; rather, they are interrelated and interdependent, because education and clinical research both de-

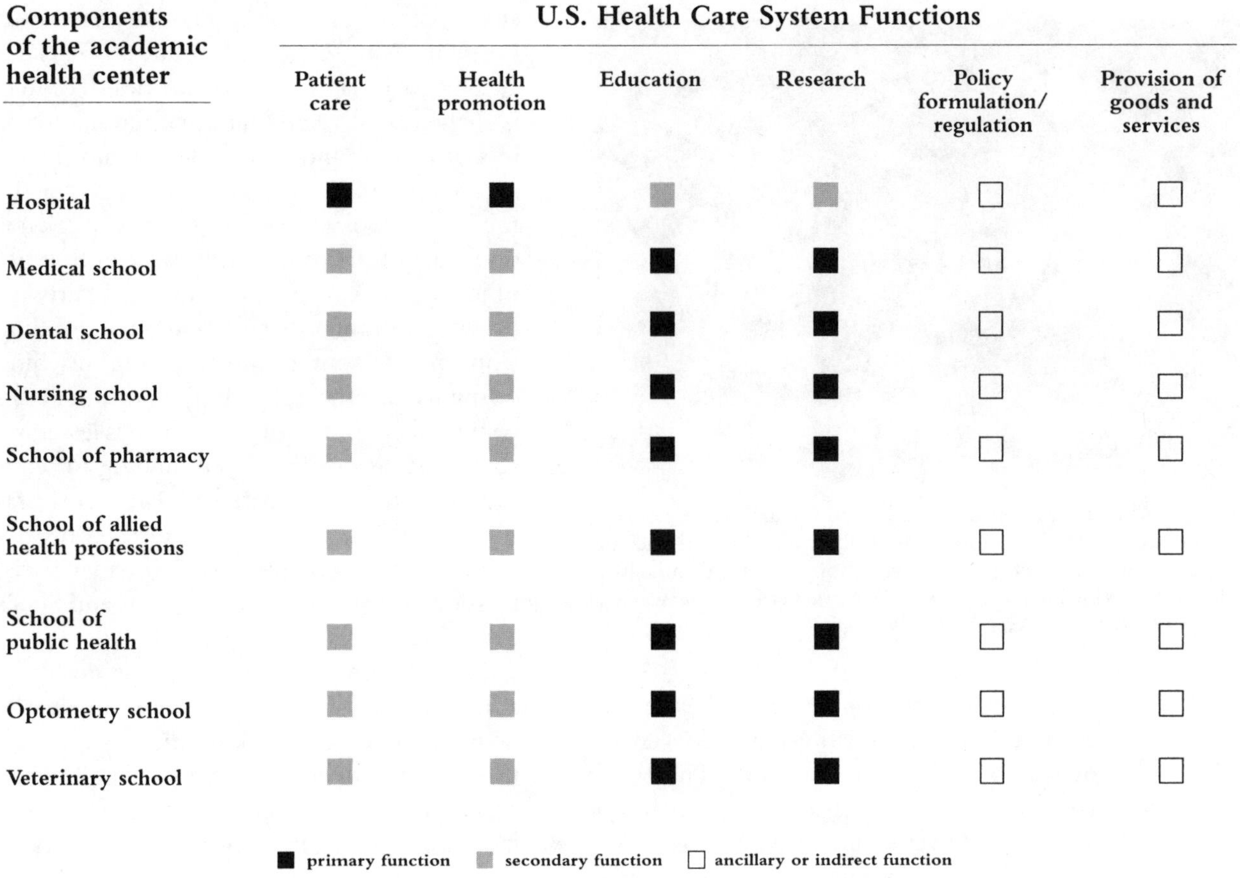

Components of the academic health center	U.S. Health Care System Functions					
	Patient care	Health promotion	Education	Research	Policy formulation/ regulation	Provision of goods and services
Hospital	primary	primary	secondary	secondary	ancillary	ancillary
Medical school	secondary	secondary	primary	primary	ancillary	ancillary
Dental school	secondary	secondary	primary	primary	ancillary	ancillary
Nursing school	secondary	secondary	primary	primary	ancillary	ancillary
School of pharmacy	secondary	secondary	primary	primary	ancillary	ancillary
School of allied health professions	secondary	secondary	primary	primary	ancillary	ancillary
School of public health	secondary	secondary	primary	primary	ancillary	ancillary
Optometry school	secondary	secondary	primary	primary	ancillary	ancillary
Veterinary school	secondary	secondary	primary	primary	ancillary	ancillary

■ primary function   ▨ secondary function   □ ancillary or indirect function

Fig. 1.1 **The role of the academic health center in the U.S. health care system.** Because academic health centers encompass most of the major functions of the U.S. health care system, they may be regarded as microcosms of the larger, overarching system.

pend on access to patient care, and advances in patient care depend on research (Lewis and Sheps 1983, 65). Thus, equal emphasis is usually placed on all three primary functions. However, affiliated teaching hospitals, in contrast to university-owned hospitals, often view patient care as their primary function and view education and research as secondary functions, an attitude that may lead to conflict.

Academic health centers have no single pattern of organization and governance. Most are part of public or private universities; a few (e.g., Thomas Jefferson University) are autonomous universities concerned only with health. An academic health center that is part of a university may be located in the same city as the rest of the university or may be some distance away, in a different part of the state. For example, the University of Connecticut Medical Center is located in Farmington, and the main campus of the university in Storrs. An academic health center that is part of a university is generally considered to be administratively separate from the rest of the university, but the relationship of an academic health center to its parent institution can vary from close physical proximity and administrative control to significant physical distance and virtual administrative autonomy. Furthermore, because of the variety in administrative organization, a job title may not indicate the same responsibilities in one academic health center that it does in another.

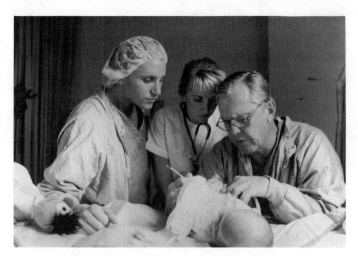

Fig. 1.2 **The confluence of teaching and health care delivery at an academic health center.** Dr. Robert Jeffs, a pediatric surgeon, combines patient care with instruction of medical students at the Johns Hopkins Hospital. *Source: Permission of* Hopkins Medical News, *Fall 1992; photograph by Bill Dennison.*

The organization of academic health centers hinges on the relationship between the medical school and the hospital. The classic structure is one in which a tertiary care hospital is owned by the university or has a close relationship to it; in this case, most of the hospital's chiefs of service chair clinical departments in the medical school. In many cases, other hospitals are also affiliated with the medical school, but in a more distant fashion.

The academic health center is the main model for the organization of academic medicine because universities find it expedient for purposes of policy making and administration to unite their health care components; however, other models also exist. Harvard University's medical school, for example, is affiliated with eleven teaching hospitals (and seven other research and patient care institutions), none of which it owns. Although the university has a dental school and a school of public health, these schools are semiautonomous and independent, respectively, and there is no overall health center administration. Harvard is one of the few exceptions to the rule, and its decentralized pattern is unusual outside of New England. The trend since World War II clearly has been for univer-

sity medical schools to build or buy their own hospitals (Munson and D'Aunno 1987, 1).

The governance of academic health centers is shaped by diverse sources of funding, centers of power, and aims of leadership (Lewis and Sheps 1983, 191). Bringing together the medical school and the teaching hospital(s) is only part of the problem, because both types of institution comprise a number of fairly independent units that also receive funding from many sources. In addition, teaching hospitals face the added burden of public accountability, although this burden is lessening somewhat as governmental funding for education wanes. Compared to large corporations, which they resemble in other ways, academic health centers have a broader social mission and are not unified (Lewis and Sheps 1983, 192).

No standard exists for the governance of academic health centers because universities do not agree on the level of authority and control that should be delegated. Generally, if an academic health center is on its own campus in a different city from the parent university, the center is significantly autonomous. A center is most often overseen by a special board or by a subcommittee of the university board, and its chief administrative officer is usually a vice president or vice-chancellor for health affairs who reports to the university's president or chancellor. If an academic health center's hospital is owned by the university, the hospital director usually reports to the academic health center's chief administrative officer. Currently, however, the trend seems to be to organize academic health centers so that their schools and their university-owned hospital(s) are governed by separate boards. The directors of affiliated hospitals, in contrast, report to the boards of their own hospitals. In an academic health center with several affiliated hospitals, a joint committee or board may be formed to set policy relating to functional divisions and clinical services. Usually the heads of an academic health center's health schools also report to the center's chief administrative officer, and an academic health center committee may be formed with representatives of the center's schools. The relationship of the deans of a center's health schools to the administrator of a university-owned hospital is often ambiguous.

Although the governance of academic health centers appears centralized, in reality it is fragmented. Because academic health centers are organized into schools and departments that are highly specialized and generate most of their funding through grants and patient care fees, the faculty members expect—and, for the most part, get—departmental control. In the past, administrators of academic health centers were expected to provide support services and little else. More recently, however, faculty members have begun to realize the need to approach problem solving at the institutional level; thus adminis-

trators whose interests are not confined to a specific department or unit are now playing an expanded role.

CONCLUSION

Academic health centers are complex conglomerates of institutions of two main types: educational institutions and health care delivery facilities. Documenting them is challenging, in large part because of their size, their composition, and their interconnections with other institutions and organizations. To document an academic health center, one must have not only an understanding of the U.S. health care system and of academic health centers in general but also an in-depth knowledge of the particular center to be documented. The checklist for analyzing academic health

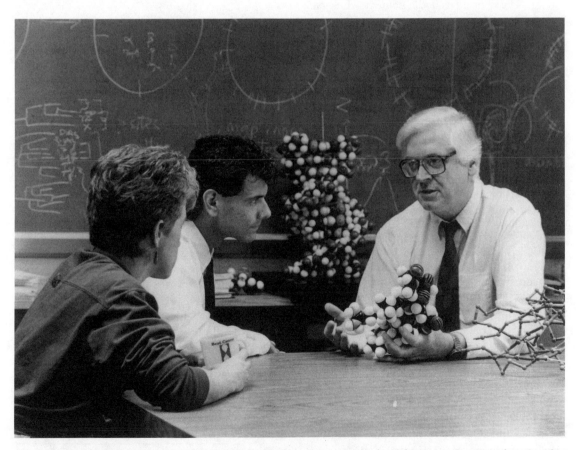

Fig. 1.3 **The confluence of teaching and research at an academic health center.** Dr. Hamilton Smith, a Nobel laureate, directs the research of students at the Johns Hopkins University School of Medicine. *Source: Permission of* Hopkins Medical News, *Fall 1992; photograph by Rob Smith.*

centers presented in Table 1.1 provides an overview of the information that academic health center archivists need before they can construct documentation plans.

BIBLIOGRAPHY

AMERICAN HOSPITAL ASSOCIATION (AHA). 1991. *Hospital Statistics*. Chicago: American Hospital Association.

ASSOCIATION OF ACADEMIC HEALTH CENTERS (AAHC). 1992. *Academic Health Centers Directory*. Washington, D.C.: Association of Academic Health Centers.

ASSOCIATION OF AMERICAN MEDICAL COLLEGES (AAMC). 1992. *COTH Directory*. Washington, D.C.: Association of American Medical Colleges.

CHOI, T., R.F. ALLISON, AND F.C. MUNSON. 1986. *Governing University Hospitals in a Changing Environment*. Ann Arbor, Mich.: Health Administration Press.

KRIZACK, J.D. 1993. Hospital documentation planning: The concept and the context. *American Archivist* 56:16–34.

————, ED. 1994. *Documentation Planning for the U.S. Health Care System*. Baltimore: Johns Hopkins University Press.

LEWIS, I.J., AND C.G. SHEPS. 1983. *The Sick Citadel: The American Academic Medical Center and the Public Interest*. Cambridge, Mass.: Oelgeschlager, Gunn, and Hain.

MUNSON, F.C., AND T.A. D'AUNNO. 1987. *The University Hospital in the Academic Health Center: Finding the Right Relationship*. Vol. 2. Washington, D.C.: Association of Academic Health Centers and Association of American Medical Colleges.

ROSENBERG, C.E. 1987. *The Care of Strangers: The Rise of America's Hospital System*. New York: Basic Books.

SAMUELS, H.W. 1992. Improving our disposition: Documentation strategy. *Archivaria* 33:125–40.

STEVENS, R. 1989. *In Sickness and Wealth: American Hospitals in the Twentieth Century*. New York: Basic Books.

Table 1.1. Checklist for analyzing academic health centers

1. Is the academic health center publicly or privately owned?
2. What educational institutions or schools are included in the academic health center?
3. What health care delivery facilities are included in the academic health center?
4. Are other centers or institutes affiliated with the academic health center?
5. What is the relationship of the academic health center to the university? Is it
   a. related and geographically close?
   b. related but geographically distant?
   c. independent but part of a state system?
   d. independent?
6. What is the relationship of the academic health center to the university's board? Does it
   a. have a separate board?
   b. have a special subcommittee of the university board?
   c. have neither of the above?
7. How many hospitals does the academic health center own, and with how many is it affiliated?
8. What is the relationship of the principal teaching hospital to the academic health center? Is the relationship one of
   a. ownership?
   b. affiliation?
9. What is the relationship of the academic health center to its other hospitals?
10. Do the affiliated hospitals have archival programs?
11. How is the university's board related to the principal teaching hospital?
    a. There is a separate board for the hospital.
    b. The hospital is governed by a special subcommittee of the university board.
    c. Neither of the above.
12. How is faculty governance organized?
    a. The health science faculty is part of a university-wide governing body.
    b. There is one faculty governing body for the entire academic health center.
    c. There is a separate faculty governing body for each health school.
13. Are clinical faculty members organized into a group medical practice?

2

Archives as Fundamental Resources for the Study and Teaching of History

Paul G. Anderson

TO BUILD HOLDINGS of archival materials that will support historical studies in a particular field, one must begin by assessing the historiography of that field.[1] The types of documentation most frequently cited in historical monographs and articles indicate the range of primary resources that an archives should acquire if its mission is to provide documentation for historical research in the field.[2] Although the sources listed in citations serve only as examples of the materials actually consulted, archivists should always be prepared to expand the horizons of collecting to include previously inaccessible documentation as well as new types of primary evidence. Citation studies nevertheless provide sound and fundamental information for planning the development of archival holdings.[3]

1. Research for this chapter involved discussion with historiographers and practitioners in the health fields. In 1987, as part of the Johns Hopkins Medical Institutions Records Project, McCall and Mix consulted a group of archivists, clinicians, historians, and records managers about the selection of documentation to be retained in archives in the health fields. The consultants' reports served as a useful resource for this chapter.
2. See Clark A. Elliott's (1981) article on citation patterns in the history of science.
3. Under the auspices of the Johns Hopkins Medical Institutions Records Project, Catherine

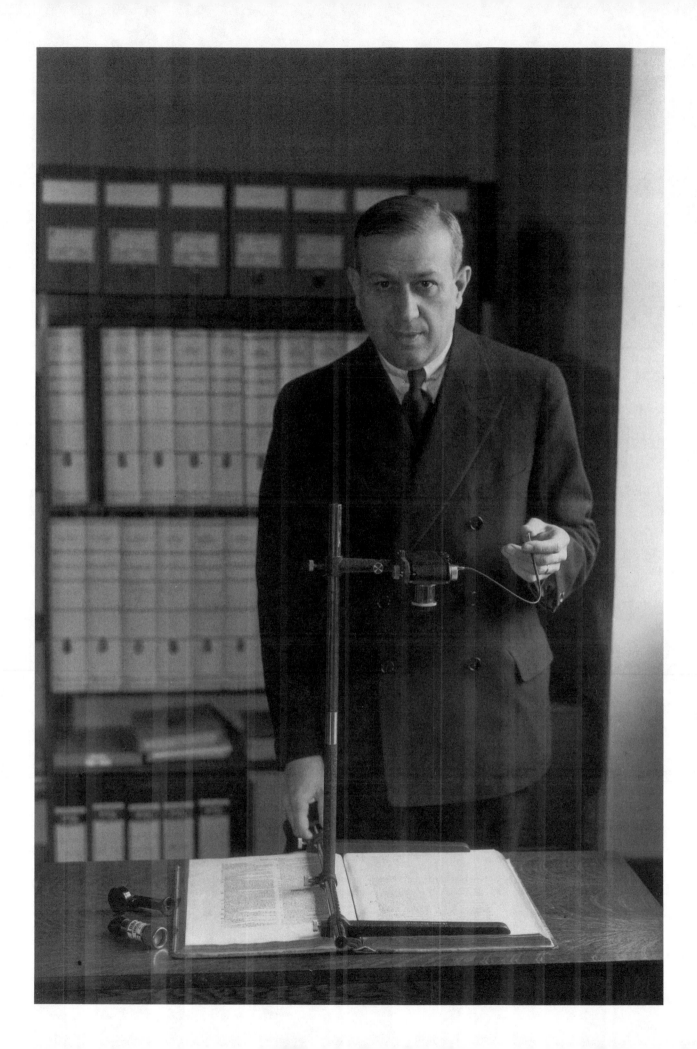

In recent decades, the historiography of medicine and the health sciences has undergone major changes. Whereas this area of historiography was once dominated mainly by practitioners in the health fields, it now engages the attention of a far wider segment of the scholarly community than ever before (Numbers 1982). In the past, physicians, nurses, dentists, and other practitioners largely produced and taught the history of their own respective fields. Today nonpractitioners are increasingly involved in historical studies of the health fields. Professional historians with many different types of specialized training are now making their mark upon the historiography of the health fields. They include economic and social historians as well as historians of science, medicine, and technology.

In contemporary studies, unpublished materials are more frequently cited as sources for the history of the health sciences—and the history of science in general—than was the case in earlier historical works. Citation studies of recent works by practitioners and nonpractitioners engaged in the history of the health fields indicate that both groups of investigators rely upon essentially the same kinds of primary source material for their research.

Because of the importance of primary source materials to the study, teaching, and writing of history, the role of archival programs in the preservation and management of these materials is a critical one for historical scholarship and education. Archival programs at institutions in the health fields occupy a particularly important position. The original records of these institutions mirror their policy and organization as well as the activities of their mandated functions. These records attest to manifold contributions to health care delivery, teaching, and research. The development of archival holdings may serve as a basis for studying an institution's past as well as a source for prospective planning. Administrators need to understand historical antecedents of institutional policy in order to plan more effectively for the future.

Because the consortia of institutions that form academic health centers include three basic types of institutions (health care delivery facilities, educational institutions, and research institutions), they provide a model for studying the range of institutional documentation in the health fields. Therefore this chapter focuses on the types of documentation that are generated at academic health centers.

THE HISTORIOGRAPHIC VALUE OF DOCUMENTATION AT ACADEMIC HEALTH CENTERS

Documentation in the health fields may be found in a wide variety of formats and media. The records that are utilized for historical research in these fields may also serve as primary source materials in other disciplines. They include both recorded documentation and material evidence. Thus, the armamentarium for historical research encompasses artifacts and specimens as well as inscriptive, visual, and aural documentation.[4]

Fig. 2.1 **Henry E. Sigerist.** This eminent scholar was a strong proponent of the use of primary source materials in the study, writing, and teaching of the history of medicine. *Source: The Institute of the History of Medicine, the Johns Hopkins University; photograph by Althausen.*

Hidalgo-Nuñez-Wohlleben, with the guidance of Clark A. Elliott, conducted a citation study of medical historical literature. The study included journal articles from 1977 and 1987 from the *Bulletin of the History of Medicine* and the *Journal of the History of Medicine and the Allied Sciences.* The results indicated a 12% increase in the use of primary source citations by journal contributors between 1977 and 1987. This increase may be attributed to changes in the methodologies of medical historians. In that span of time the training of medical historians has placed more emphasis on the use of primary source materials. In addition to the journal articles, several books in the history of medicine were surveyed. Numbers 1982 was helpful in identifying key documentation sources in the history of medicine.

4. Charles Rosenberg, of the University of Pennsylvania, noted the following in a consultant's report: "As a historian, I feel somewhat uncomfortable with a separate category for history—which, after all, includes clinical, epidemiological, and administrative aspects and is inseparable from sociology and anthropology" (Rosenberg 1987).

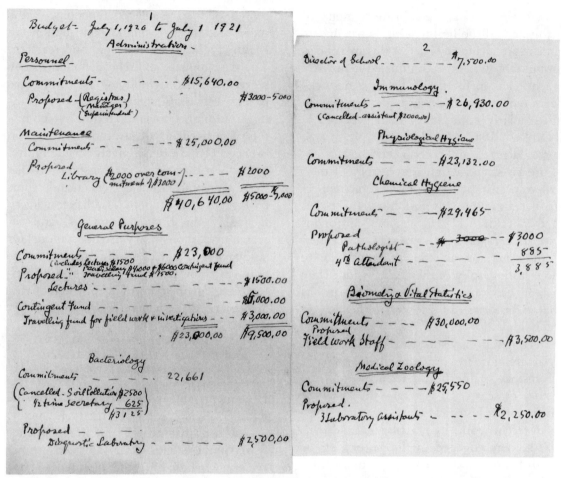

Fig. 2.2   The 1920–21 budget for the Johns Hopkins University School of Hygiene and Public Health. Inscriptive documentation (e.g. financial records) constitute important source material for historical studies. *Source: Alan Mason Chesney Medical Archives, the Johns Hopkins Medical Institutions.*

In developing archival holdings at institutions in the health fields, consideration should be given to the broad range of research activities that are to be supported by the repository. Acquisition plans and appraisal standards should revolve around the research methodologies of these various disciplines.[5]

Studying the methodologies and types of primary sources that leading contemporary scholars in the history of medicine and related fields utilize in their research offers archivists perspectives on the types of documentation that should be acquired if a program objective is to foster historical studies in these fields. The insights that are gained from citation studies of primary source materials may help

archivists to develop acquisition plans that will serve larger scholarly needs as well as the immediate and specific evidential requirements of their parent institutions.

5.   Harry Marks, of the Johns Hopkins Institute of the History of Medicine, noted the following in a consultant's report: "The question of what kinds of records are deserving of retention for historical studies is a difficult one, owing to the fact that fashions and interests in historical studies are constantly changing. In many respects, however, the kinds of data required for "historical" studies are no different than those required for contemporary clinical, epidemiological or sociological studies, differing only in the fact that they are older. Thus, clinical and epidemiological studies rely on patient records, as do historical studies of clinical practice or of patient populations. Sociological or economic studies rely on administrative or financial records similar to those which might interest historians" (Marks 1987).

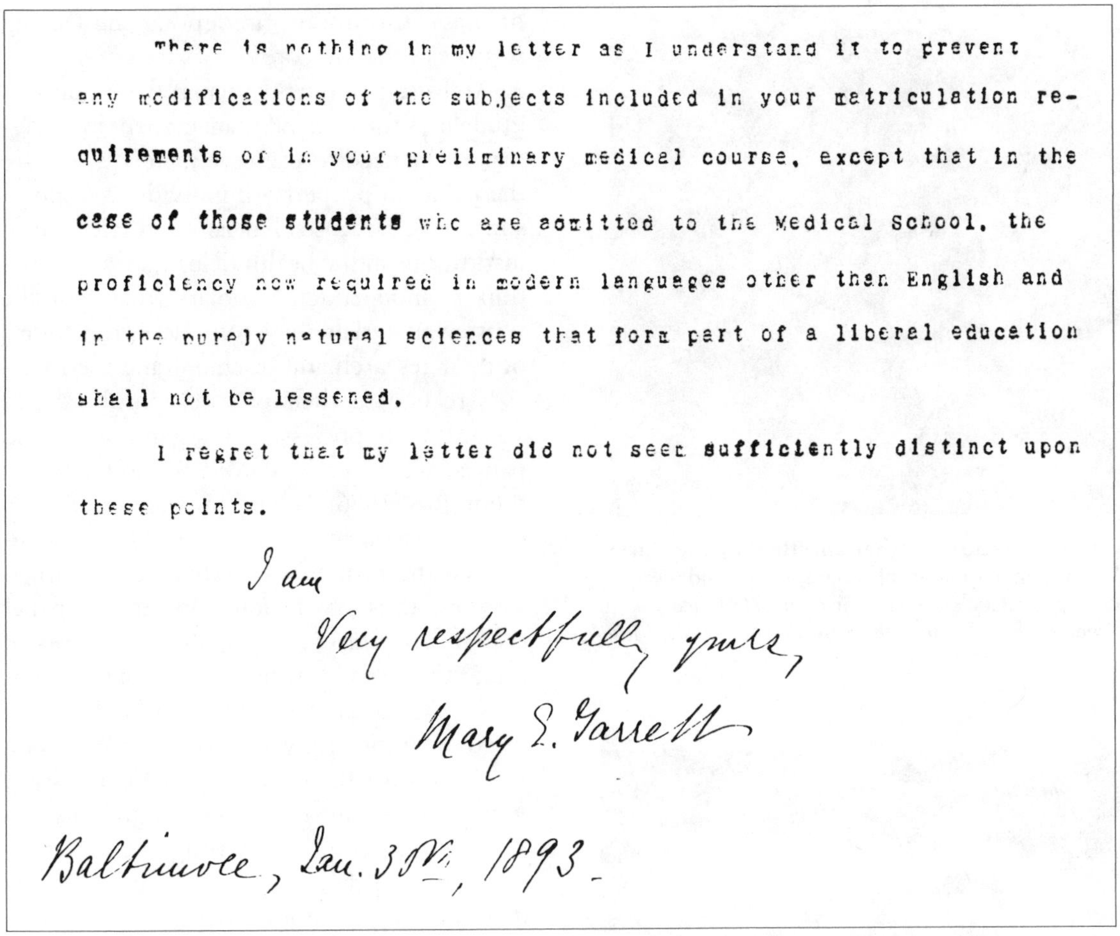

There is nothing in my letter as I understand it to prevent any modifications of the subjects included in your matriculation requirements or in your preliminary medical course, except that in the case of those students who are admitted to the Medical School, the proficiency now required in modern languages other than English and in the purely natural sciences that form part of a liberal education shall not be lessened.

I regret that my letter did not seem sufficiently distinct upon these points.

I am

Very respectfully yours,

Mary E. Garrett

Baltimore, Jan. 30th, 1893.

Fig. 2.3 **An excerpt of a letter from Mary Elizabeth Garrett, the founding benefactress of the Johns Hopkins University School of Medicine.** Correspondence with donors may reveal conditions that influenced the formulation of institutional policy. *Source: Alan Mason Chesney Medical Archives, the Johns Hopkins Medical Institutions.*

Institutional records are needed not only when an investigation focuses on the development of an institution but also when the organization serves mainly as a backdrop to the pursuit of other issues.[6] A random examination of recent historical publications on the modern American health fields, however, has indicated that despite differences in topic, perspective, and style, scholars draw upon many of the same types of documentation. The most frequently cited types of documentation in the history of the modern health fields are correspondence, minutes and agendas, narrative reports, ephemeral publications, scientific and technical reports, financial records, personnel and student records, and photographs. The central administrations of health care delivery facilities and educational institutions, together with the research departments

6. David U. Himmelstein and Steffie Woolhandler, of the Harvard Medical School, noted the following in their consultant's report: "Researchers on medical institutions and the organization of medical care will need access to institutional records on architecture, space allocation and floor plans, as well as detailed data on spending, revenues (including sources and methods of payment and billing) and personnel (including detailed job descriptions). Indications of the process of and influences on institutional decision making may be useful. Thus documents such as minutes of board meetings which record the considerations behind decisions about expansion, the range of services offered, communities served (or not served), the extent of charity care etc. may be helpful. In addition, detailed data on the demography of patients and staff including racial composition and social class should be maintained" (Himmelstein and Woolhandler 1987).

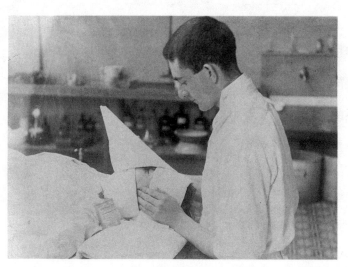

Fig. 2.4 **The administration of ether anesthesia by an intern in 1892.** Visual documentation (e.g. photographs) provides opportunities for observing the details of change in clinical practice. *Source: Alan Mason Chesney Medical Archives, the Johns Hopkins Medical Institutions.*

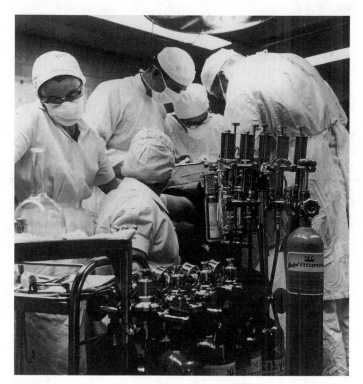

Fig. 2.5 **The administration of gas anesthesia by a nurse-anesthetist, circa 1955.** *Source: Alan Mason Chesney Medical Archives, the Johns Hopkins Medical Institutions; photograph by Richard C. Thompson.*

of these institutions, are among the leading sources of these records.

Archivists frequently depart from standard guidelines for archival management in recognizing the need to preserve materials that are the personal property of individuals (Anderson 1985). Because clinicians and scientists at institutions in the health fields may also function as independent scholars, many of the written materials they compile in the course of their research and teaching, and the materials related to their outside consulting and service with professional organizations and panels, are generally considered to belong to them (Ross 1986). Whereas in the past, the records of scientific research projects were considered the property of individual investigators (and thus may be found in personal paper collections), the ownership of records created under the aegis of institutional sponsorship is now shifting to the institutions. (Chapter 4 discusses more fully the issues surrounding research records.) Personal paper collections, which are usually acquired through individual donations rather than through regular institutional records schedules, are essential for documenting significant ties between faculty and staff, the health centers they served, and other organizations and institutions. The papers of a particular scientist, for example, might well document the social circumstances of his or her research: how projects began, how they were funded, equipped, and staffed, and how they were ultimately received by the scientific community.

In their physical characteristics, personal paper collections may differ only slightly from institutional records. The papers of physicians who serve as heads of clinical departments, for example, frequently include hospital administrative records and even selected files on patients. The papers of a director of nursing might include personnel files. Many personal paper collections, however, contain truly personal items, such as correspondence with friends and family, diaries, memoirs, scrapbooks, and other memorabilia. Personal paper collections frequently hold documents generated by professional associations and interest groups, manufacturers of equipment and supplies, public funding agencies, and private philanthropic foundations. Moreover, physicians, biomedical scientists, nurses, and public health practitioners are often among the most widely traveled professionals, and have many prolonged research sojourns and clinical or diplomatic missions abroad to their credit. Their personal effects may yield an array of documentation and memorabilia from people and institutions in many different for-

eign lands. Such individuals are often diversely cultured people with ties to other notable individuals, not only in their own fields but also in other sciences, the arts, and political affairs; and the total evidence of these interactions inestimably enriches their collections when these are deposited in an archives.

DOCUMENTATION OF HEALTH CARE DELIVERY

Archives at academic health centers, as a rule, should anticipate interest in the history of the corporate enterprises they serve (Krizack

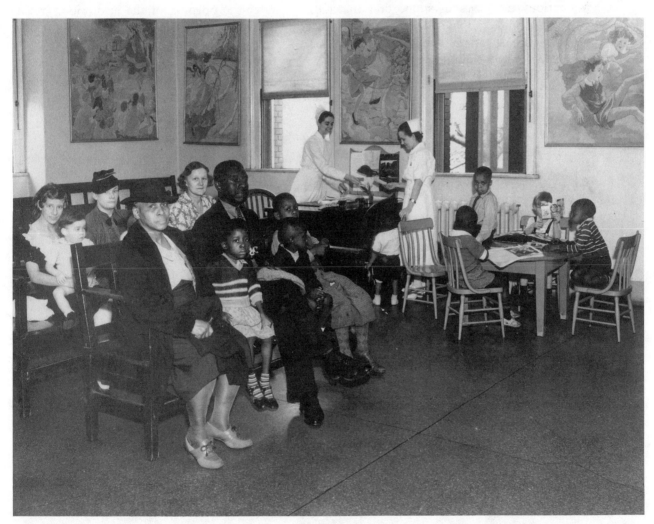

Fig. 2.6 **The Harriet Lane Home Dispensary, circa 1935.** Visual documentation is also a major resource for the study of socioeconomic conditions at health care institutions. *Source: Alan Mason Chesney Medical Archives, the Johns Hopkins Medical Institutions.*

1993; Krizack 1994).[7] Most U.S. hospitals trace their origins to the specific intention of an individual or a group to care for sick people in a given community or segment of the population. This purpose is likely to be set forth in one or more founding documents, such as bequests, deeds, charters, or legislative acts. Frequently these early records also include data and information about important social factors, such as the identities of the hospital's founders, first owners, or sponsors; these individuals' relationships to the community where the hospital is located; and their mandate to serve particular types of patients. In addition, various categories of supporting materials, such as photographs, personal statements by participants, and press coverage, augment the interpretation of founding documents.

More extensive than the body of official founding documents are likely to be materials generated during the early planning and financing of buildings, equipment, and operations. The original architectural sketches, projections, and engineering drawings and specifications for a hospital are certain to retain historical significance. Likewise, the early budgets, personnel descriptions, and transactions with equipment manufacturers may exemplify the state of hospital administration from another era.

The status and functions of the official governing board of a hospital, both before and after the opening of the institution, are in-

7. Chapter 2 in Krizack 1994 deals with documenting health care delivery facilities.

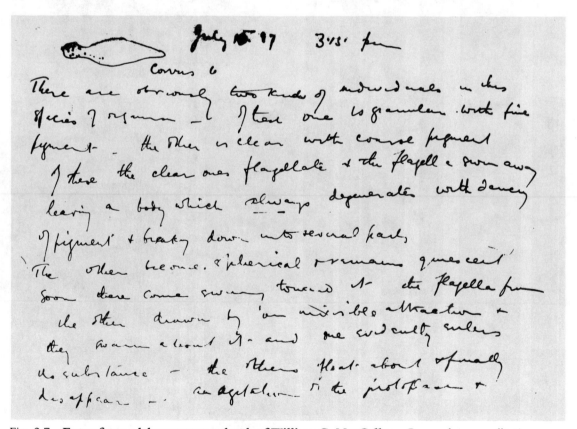

Fig. 2.7   **Entry from a laboratory notebook of William G. MacCallum.** Personal paper collections provide a finer focus on the contributions of individuals. For example, in this entry MacCallum records one of the first descriptions of the sexual conjugation of the malarial organism. *Source: Alan Mason Chesney Medical Archives, the Johns Hopkins Medical Institutions.*

herently significant to the hospital's history. How the group was selected, how it perpetuated itself, to what higher authorities it reported, and what relations it established with the medical staff, the medical faculty, and the nearest medical society are among the topics of interest to historians. The minutes and other records of this group may be expected to elucidate matters such as financial management, hospital administration, and the recruitment and competency of professional staffs.

The records of academic health centers also document the rationale for the priorities that the institution has set for clinical, research, and educational programs. Studies of shifts in institutional policies provide important insights into the histories of these institutions. For example, the records of governing boards of hospitals and clinics reflect the changing missions of these institutions. The records document the increase in the power and responsibility of the chairs of these boards, a change that made the chair's position analogous to that of a chief executive officer. Any series of records that documents the selection of the medical staff, the nursing staff, and the ancillary care staff, and the composition and functions of these staffs, is likely to have considerable historical value.

Historians frequently focus on the role of individuals who contributed to the development and reputation of the institution. Analyses of the professional specializations and the social backgrounds of the faculty and staff of these institutions provide insights into the attitudes and standards that shaped the institutions. Assessment of the historical relationships of the medical staff to the medical school faculty provides background for analyzing the dynamics of faculty and staff interaction. Records of medical staff governance, including the minutes or transcripts of business and clinical meetings, may be expected to trace the scope of the staff's activities and levels of competence. These records usually include deliberations on matters such as professional standards and credentials, the maintenance

and operation of diagnostic and therapeutic facilities, advice provided to the administration on equipment and supplies, and other issues of mutual concern to both physicians and administrators.

Records of patient rounds and of the clinical conferences of the various departments provide an overview of the institution's priorities for health care delivery. They also yield insights on the institution's clinical and therapeutic standards and ethical decision making. The committees and subcommittees that set the criteria for patient rounds and other types of clinicopathological conferences may be expected to have produced reports on their activities over the years.

Special informational value is inherent in the records concerning the house staff. The medical schools from which these physicians were selected; the specialties in which they served in internships and residencies, and the average length of such service; and the career paths they chose upon finishing this phase of their medical education all reveal much about the character of the institution: for example, certain hospitals have long traditions of sponsoring the careers of ethnic minority and women physicians through residency training. Many academic health centers sponsor alumni associations that regularly compile and maintain documentation on their former house staffs.

The records of nursing staffs and staffs in other ancillary care specialties also have a significant place in the historical armamentarium of an academic health center.[8] In addition to nurses, the dentists, pharmacists, physical and occupational therapists, and medical social workers associated with academic health centers represent the range of the various other professional cadres that staff these centers. The records of these staffs constitute vital pri-

8. Charles Rosenberg noted the following in a consultant's report: "Historians have found that the experience of nurses, patients, and workers—not to mention the growing ranks of middle management—is not well documented" (Rosenberg 1987).

mary source material for the study of the institution as well as the ancillary care professions.

The records concerning nonprofessional support staffs are the subject of increasing scrutiny by historians and other social scientists. These records provide significant details about the institutional role of the nonprofessional work force and the lives of its individual members. An examination of the nonprofessional staff of an academic health center is likely to reveal a vast and enormously varied sociological spectrum. Even in cities as large as New York, Los Angeles, or Chicago, academic health centers rank as major employers and control important economic assets.

Selected records of hospitals' business operations have lasting historical importance. In particular, the office of the chief administrator is certain to generate files and other record series that document internal policy decisions, relationships between academic health center institutions, and connections to individuals and organizations outside the center. Among the materials from a hospital's central offices that should certainly be targeted for permanent archival preservation are annual reports, endowment records, schedules of patient fees, and files on major grants and contracts. Special consideration should be given to preserving accreditation documents, and analyses of operations prepared by consultants.

To a great extent, the history of academic health centers may be studied in terms of their role over the years as leaders of scientific and technological innovations in the health fields. Because academic health centers in the United States have historically competed with one another, the records of these institutions constitute a major resource for comparative studies. The academic, clinical, and research programs that are hallmarks of academic health centers may also be assessed in terms of their historical role in promotional strategies for their institutions. The history of academic health centers may be seen through the images they have striven to project for teaching, research, and health care delivery.

Revolutionary developments in science and technology have led to major changes in the organization and the operation of academic health centers. For instance, the diagnostic significance of x rays was rapidly grasped throughout the industrialized world following their discovery by Roentgen in 1895, and by the second decade of this century leading hospitals had acquired radiological equipment and instituted new forms of diagnostic procedures. By the close of World War II, very substantial expansion or alteration of existing physical plants was necessary for hospitals to keep pace with the therapeutic as well as the diagnostic techniques that radiologists were developing. As we near the end of the twentieth century, radiology has evolved to embrace a host of subdisciplines, ranging from radiation oncology to nuclear magnetic resonance imaging, all of which require an enormous investment of capital and extensive facilities. Numerous analogies to these developments in radiology may also be found in each of the clinical sciences.

To build a body of records that representatively documents the history of an academic health center, the holdings should encompass records regarding the endowment, the financing, the administration, the architecture, and the mandated functions of each component institution, past as well as present. This body of documentation would include the records of any defunct hospital, institute, or clinic (or, to recall less current terminology, any asylum, dispensary, infirmary, or sanatorium) with past connections to an ongoing center. Documentation pertaining to the military hospitals sponsored by academic health centers during the two world wars may be of special significance. It should be noted that the records of certain defunct institutions may have ongoing importance for historical studies as well as for the current administration of related institutions. Some now-closed hospitals, for example, were established on endowments that continue to yield support for current programs. The buildings that formerly housed clinical services that have been terminated or reorganized may subsequently be renovated to serve other functions without obliterating important historic names. Alumni traditions and their documentation may retain strategic significance long after the closing of certain units.

There are at least two circumstances in which archival programs may select and preserve clinical documentation for historical studies. The first pertains to relatively old records—dating from the early twentieth century and still earlier times—that are not needed for regular clinical or administrative activities. These records which may include operating room logs, appointment ledgers for clinics, and patient histories, constitute an important resource for medical historical and social historical research. The second circumstance concerns patient records that may be included in the personal paper collections of clinicians whose work is of historical interest. These records may be used to study the treat-

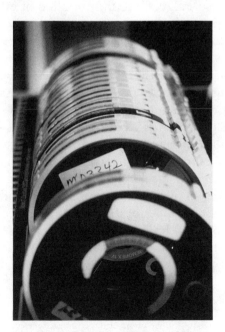

Fig. 2.8 **Memorex IV tape files.** In the last half of the twentieth century the inscriptive record has shifted primarily from paper-based media to machine-dependent media. *Source: Alan Mason Chesney Medical Archives, the Johns Hopkins Medical Institutions.*

ment modes of the physicians. Historical patient documentation may also serve as an important resource for ongoing clinical research. Epidemiological, genetic, and etiological studies frequently begin with reviews of historical patient records. Specific issues concerning access to patient records for purposes of clinical and historical research are discussed in chapters 3 and 8 of this volume.

Some of the official publications of academic health centers may provide data and information about the overall patient population in abstract form. Annual reports and special statistical publications are especially important resources for obtaining an overview of clinical activities. Because such published reports and studies are usually not collected by libraries, they should be designated for archival selection. These publications are usually highly reliable sources of basic information about the institution's health care delivery activities.

DOCUMENTATION OF EDUCATION

To understand the documentation base of academic health centers, one must gain an overview of the administrative dynamics of these institutions.[9] From the point of view of the community in which an academic health center is located, the biggest hospital among the member institutions is likely to claim the dominant profile. Yet in significant respects the medical school sets the tone for the entire academic health center: the quality of the research and teaching at the principal academic unit determines the center's reputation outside its immediate locality. This reputation, in turn, is a powerful factor in attracting new faculty and staff members and funding for research. The connections between the hospital and the school also exist at other levels, of course. The heads of academic clinical departments are, or have the right to appoint, the heads of clinical services. At most centers clini-

9. Chapter 6, by McCall and Mix, in Krizack 1994, provides a context for documenting educational institutions in the health fields.

cal income supports the teaching departments and a major portion of the research budget. The full-time faculty members, moreover, make up a large proportion of the hospital's attending physicians. Because of the strategic role of the medical school in shaping health care delivery programs throughout the academic health center, it tends to dominate the other professional schools that may be part of the institutional consortium.

Educational institutions and instructional programs in the health fields vary enormously in terms of their organization and administration. Colleges and professional schools are generally headed by deans; programs commonly have directors. The overall institutional entity may be led by officials bearing titles such as president or chancellor. The relative power that each of these officials wields depends upon a number of factors, including the constitution and bylaws of the parent university and the academic health center corporation, the amount of the endowment, the clinical income and grant revenues, the size and complexity of the subordinate administrative staff, and the collective influence of the faculty.

Until relatively recently, the administrative duties of the deans of even the largest health science schools amounted to part-time responsibilities: that is, an individual could teach, do research, or engage in clinical practice while serving as the head of a medical, nursing, dental, or public health school. Although many deans today continue in their professorial specialties, it is becoming more common for educational administration to claim full-time attention from its executives. Administrative tasks, furthermore, may require the services of several associate or assistant deans, each responsible for one or more areas such as student affairs, curricula, continuing education, finance, personnel, instructional and research facilities, and the care of laboratory animals.

The degree of authority and self-governance exercised by the chairs of academic departments is a factor that often sets medical schools dramatically apart from other teaching bodies at universities or academic health centers. The heads of clinical departments play key administrative roles because income from their health care delivery services constitutes a major source of revenue for the institution. For their part, basic science departments often conduct research and teaching programs that are so well funded as to afford their heads considerable power.

Medical schools as corporate bodies inevitably blend elements of oligarchy and democracy. Since the opening in 1893 of the Johns Hopkins University School of Medicine, the faculty governance of that school has served as a model for institutions throughout the country. At Johns Hopkins, the major department heads comprise the advisory board (known at some other institutions as the executive faculty), which is the primary decision-making authority for the school. Its powers extend directly to the appointment of the dean and the approval of all professorial tenure, and indirectly to the operation of every constituent health center institution.[10] Board meetings, therefore, may be arenas where issues vital to the entire center are reviewed and debated. Records of these conclaves, notably the agendas and minutes compiled before and after each session, are of prime historical importance. Associated documents, such as the minutes of committees and subcommittees, consultants' reports, and memorial tributes to deceased faculty members may also be sources of significant information. In addition, the faculties of the various professional schools may have joint meetings and assemblies from which significant records result.

10. Kenneth M. Ludmerer, of the Washington University School of Medicine, noted the following in a consultant's report: "The history of nineteenth- and early twentieth-century medical schools can be written from centralized records from the dean's office, but the history of the second half of the twentieth century will rely increasingly on departmental and even on divisional records. The most useful records, at least to historians, will probably come from deans' offices and departmental offices. Keep in mind, however, that what must be preserved are not just official documents, reports, and grant applications but correspondence, laboratory notebooks, diaries, and records of seminars and meetings" (Ludmerer 1987).

Records pertaining to the programs of the educational divisions are of significant historical interest. Through most of this century, educational institutions at academic health centers have focused their curricula around the latest advances in science and technology. One strong implication of this trend, either explicit or implied, has been that all graduates are expected to make their careers in specialty practice or in research. Another implication has been that there is little room in the curriculum of these schools for serious consideration of the humanistic and sociological issues in the health fields. The files of administrators and the minutes of committees that have addressed curriculum issues touch the very heart of the history of education in the health fields. Some distinguished schools, it is fair to say, have always strongly emphasized medical humanism or have promoted general practice as a career option. More recently, at other institutions, there seems to have been a reappraisal of the value of instruction devoted to the cultural context of the health sciences.

Medical schools have long structured the M.D. curriculum in two parts: an introduction to the basic scientific disciplines, and an introduction to the basic clinical disciplines. The basic science departments generally perpetuate titles and administrative traditions that have their roots in the medical academia of fifty years ago or more: for instance, they are known by traditional names such as anatomy, biochemistry, genetics, microbiology, pharmacology, and physiology. Some of the courses they offer, such as gross anatomy, are essential to the medical curriculum, and variations on these courses are mandatory as well for students of dentistry, nursing, and certain other allied health disciplines. However, considerable disparity may exist between tradition-bound areas of the curriculum as presented to students, on the one hand, and the actual research priorities of the institution, on the other.

Faculty members in professional schools at academic health centers instruct and advise students working toward single and joint advanced degrees. The programs may combine study toward both the M.D. and Ph.D. degrees (often under the auspices of the Medical Scientist Training Programs, funded by the National Institutes of Health), or may be concentrated solely on work in a particular field of natural science (Bickel et al. 1981). To address the needs of students in these categories, certain universities have created special divisions that reside within their medical schools or are administered jointly by the medical schools and by the graduate faculty in the universities' natural science departments. The faculty committees and administrative offices involved may create important historical records, particularly when they are assigned to examine factors that define the place of biomedicine in the larger world of science. Senior faculty members commonly hold at least one joint appointment that may extend across collegiate or health center lines. Overlapping also occurs as a result of faculty involvement in continuing education programs and various other special instructional programs.

If curriculum documentation is a matter of historical significance, so also are the personnel records of the faculty and staff of the professional schools. It should perhaps be acknowledged in this context that members of the basic science departments often do not have hospital positions and privileges but hold appointments that are essentially analogous to those held by their colleagues in the "pure" academic disciplines. Nevertheless, any attempt to measure the quality of an academic health center—let alone the caliber of instruction in a given school—must take into account the recruitment, qualifications, and performance of the entire faculty. The criteria for promotion and for the granting of tenure and emeritus status are prominent among the issues certain to be deeply etched into the history of an institution. Other important matters might include how embracing the definition of professional status was: Did it include long-employed but unranked researchers, as well as professors? Did it include auxiliary specialists such as business managers, librarians, and technical writers?

Student records, both official and unofficial, afford a rich variety of historical information. They begin with materials relating to recruitment. Although for decades many more U.S. undergraduates have applied to study medicine than have been accepted, medical school administrations have nevertheless endeavored to "balance" their enrollments in some manner. Geographic balancing has traditionally been a major concern for private schools. More recently, civil rights legislation has prompted schools to strive for a wider representation of minorities and women among their student bodies. The task has not been easy, for competition and the intrinsic scholarly demands on students in medical training have required that academic standards remain high. In some instances, administrations have established special offices (e.g., offices for minority student affairs) dedicated to the planning and encouragement of affirmative action programs. The records of these special offices are of considerable historical interest.

The records of students in the health sciences provide a major source of information about the way in which academic programs were operated and the students to whom they appealed. Of course, access to such materials is governed by constraints fully as complex as those concerning data on patients (Elston 1976; Barritt 1986; Greene 1987). The confidentiality of student records is enforced by the Family Education Rights and Privacy Act of 1974, which was amended in 1982. Experts in the administration of collegiate archives generally argue, however, that the act does not preclude all historical research, even during the lifetimes of the individuals named, provided that the identities of the individuals are protected (see chapter 8 for further discussion of this legislation and of the ways in which these materials may be made available for research).

Informal documentation pertaining to student life is also an important resource for his-

torical research. Student societies and fraternities in medicine, dentistry, nursing, and public health have long held traditions that combine academic pursuits with purely social functions. Academic groups ranging from honor societies to informal journal clubs produce a variety of documentation. At most campuses students are involved in a host of social, political, ethical, and religious activities for which posters, leaflets, programs, and other ephemera are distributed. Not to be forgotten either are the various bulletins, newspapers, and yearbooks published during the academic year. These sorts of material, when consistently collected over the years, will yield an overview of the experiences of student life—evidence of a kind that is usually not found in administrative records.

DOCUMENTATION OF RESEARCH ACTIVITIES

The function generally considered to be the hallmark of academic health centers is scientific research.[11] Although hospitals and other health care delivery facilities may be the locus of clinical investigation, research is generally administered under the auspices of the teaching departments of the educational institutions. A portion of the revenues from grants and contracts involving faculty research reverts to help cover administrative overhead costs. As is discussed in chapter 4, archives at academic health centers may contribute a scientific as well as a historiographic service by preserving selections of research data. The historical importance of retaining some types of research documentation, however, deserves comment here.

Archival projects documenting the activities of research owe much to precedents set by archives in the sciences, notably physics. The idea of a *discipline history center* developed out of efforts led by the American Institute of Physics to rescue early data sets pertaining to atomic energy research, among other fields

---

11. Chapter 4, by Anderson, in Krizack 1994, provides a context for documenting research in the health fields.

(Warnow-Blewett 1989; AIP 1992). A general analysis of methods and goals in discipline history is presented in *Understanding Progress as Process* (Elliott 1983), a study by the Joint Committee on Archives of Science and Technology (JCAST), a task force sponsored by several related interest groups, including the History of Science Society and the Society for the History of Technology.

The concept of *process* cited in the title of the JCAST report is most appropriate for defining the historical dimension of research records in the health fields. An ideal common to academic archives is the documentation of significant activities from beginning to end. Whereas it is true that the actual intellectual genesis of research may be difficult to pinpoint on paper, the official beginnings of any particular project in this age of "big science" are almost invariably set forth in funding proposals and other bureaucratically generated series of records. Thus, every academic health center archives has an opportunity to chart the inception of research that may be of special historical significance.[12]

The granting agencies of the National Institutes of Health and other governmental institutions, private foundations with interests in the health sciences, and other outside sources of funding require detailed statements of objectives and project budgets in applications for research funding. Even projects supported completely by internal sources are delineated in budgets and statements required by auditors. If awards are made that enable the full realization of the research designs for a particular project, progress reports and revised budgets are likely to be added to the record at various intervals, and a summation and final fiscal accounting rendered at the end of the project. These funding documents may reveal significant details about the history of the project and the individuals who conceived it and carried it out.

Throughout the course of a project, but especially in its early phases, many auxiliary types of record are created by or at the behest of investigators and the authorities to whom they must report. Additional personnel are likely to be hired, and files relating to their qualifications, job performance, and exposure to hazards must be compiled by their supervisors. Equipment is likely to be purchased or leased for the project, leading perhaps to modification of the original budget and specifications. The acquisition and the use of dangerous or controlled substances require meticulous logging and appropriate reporting to regulatory agencies. Plans to use human subjects and laboratory animals result in correspondence with institutional review boards. Such materials reveal a great deal about the experiences, judgments, and value systems of scientists, and thus may serve as significant historical resources (Grover and Wallace 1979).

CONCLUSION

The preservation of empirical evidence in the health fields is crucial to the study, teaching, and writing of history. The types of materials that chart the course of institutions from their founding to the present include selections of records that document major institutional functions such as health care delivery, teaching, and research. Special "monuments"— documentation that represents key events in an institution's history and the institution's most important contributions—must be preserved, as must other, less obvious types of documentation—materials that represent the routine and the ordinary.

Historical evidence cannot be drawn exclusively from monumental documentation. Ubiquitous materials are also needed to demonstrate the commonplace and to serve as a barometer or a baseline. The principal challenge in developing a body of archival holdings to support a broad range of historical

---

12. In a consultant's report Harry Marks noted, "One area sure to be of interest to future historians is the development of policies for dealing with commercial enterprises or for developing and marketing products/services which come about as the result of in-house research. These records are likely to be both institutional (committees, etc.) and individual, and institutions should be encouraged to identify and collect them" (Marks 1987).

studies is to provide a balance between monumental and ubiquitous documentation.

The selection of documentation for inclusion in archival repositories should be guided in part by their value for historical research. However, final decisions regarding selection should always be directed by the broader institutional, scientific, and social context of the materials.

In conclusion, it is hoped that this chapter will serve as a helpful guide not only to archivists and institutional administrators as they develop acquisition plans for archival programs but also to historians and other researchers who are embarking on studies of the health fields. The selectors as well as the potential users of the documentation stand to benefit from an overview of the range and types of materials that are relevant to historical studies.

BIBLIOGRAPHY

AMERICAN INSTITUTE OF PHYSICS, CENTER FOR HISTORY OF PHYSICS. 1992. *AIP Study of Multi-institutional Collaborations, Phase I: High-Energy Physics*. New York: American Institute of Physics.

ANDERSON, P.G. 1985. Appraisal of the papers of biomedical scientists and physicians for a medical archives. *Bulletin of the Medical Library Association* 73:338–44.

BARRITT, M.R. 1986. The appraisal of personally identifiable student records. *American Archivist* 49:263–75.

BICKEL, J.W., C.R. SHERMAN, J. FERGUSON, L. BAKER, AND T.E. MORGAN. 1981. The role of M.D.-Ph.D. training in increasing the supply of physician-scientists. *New England Journal of Medicine* 304:1265–68.

ELLIOTT, C.A. 1981. Citation patterns and documentation for the history of science: Some methodological considerations. *American Archivist* 44:131–42.

———, ED. 1983. *Understanding Progress as Process: Documentation of the History of Post-War Science and Technology in the United States*. Final report of the Joint Committee on Archives of Science and Technology. Chicago: Society of American Archivists.

ELSTON, C. 1976. University student records: Research use, privacy rights, and the Buckley law. *Midwestern Archivist* 1:16–32.

GREENE, M.A. 1987. Developing a research access policy for student records: A case study at Carlton College. *American Archivist* 50:570–79.

GROVER, F., AND P. WALLACE. 1979. *Laboratory Organization and Management*. London: Butterworths.

HIDALGO-NUÑEZ-WOHLLEBEN, C. 1988. Citation study.

HIMMELSTEIN, D.U., AND S. WOOLHANDLER. 1987. Consultant's report to the Johns Hopkins Medical Institutions Records Project.

KRIZACK, J.D. 1993. Hospital documentation planning: The concept and the context. *American Archivist* 56 (1): 16–34.

———, ED. 1994. *Documentation Planning for the U.S. Health Care System*. Baltimore: Johns Hopkins University Press.

LUDMERER, K.M. 1987. Consultant's report to the Johns Hopkins Medical Institutions Records Project.

MARKS, H.M. 1987. Consultant's report to the Johns Hopkins Medical Institutions Records Project.

NUMBERS, R.L. 1982. The history of American medicine: A field in ferment. *Reviews in American History* 10:244–63.

ROSENBERG, C.E. 1987. Consultant's report to the Johns Hopkins Medical Institutions Records Project.

ROSS, R.S. 1986. Academic research and industry relationships. *Clinical and Investigative Medicine* 9:269–72.

U.S. DEPARTMENT OF LABOR, BUREAU OF LABOR STATISTICS. 1986. *Occupational Outlook Handbook*. Bulletin 2250, 1986–87 ed. Washington, D.C.: U.S. Department of Labor.

WARNOW-BLEWETT, J. 1989. Saving the records of science and technology: The role of a discipline history center. *Science and Technology Libraries* 7:29–40.

3

Preserving Patient Records to Support Health Care Delivery, Teaching, and Research

Joel D. Howell

ORIGINALLY INTENDED to assist in the management of patient care, the patient record has been subject to an increasing number of secondary uses during the twentieth century. Whereas the patient record constitutes a vital body of data and information for both medical and historical research, it has also come to serve numerous other important functions, from helping to measure the quality of patient care, to determining fiscal reimbursement, to serving as an important teaching tool at academic health centers.

Because more people in the United States are receiving health care, the number of patient records that are being produced is unprecedented. Moreover, the average size of the individual patient record has

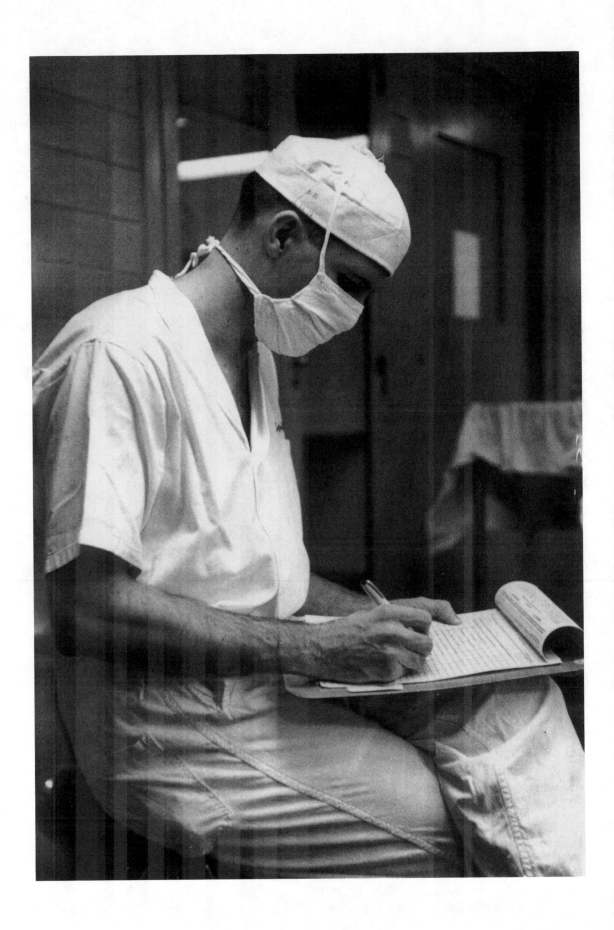

also grown significantly because of many factors, including increases in regulatory requirements and greater reliance upon ancillary care and diagnostic technology. The patient record has become cluttered with the paperwork of accountability. A myriad of forms must be included to measure various regulatory processes, the services provided by many new types of ancillary care personnel, and the use of many new types of diagnostic procedures. As both the quantity and the scope of patient records have expanded over the course of the century, the cost of their storage and retrieval has grown at a commensurate rate. During the early years of the twentieth century, most hospitals attempted to retain patient records, either on a permanent basis or at least for the lifetime of the patient. However, faced with budgetary restraints, today's hospital administrators are being forced to regard patient records in terms of their immediate administrative usefulness more than their long-term research and teaching value. An increasing number of hospitals are choosing to dispose of older records. Some hospitals are even beginning routinely to eliminate relatively recent records.

This chapter weighs the clinical, research, and teaching value of patient records against the economic realities that beset health care delivery facilities. It recommends practical and affordable ways to reduce the overall scale of patient records in storage and to retain core selections of records that will be relevant to the institution's ongoing need for patient care, research, and education. In this way, a significant segment of materials may be preserved so that they may be utilized for ongoing reference and study. Because patient records follow the course of both diagnosis and treatment,

they provide a direct means for observing the modes of clinical intervention. They also provide a means of assessing the patient population and the health personnel who are involved in patient care. The confluence of many different types of primary evidence (clinical, scientific, technological, and socioeconomic) that is found in patient records makes them a rich and unique resource for study and for the advancement of knowledge in many areas.

THE EVOLUTION OF CONTEMPORARY PATIENT RECORDS

The patient record is designed to serve as a documentary intermediary between the patient and health professionals (Pettinari 1988). At most health care facilities, the patient record usually consists of the unit medical record and ancillary diagnostic media.

The Unit Medical Record

Origins and Standardization   A unit record consists of a single file that contains all the data and information generated in each staff encounter with a given patient in any of the divisions of a hospital. The unit record system was created to deal effectively with the proliferation of different departments in the early twentieth-century hospital, in part because units such as x-ray and social work departments were producing increasing numbers of records. Assigning each patient a unique number and a single file made it easier to collect and compare patients' records; the new record-keeping system may thus have been an important impetus for clinical research.

Most of the major U.S. hospitals adopted the unit record system in the first few decades of this century (Howell 1987). Since 1965, the Medicare-Medicaid system has recommended it for participating hospitals (Waters and Murphy 1979), and it is now the prevailing medical record-keeping system in U.S. hospitals.

Components   The unit medical record file is composed of sections and subsections.

Fig. 3.1 **A surgeon preparing postoperative notes at the Johns Hopkins Hospital, 1952.** A physician's notes for the patient record are usually prepared in proximity to the site of examination and treatment. *Source: Alan Mason Chesney Medical Archives, the Johns Hopkins Medical Institutions; photograph by Werner Wolff, Black Star.*

The choice of these multiple components needs to meet the information requirements for the management of both low-severity and high-severity cases. The average inpatient unit record for an individual undergoing a standard, uncomplicated operative procedure (such as an appendectomy) is several inches thick, whereas the thickness of the average inpatient unit record documenting a complex operative procedure (such as a heart-lung transplant) may be measured in feet.

According to guidelines established by the Joint Commission on Accreditation of Healthcare Organizations (JCAHO), the basic components of the unit medical record should include, among other items,

- identification data;
- the medical history;
- a summary of the patient's psychosocial needs;
- reports of the relevant physical examinations;
- diagnostic and therapeutic orders;
- evidence of appropriate informed consent;
- clinical observations;
- progress notes made by members of the clinical staff;
- consultation reports;
- nursing notes and entries by nonphysicians that contain pertinent, meaningful observations and information;
- reports of procedures and tests, and their results;
- reports of pathology and clinical laboratory examinations, radiology and nuclear medicine examinations or treatment; anesthesia records; and any other diagnostic or therapeutic procedures;
- medical records of donors and recipients of transplants; and
- conclusions at the termination of hospitalization (JCAHO 1993).

Other components of the record are included for other specific clinical settings.

Size   Much of the increase in the size of the unit record occurred early in the twentieth century. For example, the median length of a patient record at New York Hospital went from one page in 1900 to eight pages in 1910 to eleven pages in 1920 (Joel D. Howell, unpublished data, 1993). The expansion at New York Hospital and elsewhere largely resulted from additional reports, often presented on separate forms, produced by the growing number of distinct units in the increasingly bureaucratic hospital (Howell 1986; Howell 1988).

The scope of U.S. medical documentation also expanded dramatically in the second half of this century, largely because of major changes affecting the funding, practice, and study of medicine in the United States. These changes include the rise of complex, highly bureaucratic systems of third-party payment, as well as the expansion of regulatory procedures and the rapid introduction of new technologies.

Originally hailed for streamlining both the recording and the filing of patient information, the unit record system in the 1990s has grown to unwieldy proportions. A significant increase in the number of component parts, as well as greater frequency of use and longer transit time, have impeded the effectiveness of this system.

Ironically, some of the very features that made the unit record concept so practical for clinical management, teaching, and research have also contributed to its ungainly growth. The demand that the unit record serve a greater variety of functions has led to the inclusion of more forms and component parts. The federal Medicare-Medicaid bureaucracy and private third-party insurers have seized upon the unit record as a mechanism for recording the information they require for reimbursement purposes. Academic medicine has also contributed to the size and complexity of the unit record, requiring additional forms to collect data for teaching and research purposes.

Quality of Information   The unit medical record contains a vast array of data and information, ranging from highly technical facts and figures (e.g., laboratory test results and diagnostic reports) to descriptive prose (e.g., personal observations, short biographies, and family histories). Initially, the level of accuracy of the data and information generated for the unit medical record is generally quite high; however, a number of factors involving production and maintenance of component parts frequently compromise the overall quality of the unit record (Burnum 1989). Because medical records are used so frequently for insurance purposes, quality assurance, and cost reviews, as well as for teaching and research, parts of the record are occasionally lost or misfiled. Other problems that impair quality are poor handwriting, inaccurate transcription of dictated notes, faint carbons, and low-resolution printouts of computerized data.

Ancillary Diagnostic Media

A wide variety of ancillary diagnostic media is stored outside the unit medical record. These items include images (such as x rays, computed tomography [CT] scans, and magnetic resonance imaging [MRI] scans), pathological specimens and documentation, the results of clinical laboratory tests, the output of in vivo tests (such as electrocardiograms [ECGs] and electroencephalograms [EEGs]), and photographs. Generally, the department of origin (e.g., radiology, pathology, or laboratory medicine) retains control of the actual test medium (the strip chart, image, or specimen) and prepares a report of the test results for inclusion in the unit record.

THE ROLE OF PATIENT RECORDS
AT ACADEMIC HEALTH CENTERS

Health Care Delivery

Patient records are important for health care delivery as long as the subjects of those rec-

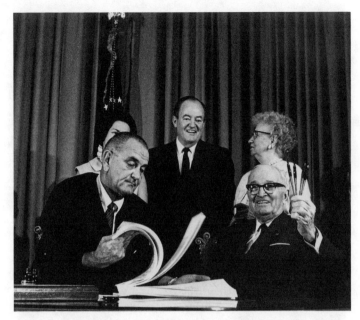

Fig. 3.2   **President Johnson signing the Medicare Bill.** Medicare legislation has transformed the generation of patient records in terms of format, content, and quantity. *Source: Lyndon Baines Johnson Library, by permission; photograph by Okamoto.*

ords are alive—provided that the patients know where their records are stored. Records are, for instance, important for establishing whether or not a person has had prior surgery, particularly if that person is unable to provide the information. They are also useful for identifying medications and their dosages, as well as noting the responses to particular drugs, especially if there is a question about a true drug allergy.

One may also make a case for keeping a patient's records after the patient's death to benefit his or her relatives. Such records could be important when advice is sought regarding hereditary disorders. For example, a person at risk for developing a late-onset autosomal disorder would benefit from knowing if his or her parents had that disorder. Knowing whether the poorly remembered neurological disorder of a patient's father was Parkinson's disease or Huntington's disease would help a physician advise that patient on the risks of developing a neurological disease. However, the rapid pace of research on the molecular diagnosis of genetic diseases makes speculation on the future role of patient records in the study of inherited conditions difficult.

Ancillary media are also important to the ongoing delivery of health care. The rationale for preserving diagnostic data in the original form rests upon the fact that the interpretation of such information may change with time and is not totally captured by any summary report. Clinical studies of disease processes, as well as the diagnostic process itself, require analysis of the actual diagnostic media. Patterns thought to be unimportant on first reading may later come to be seen as significant, both for health care delivery and for research. If a subtle nodule is noted on a chest x-ray image, it may not be clear whether the nodule ought to be a source of concern. The availability of a previous chest x-ray image may reveal that the nodule had been present several years earlier but had not been remarked upon. If comparison reveals that the nodule has not changed, the patient may be reassured and may also avoid an unnecessary operation. Similarly, the initial interpretation of a biopsy specimen may be called into question by a patient's subsequent clinical course. A rereading of the tissue specimens, combined with the knowledge gained by a year or two of clinical observation, may lead to a change in diagnosis and treatment.

Administrative Functions

Historically, the patient record has been the source document for clinical review (Pettinari 1988). In addition, patient records currently play a critical role in the quality assurance process. Analysis of patient records can aid in the evaluation of the clinical management of patients, the performance of health care professionals, and the distribution of health care services. It can identify problems and indicate areas in which improvement is needed. This type of analysis may be used for internal review within the organization, or it may be mandated by organizations external to the hospital.

A quality assurance program consists of the following components:

- Ongoing evaluation of medical care to identify deficiencies in the quality or administration of health care services
- Ongoing programs to ensure the appropriate use of hospital services
- Periodic retrospective analysis of the performance of the health care delivery system

The Joint Commission on Accreditation of Healthcare Organizations requires hospitals to conduct medical care evaluation studies. These standards are frequently being revised in the 1990s (JCAHO 1993).

Research

Biomedical Research   Even if a patient is known to be dead and to have left no relatives, his or her record may still be valuable for clinical research. Some clinical studies, such as prospective, double-blind studies—the "gold standard" for clinical research—do not depend on the records of patients who are not explicitly enrolled in the study. However, to design a prospective study, researchers need to know what it is they wish to study and how they wish to design their study. Knowledge of the relevant variables and outcomes is usually obtained from a retrospective review of patient records. Registers of patients having specific diseases or undergoing certain procedures are useful in selecting cases for a prospective study.

In many instances a prospective study is not possible or practical, and investigation depends on an analysis of patient records that were not originally created to serve a research purpose. Sometimes the rarity of the disease requires researchers to gather records from a wide range of institutions or over a long span of time. In other instances deliberate randomization of a study population is not possible, and investigators who wish to compare two groups of patients need to compare cases from the present with cases from an earlier period.

For such case-control studies, researchers attempt to construct a control group that is as similar as possible to the case group with respect to whatever variables are known to be relevant to the disease in question.

Epidemiologists have long been aware that some of the difficulties of the prospective design might be circumvented if the subjects could be traced not in life but in the medical records of a large population (Kurland and Molgaard 1981). Some diseases may not appear for many years after exposure to the causative agent. For example, the epidemiological studies that established a relationship between mothers who took diethylstilbestrol (DES) and their daughters who developed cervical carcinoma a generation later required medical records that had been saved for several decades. Case reports may provide evidence that a "new" disease, such as Legionnaires' disease or AIDS, was present before it was first recognized as a distinct entity, though it may have been diagnosed as something else. Finally, retrospective studies, which attempt to characterize how the manifestation and character of particular diseases have changed over time, depend on clinical records. Examples of such studies include historical analyses of patients having endocarditis or difficult-to-diagnose fevers.

To estimate how often patient records are now used retrospectively for clinical research, I reviewed one year (1988) of two major clinical journals: the *New England Journal of Medicine* and the *Annals of Internal Medicine*. I analyzed the articles that presented original research, and found that 13 percent used information based on patient records from patients not originally identified as part of the study. (The percentage was almost exactly the same in both journals.) Obviously, these results would vary depending on what journal was surveyed. Nonetheless, it is clear that patient records are being used to a measurable extent in clinical research.

If patient records were well managed and records covering a long span of time were available, patient records might be used in retrospective studies more often, especially if most of the population from a given area obtained health care at a single site. As Kurland and Molgaard described (1981), such a scenario exists at the Mayo Clinic in Rochester, Minnesota. These authors gave several examples of epidemiological studies using Mayo Clinic records.

In addition to the unit record, the original ancillary media are also important for many studies, because much of the information contained cannot be captured easily in the numbers or words that become part of the unit patient record. The retention of these materials may be especially valuable for academic health centers, because more research involving the use of new imaging methods may be carried out at these centers than elsewhere.

Historical Research   Widespread use of patient records for research in medical history is a recent phenomenon that reflects a general shift in what historians of medicine choose to study. The history of medicine was once a field devoted primarily to a litany of important men and their deeds, focusing attention on the key events in a field. Usually these key events were defined by their publication in medical journals, and the historian, who usually had medical or scientific training, took the description of an event solely from the published account. The actual patient record from a particularly important event, such as the introduction of graphic records for anesthesia, was occasionally the subject of attention (Beecher 1940). However, there was little interest in systematically studying a wide range of patient records.

This situation has changed, largely as a result of increased interest in social history. Social historians have attempted to understand life as it was experienced by the majority of people in a society, not simply by the elite. They have consulted documents such as birth records and parish records to study where ordinary people were born and how they lived. This has led to an increased interest in the use of hospital records to study how people received health care (Risse and Warner 1992). Patient records have recently been used to study a wide range of topics, including eighteenth-century care at the Edinburgh Infirmary (Risse 1986), nineteenth-century anesthesia and therapeutics (Pernick 1985; Warner 1985), and twentieth-century use of medical technology (Howell 1986).

Hospital records are particularly important for the history of twentieth-century medicine, because during this century the hospital became a site for routine medical care for most people, as well as a place where almost all physicians receive a large part of their training (Rosenberg 1987). Hospital records offer the historian the ability to study care as practiced by a wide range of physicians, as well as to study the interaction between hospital organization and medical practice. Patient records also offer researchers the opportunity, as summaries found in hospital annual reports (and elsewhere) do not, to associate specific attributes with individual patients. For example, patient records would allow a historian to study differences in social class or gender between patients receiving and not receiving x-ray examinations for leg injuries that might be fractures; summary reports would not. Similarly, one could use patient records to analyze how different physicians treated patients at the same hospital. If one were interested in the relationship between the theory and the practice of medicine, one could use patient records to establish when taking the blood pressure became routine, on which patients the procedure was performed, for which diagnoses it was used, and when physicians started to record both the systolic and the diastolic pressure.

AN OVERVIEW OF PATIENT RECORD–KEEPING PROCEDURES AT ACADEMIC HEALTH CENTERS

Although there is a high degree of standardization in U.S. patient record-keeping systems as a result of the widespread use of the unit record system, there is no well-established standard in the United States for the length of time that patient records should be retained. There is a great deal of confusion among medical institutions about the question of retention time; as a result, patient records are kept or discarded on an ad hoc basis, often with little thought given to their long-term value. The American Hospital Association has advised hospitals to store each record for ten years after the most recent date of patient care (AHA 1990). They also note that the retention period for patient records is dependent on the purposes for which the record is being kept. The legal retention requirements, as established by state law, vary from three years' retention to permanent retention (Ator 1981). Not surprisingly, U.S. academic health centers vary widely with respect to their retention of patient records.

An extensive overview of retention practices concerning patient records at academic medical centers comes from the National Records Survey of Academic Medical Centers (Nancy McCall and Lisa A. Mix, unpublished data, 1987) carried out by the Johns Hopkins Medical Institutions Records Project. From the seventy-eight responses provided by the 116 U.S. medical centers surveyed (see Appendix), one can obtain a sense of the diversity of standards.[1] Overall, the survey documents a striking lack of agreement among teaching hospitals regarding retention policies, procedures, and definitions.

Figure 3.3, based on this survey, shows that the lifetime of an "active" patient record varies tremendously from hospital to hospital. Some hospitals designated a record as "inactive" at the time of discharge; others did so six months after a patient last had contact with the hospital, and still others designated records as "active" until twenty-five years after the patient's last contact with the hospital. Most centers declared all records more than five years old inactive. This situation can present a problem for researchers wishing to use

1. The response rate for each question was less than 100%, so the totals for each item are less than seventy-eight.

records from a wide range of years or to consult patient records more than ten years old. Such records are not universally available, and a researcher needing to use them will have to find a medical center with a long retention period.

The survey also asked about retention policies for diagnostic data not kept in the unit record. Here there is even less agreement than there is for written records. Figure 3.4 shows a histogram of the retention time for x rays, and Figure 3.5 shows a similar histogram for computed tomography (CT) scans. Most centers reported that they discard these two diagnostic media after seven years, usually recycling x-ray films to recover the silver content. Researchers wishing to use older images, either for research or for health care delivery, will probably find that they have been destroyed.

The Johns Hopkins survey indicated that the records retained at academic medical centers are largely open to research. All the centers surveyed said that their records were, or could be, used at least occasionally for clinical, biostatistical, epidemiological, or historical studies. When asked if their records were used for research, some responded "yes" and some "occasionally," but information on how intensively records were actually used was not collected in the survey.

All but three of the responding centers retain active unit records in their original form and not on microfilm or some other medium. Records recently declared inactive were preserved only on microfilm at 41 percent of the institutions. Some states regulate the precise form of microfilming, or even the site at which the microfilming must be performed. Prospective microfilming of patient records may be a viable option if a well-organized system with good quality controls is established and if the microfilming is done in accordance with proper archival standards.[2] However, this process can be very expensive, and many hospitals are not willing to take on such an expense. Unfortunately, several hospital record–microfilming projects undertaken in the 1950s

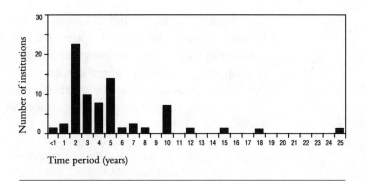

Fig. 3.3 **Duration for active patient record.**

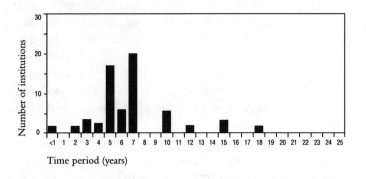

Fig. 3.4 **Retention period for x rays.**

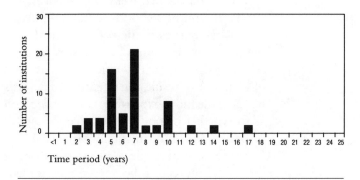

Fig. 3.5 **Retention period for CT scans.**

and 1960s, which were not guided by such standards, produced poor-quality images that are virtually unusable today. Retrospective microfilming of existing paper records is even more expensive because the documents must

2. It should be noted that the linear access feature of microfilm inhibits easy access to and use of data and information. Clinicians as well as researchers who actively use patient records on microfilm complain about the problems and limitations of the medium.

first be put into good clerical order—a very labor-intensive, time-consuming process. Similarly prohibitive costs are inherent in the retrospective conversion of records into computer format. In addition, one must also consider the long-term stability of the computer media (Reed 1987).

THE FEASIBILITY OF LONG-TERM RETENTION OF PATIENT RECORDS

Since patient records are potentially useful for research and health care delivery, why discard them? Almost all researchers would like to have a complete set of patient records available. If necessary, they could choose a sampling method that suited the particular requirements of their research. Thus, if all of the records could be saved, all of the users could, at least in principle, be satisfied.

However, the bulkiness of hospital records makes such an idealistic approach difficult. Since the early twentieth century, patient records have grown increasingly large, a trend driven by the standardization of records, the increasing numbers of hospital employees who make entries in the patient record, and the proliferation within hospitals of separate specialized units, each of which has its own set of forms. As a result, the retention of records has become more expensive, and the decision as to whether or not it is possible to save all records is often fundamentally a financial one.

Some institutions decide to save complete sets of patient records because money is plentiful and/or storage space is inexpensive. Others choose to retain all of their records because they feel a particularly strong sense of history. Still others choose to save all records for those patients involved in important research projects or path-breaking clinical attempts. All of those institutions that save complete sets of records must realize, however, that without proper archival management, their patient records, even if saved, will be of little use.

For the remaining institutions, and this includes most hospitals, records managers will at some point be forced to make decisions about what to discard. However that decision is made, two general guidelines should be followed if the records that remain are to be of maximal research value: (1) the process by which records are selected to be saved must be documented; and (2) a list should be retained of all patients seen at the institution, together with some basic details. Even a rudimentary tabulation summarizing such factors as age, sex, and diagnosis could be used later to improve upon the accuracy of estimates made from the sample.

Those who elect to discard some subset of hospital records while attempting to maintain a useful research resource should be aware of the consequences of that decision. First, they will eliminate the possibility of some types of research, such as the tracing of genetic linkages. For this type of research, the investigator needs access to virtually all of the records. There is no way of predicting which records will be of interest for future family studies, and a sample of the original set of patient records simply will not allow scholars to trace genetic linkages. Second, if one wishes to preserve records so as to be able to document specific events, and if one cannot predict in advance exactly which records document those events, one will be forced to save all of the records. Third, if the aim is to preserve the possibility of research on low-frequency events, large samples will be needed. If the frequency of the events is very low, it may be necessary to retain all the records. The act of selecting only a sample of records to be kept necessarily eliminates some research possibilities. However, if the sampling is done in an appropriate way, it can allow researchers to document broad characteristics of a population and to fulfill some of the goals of social history, but not to follow specific people or events.

The Massachusetts court system sponsored a study of what to do with its court records (Hindus, Hammett, and Hobson 1980). Although this research dealt with judicial records rather than patient records, the results are instructive. First, the authors of the study found that records dated later than 1859 were causing most of the space problem. Although the corresponding date for hospital records is somewhat later (probably sometime after 1900), the general observation is the same: later records tend to be bulkier and more difficult to use and store than earlier ones. Hindus, Hammett, and Hobson also found that many records had been destroyed by local units without notice to or consultation with the scholarly community. Similarly, many hospitals have already started to discard early twentieth-century records.

The analysis of records from the Massachusetts courts (using standards from the 1970s) revealed that about 7 percent of randomly destroyed files would contain historically interesting information. Whether this estimate is too high or too low is, of course, a matter for debate. The advisory group did a systematic and insightful study to find ways of predicting which records were historically interesting, and found this a surprisingly difficult task. They concluded that three criteria correlated with the historical interest of a given file; of the three, the only criterion applicable to hospital records was simply the thickness of the file. The group eventually recommended systematic sampling, with oversampling of files on the basis of predictors of historical interest. Systematic sampling is likely to be the best method for saving medical files as well.

Options for Long-Term Retention

When deciding what to save, hospitals have a number of options. This section will explore the advantages and disadvantages of the following approaches to the retention and disposal of unit records:

- Permanent retention of all patient records by certain hospitals
- Selective retention by year
- Selective retention of portions of patient records
- Systematic sampling
- Selection by size ("fat file" selection)

Permanent Retention Some hospitals might choose to save all of their patient records, whereas others would discard their records after waiting a sufficient interval to make clinical use of the records unlikely. This method would allow detailed analysis of those hospitals that saved their records. If the decisions about which hospitals would save all of their records and which would discard their records could be coordinated nationally, using a method that randomly designated certain hospitals to save their records, a meaningful analysis could be performed. However, such national coordination is unlikely. In the absence of national coordination, those hospitals that voluntarily chose to save all records would probably be quite different from those that discarded records. The former would be more likely to be larger, more distinguished centers, whereas the latter would be more likely to be small community institutions. Scholars would be left with a picture of hospital care skewed toward one particular kind of institution.

Selective Retention by Year Another possibility would be to save all records from certain years, such as every fifth or every tenth year. Whereas this method would allow a broader base of sampling institutions, it would be influenced greatly by the choice of years to be sampled. In addition, it is not clear how one would define whose records would be included in the sample. Would the sample include all patients first admitted during that year? all patients who died during that year? those whose records were declared inactive during that year as a result of death or on the basis of some other criterion? Some changes, such as the diffusion of a new technology or the impact of a change in the reimbursement structure, would occur too rapidly to be well represented by a selection process that retained records at intervals several years apart. This method might be useful for some specific issues or hospitals but would not be the best for broad application.

Selective Retention of Portions of Patient Records   A third approach would be to save only selected portions of all patient records. Twentieth-century inpatient hospital records contain a staggering array of discrete forms and entries. A single patient record may include (as a partial listing) admission and discharge notes (written, in some instances, by the attending physician, a resident, and an intern); notes by medical students; consultants' notes; progress notes by all physicians concerned; procedure and operative notes; nursing administrative, admission, progress, and discharge notes; social work notes; medication records; order sheets; pathology and autopsy records; laboratory and x-ray results; photographs; and demographic and financial data concerning the patient. One could save the admission note and the discharge summary, throwing away the parts of the record deemed less essential. Such an approach might seem appealing because it would allow one to save only the interesting parts of the record, eliminating those portions with little information content or historical value.

The problem is that this approach presupposes that one has the ability to predict what will be interesting to researchers of the future. Some of that information may seem mundane to us now. For example, medical history at one time focused on the great moments in medicine and the eternal search for truth. Now, however, many medical historians are interested in understanding how people in the past reached their conclusions, whether or not we would now think them correct. For example, researchers are interested in analyzing how physicians in the past used information about a patient's temperament in making decisions about how to treat that individual (Warner 1985). Such information might well have been eliminated from a record if only the information considered most important at that time were kept. Similarly, parts of the record that may at first glance seem less illuminating, such as the order sheet or the nursing notes, contain considerable information about how the patient was cared for and how

nurses were trained. Thus, rather than try to predict what parts of the record are likely to be useful in the future, it is advisable to save a complete record whenever possible. Moreover, the cost of going through each entire record to save only certain parts is likely to be prohibitive.

Systematic Sampling   When hospitals find it necessary to discard patient records, systematic sampling—a specific type of probability sampling (Kalton 1983; Kish 1965)—is likely to be the best approach. With probability sampling, each element of the population (in this case, each patient record) has a known and nonzero probability of being sampled. By using probability sampling, the researcher can draw upon a large body of statistical theory to make inferences from the sample results to the entire population of all such records. In other words, one can predict from the sample what the entire population would have been like, had one been able to study it; in addition, one can estimate the accuracy of those predictions.

Systematic sampling is a form of sampling that involves taking every kth record to arrive at the total number desired. For example, if there were one thousand records and one wished to save one hundred, one would pick a random starting point among the first ten records and then save that record and every tenth record thereafter. Every record would therefore have an equal probability of being selected.

During the sampling process, if one were using a master list of admissions, one might encounter a situation in which the record to be sampled does not exist, either because it is lost or for some other reason. In such instances, the correct response would not be to take the next record in the sequence, because that record would then have twice the probability of being sampled as any other record (it could be sampled either because its own number came up or because the missing record before it was selected); instead, the commonly accepted procedure would be to skip that record and go on to the next record that would normally be sampled. Also, if one were attempting to save a certain number of records, rather than a certain percentage of records, a nonintegral value for k could be chosen. For details on techniques for dealing with this situation, as well as other matters of sampling methodology, the reader is referred to the texts listed in the Bibliography, below (Kalton 1983; Kish 1965).

Systematic sampling may not preserve even a single record of a low-frequency event. The more records are saved, the greater the probability that a low-frequency event will be documented, as Table 3.1 illustrates: When only 40 records in a set of 40,000 patient records document a particular disease, 1,609 records must be saved to give an 80-percent probability that at least 1 record documenting that disease is saved; to achieve a certainty of 99.9 percent, 6,905 records must be saved.

Even though a single record of a rare event is useful, it is hardly ever sufficient—one can almost never generalize from a single record. A larger sample of records is needed to allow researchers to draw useful statistical inferences from the results.

Table 3.2 illustrates some of the variables that determine the accuracy of predictions made on the basis of a subgroup sample of records. A major factor is the relative size of the subgroup sampled: whenever a selected sample of records is used to make predictions about a larger population, the size of that subgroup sample directly affects the accuracy of the estimates that are made—the larger the size of the subgroup sample, the higher the accuracy of the estimates.

Consider an example: suppose a group of historians was interested in studying how often x-ray examination had been used to diagnose fractured legs. Suppose further that the historians' research covered ten years' worth of records from a hospital that admitted about forty thousand patients each year and used systematic sampling to save every tenth record. Table 3.2 gives a measure of the precision of the estimates that the researchers could make from the available sample of four thousand records that had been saved from the original universe of forty thousand records.

Suppose the historians examined only one hundred of the four thousand available records and found that 10 percent of the patients with a final diagnosis of fractured leg had been x-rayed. According to Table 3.2, there is a 95-percent chance that the actual percentage of x-rayed patients among the entire popula-

Table 3.1. The effect of sample size on the probability of saving a record of a low-frequency event

Sample Size (No. of records)[a]	Probability (%)
1,609	80.0
2,302	90.0
2,995	95.0
6,905	99.9

[a] Assuming a set of 40,000 patient records, of which 40 (0.1%) document a rare disease. The values given indicate the number of records that must be saved to achieve a given probability that the records of at least one patient with that rare disease will be preserved.

Table 3.2. The effect of subgroup sample size on the precision of estimates made for a larger population

Size of Subgroup Sample	95% Confidence Interval[a] for an Observed Frequency of		
	10%	20%	50%
100	± 5.7	± 7.6	± 9.5
400	± 2.9	± 3.8	± 4.7
1,000	± 1.8	± 2.4	± 3.0
4,000	± 0.9	± 1.2	± 2.5

Note: These calculations are based on the assumption that the subgroup sample was selected by simple random sampling from a set of 40,000 patient records.

[a] Given a particular frequency (e.g., 10%) of an event or characteristic in a subgroup sample of particular size (e.g., 100 records), there is a 95% probability that the frequency in the entire population of 40,000 records would fall within this range (e.g., 10% ± 5.7%).

tion of forty thousand patients at that hospital was between 4.3 and 15.7 (that is, 10% ± 5.7%—the 95% confidence interval [Kish 1965; Kalton 1983]). Because the size of the subgroup population studied (one hundred patients) was very small, the accuracy of the estimate for the entire population of forty thousand patients was not very high. If a much larger subgroup had been studied, the estimate made for the entire forty thousand patients would have been more accurate: for example, if all four thousand available records had been studied and a value of 10 percent obtained, then (as Table 3.2 indicates) there would be a 95-percent chance that the true percentage for the entire forty thousand patients was between 10.9 and 9.1 (10% ± 0.9%).

Table 3.2 further indicates that the predictability is also influenced by the percentage distribution. The estimates are more accurate when only a small percentage of the patients sampled show a particular characteristic: as the percentage with a particular characteristic approaches 50, the standard errors become larger and the predictability worsens.

One potential solution to the difficulty of studying low-frequency events is disproportionate stratification: selecting a sample that includes relatively fewer records from homogeneous groups, such as patients with common diagnoses, and more from other groups, such as patients with rare diagnoses. The precision of the results for the low-frequency events can be increased by sampling them at higher rates.

There are a number of different ways in which one could apply disproportionate stratification. One might stratify according to disease characteristic, such as diagnosis. Within diagnoses, one might stratify by the level of severity, attempting to sample fewer routine cases and more complex cases. However, we do not yet have a simple, reliable, and valid method for measuring the severity of illness, even for records of the recent past (McMahon and Billi 1988). If, instead, the research question concerned determinants of how physi-

cians practice medicine, one might base stratification on characteristics of the physician: date of graduation from medical school, type of residency, age, and gender. To study the types of patient entering the hospital, one might stratify on the basis of the patient's social class, insurance status, or personality type. (The latter approach was used in the past and is now making a minor comeback in the study of the "type A" personality and its possible relationship to coronary heart disease.) This list of possibilities for disproportionate stratification should make it obvious that there are many ways to choose groups to be oversampled. The difficulty is that one needs to know in advance which groups one will want to sample at higher rates. Because one does not have such knowledge when records are sampled for unknown clinical and historical studies to be performed in the future, disproportionate stratification is not in general a desirable strategy. Considering our inability to predict future understanding of health and disease, as well as to identify future research interests, it quickly becomes obvious that any disproportionate stratification sampling system would unduly constrain research.

The physical process by which a record is identified as being part of the sample may vary, depending upon the sampling process used and the way that records are stored at a particular institution. The record could be identified by at least three distinct methods: (1) it could be identified directly on the shelf, as through systematic sampling; (2) it could be identified through an index of all admissions and then located on the shelf; and (3) it could be identified only after examining its contents to see if it should be part of the sample (e.g., when the disproportionate stratification approach is being used). Obviously, the second of these methods requires more skill on the part of the person doing the sampling, and involves more expense, than does the first; and the third method requires more skill and involves more expense than does the second.

A basic sampling question is, what size should the sample be? In theory, the answer is determined by the events to be measured and the statistical precision of the estimates one wishes to compute.[3] For a sampling of patient records for future historical research, the estimates that will be required are unknown, and hence a theoretical solution to the question of sample size is impossible to provide. As a result, the answer to "How many records should we save?" cannot be given in a statistically sophisticated sense. Instead, the decision must depend primarily on the financial resources available, together with a general sense of the kinds of precision that may be attained for some general types of question.

One common fallacy should be mentioned: On an intuitive basis, it may seem reasonable that the precision of sample estimates should be largely a function of the proportion that the sample represents of the total group from which the sample is drawn (i.e., that a sample of four hundred will give a more accurate estimate when drawn from a population of five thousand than when drawn from a population of five hundred thousand). However, this is not the case. The precision of the estimate depends primarily on the total number in the sample, not on the fraction that is sampled. The percentage of the total universe that is sampled has a negligible effect on the precision of estimates when the fraction sampled is less than about 10 percent, as is usually the case in practice.[4]

Selection by Size ("Fat File" Selection)
All of the discussion thus far has been focused on using probability sampling. However, considering the findings of the survey of legal records discussed earlier (Hindus, Hammett, and Hobson 1980), it seems reasonable to recommend a final group of files to be saved—the thick ones. Though not in any sense a statistically valid group, the thickest files in a collection may contain unique information. Furthermore, they are easy to identify during the sampling process. The definition of the "thickest" files will vary from site to site but

should encompass approximately 1 percent of all files from a given decade.

Long-Term Retention of Ancillary Diagnostic Media

Throughout most of the nineteenth century, hospital patient records were almost completely composed of paper. In addition to the entries by nurses and physicians, other information, such as the results of urinalysis, or the patient's temperature chart, was also recorded on the same types of paper as the patient record. Pathological specimens, the main exceptions to this generalization, were often stored in special museums.

The invention of the x-ray machine in 1895 forced those who stored hospital records to face a new set of issues. However, there was not an immediate need for space to store x-ray images, both because it took time before the use of the x-ray machine became routine and because there was at first considerable debate over whether radiologists should simply visualize the body using fluoroscopy or whether they needed as well to produce a permanent

3. When sampling patient records from the early twentieth century, I wished to compare the use of medical technology in two hospitals. On the basis of a pilot study, I estimated the percentage of patients who would receive a particular technological intervention at between 1% and 25%. I then decided that I wanted to be able to detect, 80% of the time, a true 10% difference between the incidence of use at one hospital and the corresponding figure at the other. On the basis of these estimates, I calculated that a sample size of four hundred records would be needed from each hospital. Two important caveats about this estimate must be stressed. First, it is based on a specific set of questions and a specific series of estimates: if any of the above numbers were to change—if, for example, I were to decide that I wanted to be not 80% but 90% certain of seeing a difference, or if I decided that I cared only if the difference between hospitals was greater than 25%, not 10%—the estimated sample size would change. Second, the estimate is independent of the total number of admissions to the hospitals. For details of this calculation, see Kalton 1983 or Kish 1965.

4. In the calculation for standard error, the sampling fraction (f) enters only into the multiplier:

$$\sqrt{1 - \frac{\text{number sampled}}{\text{total number in population}}}$$

The value of this multiplier is 0.975 for a 5% sample and 0.95 for a 10% sample, and it remains very close to 1 until the fraction becomes relatively large (Kalton 1983; Kish 1965).

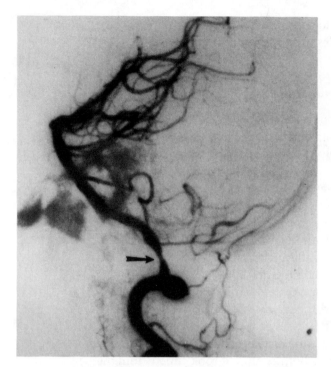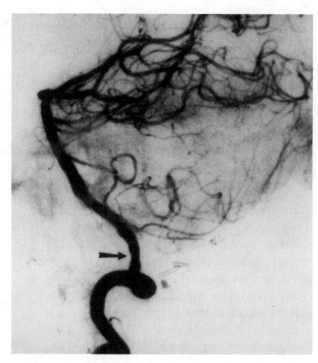

Fig. 3.6 **Arteriograms demonstrating the result of surgery of the left vertebral artery, 1981.** Visual diagnostic formats have become prevalent in the twentieth century. *Source: Alan Mason Chesney Medical Archives, the Johns Hopkins Medical Institutions.*

image on an x-ray plate. But even from the time of the very first x-ray pictures, physicians and hospitals saved some images. With the advent of high-speed film and more powerful machines in the 1920s, the trend shifted toward routinely recording a permanent image for many types of patients. Permanent images could be reviewed by more than one person (e.g., the person who took the image, the referring physician, and, at times, the patient) and could be easily assembled for teaching purposes.

Saving x-ray images presented hospitals with a new set of problems. The images were at first recorded using film based on cellulose nitrate, a highly flammable substance. The danger of storing x-ray films was reduced by substituting more expensive but less dangerous cellulose acetate film. Although this change eliminated the physical danger of storing x-ray images, the problem of what to do with the increasing bulk of images remained. As the amount and variety of diagnostic me-

dia have continued to expand throughout the twentieth century, hospital records managers have confronted a problem of increasing magnitude.

The selection of media to save should be guided by a line of reasoning similar to that used for the selection of written records. Systematic sampling holds the greatest promise for meeting the needs of historians of the future. Thus, as a supplement to systematic sampling, the largest sets of diagnostic records—like the largest sets of written records—should be saved. If possible, the selection of diagnostic records should be linked to the selection of written records (i.e., the written records should be sampled first, and those diagnostic records associated with each written patient record should then be saved). Matching the two types of record will, of course, entail additional time and expense. If this matching is not possible, or if the written records either cannot be located or never existed (as in the case of screening chest x rays), then the best

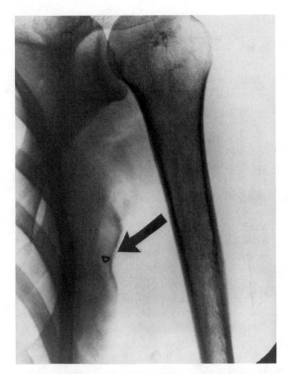

Fig. 3.7 **X ray showing subcutaneous implantation of pellets of crystalline synthetic adrenal hormone in the scapular area, 1939.** *Source: Alan Mason Chesney Medical Archives, the Johns Hopkins Medical Institutions.*

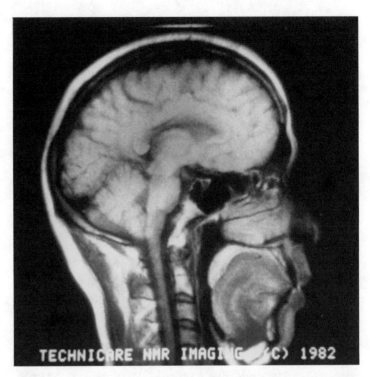

Fig. 3.8 **Magnetic resonance imaging scan of the head, 1982.** *Source: Alan Mason Chesney Medical Archives, the Johns Hopkins Medical Institutions.*

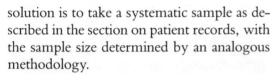

solution is to take a systematic sample as described in the section on patient records, with the sample size determined by an analogous methodology.

The results of many diagnostic procedures, such as CT scans, are now recorded and used in electronic form, and many more may be routinely recorded electronically within the next few decades. This advance presents a second question regarding diagnostic media: should the physical image or the electronic record be retained, or both? For at least a subset of records, it will be essential to retain the electronic record, and in some instances the equipment that is needed to read the format. Although the physical images are easier to store and to examine, radiologists can often make most effective use of a CT scan by electronically manipulating the image. Future historians will wish to have access to that means of interpretation to study how medical

technology such as the CT scan was actually used. Similar arguments could be made for storing other types of electronically encoded diagnostic media. See chapter 9 for a discussion of the strategies for retaining and interpreting electronically encoded data and information.

CONCLUSION

There is now little consensus concerning when, how, and how often to save records of clinical care for patients in teaching hospitals. The ever-increasing bulk of patient care material makes it inevitable that, in the next decade or so, almost every institution will face major decisions about what to do with its records. This chapter has suggested systematic sampling as one feasible way in which medical institutions can deal with the problem of the need for space and yet retain as much valuable data as possible for the generations of scholars to come. Other sampling options, however, may be appropriate for some institutions. For example, an institution with ample space and resources for both the storage and the management of records may choose to retain all its records permanently. There are a variety of answers to the question of effective record selection; each eliminates certain options both for health care delivery and for historical research. The individuals who make these decisions should be aware of the advantages and disadvantages of each approach. Having saved the records, the archives staff should then not only catalog and preserve them but also encourage their use, within the ethical and legal constraints applicable to patient records.

ACKNOWLEDGMENTS

I would like to thank Harry Marks, Martin Pernick, and Jack Pressman for their reactions to an earlier draft of this chapter, and Graham Kalton for his comments on the section on sampling. Comments from anonymous reviewers were particularly useful.

The preparation of this chapter was supported in part by a grant from the National Endowment for the Humanities.

The discussion of sampling strategies was informed by two meetings on sampling held at the Johns Hopkins Medical Institutions on July 7 and November 10, 1988, under the auspices of the Johns Hopkins Medical Institutions Records Project.

BIBLIOGRAPHY

ALDRICH, R.F., AND J.A. TURNER. 1977. *Dilemma: A Report of the National Conference on the Health Records Dilemma.* Washington, D.C.: National Commission on Confidentiality of Health Records.

AMERICAN HOSPITAL ASSOCIATION (AHA). 1990. *Preservation of Medical Records in Health Care Institutions.* Chicago: American Hospital Association.

ATOR, N.E. 1981. Retention of medical records: Legal requirements and practical constraints. *Topics in Health Records Management* 2:31–40.

BEECHER, H.K. 1940. The first anesthesia records (Codman, Cushing). *Surgery, Gynecology, and Obstetrics* 71:689–93.

BRUCE, J.A. 1984. *Privacy and Confidentiality of Health Care Information.* Chicago: American Hospital Publishing.

BURNUM, J.F. 1989. The misinformation era: The fall of the medical record. *Annals of Internal Medicine* 110:482–84.

CRAIG, B.L. 1985. The Canadian hospital in history and archives. *Archivaria* 21:52–67.

HAYT, E. 1977. *Medicolegal Aspects of Hospital Records.* 2d ed. Berwyn, Ill.: Physicians' Record Co.

HINDUS, M.S., T.M. HAMMETT, AND B.M. HOBSON. 1980. *The Files of the Massachusetts Superior Court, 1859–1959: An Analysis and a Plan for Action.* A report of the Massachusetts Judicial Records Committee of the Supreme Judicial Court, 1979. Boston: G. K. Hall and Co.

HOWELL, J.D. 1986. Early use of x-ray machines and electrocardiographs at the Pennsylvania Hospital, 1897–1927. *JAMA* 255:2320–23.

———. 1987. Machines, meanings: British and American use of medical technology, 1890–1930. Ph.D. diss., University of Pennsylvania.

———. 1988. Patient care at Guy's and the Pennsylvania Hospital, 1900–1920. *British Society for the History of Science and the History of Science Society Program, Papers and Abstracts for the Joint Conference,* pp. 247–54.

HUFFMAN, E.K. 1990. *Medical Record Management,* 9th ed., ed. R. Finnegan and M. Amatayakul. Berwyn, Ill.: Physicians' Record Co.

JOINT COMMISSION ON ACCREDITATION OF HEALTH-CARE ORGANIZATIONS (JCAHO). 1993. *Accreditation Manual for Hospitals.* Oakbrook Terrace, Ill.: JCAHO.

KALTON, G. 1983. *Introduction to Survey Sampling.* Beverly Hills, Calif.: Sage Publications.

KEARSEY, I. 1988. To keep or not to keep, that is the question addressed by the General Disposal Schedule. *Australian Medical Records Journal* 18:107–10.

KISH, L. 1965. *Survey Sampling.* New York: John Wiley and Sons.

KURLAND, L.T., AND C.A. MOLGAARD. 1981. The patient record in epidemiology. *Scientific American* 245:54–63.

LIEBLER, J.G. 1980. *Managing Health Records: Administrative Principles.* Germantown, Md.: Aspen Systems Corp.

LUDMERER, K.M. 1982. Writing the history of hospitals. *Bulletin of the History of Medicine* 56:106–9.

MCMAHON, L.F., JR., AND J.E. BILLI. 1988. Measurement of severity of illness and the Medicare prospective payment system: State of the art and future directions. *Journal of General Internal Medicine* 3:482–90.

NICOL, A., AND J. SHEPPARD. 1985. What records are kept now? The present scene. Discussion paper C, presented at the symposium "Hospital Clinical Records," King's Fund Centre, London, May 8.

PERNICK, M.S. 1985. *A Calculus of Suffering: Pain, Professionalism, and Anesthesia in Nineteenth Century America*. New York: Columbia University Press.

PETTINARI, C.J. 1988. *Task, Talk, and Text in the Operating Room: A Study in Medical Discourse.* Advances in Discourse Processes, ed. R. O. Freedle, Vol. 33. Norwood, N.J.: Ablex.

REED, B. 1987. Retention of medical records at Sydney Hospital. *Australian Medical Records Journal* 17:6–10.

RISSE, G.B. 1986. *Hospital Life in Enlightenment Scotland: Care and Teaching at the Royal Infirmary of Edinburgh*. Cambridge: Cambridge University Press.

RISSE, G.B., AND WARNER, J.H. 1992. Reconstructing clinical activities: Patient records in medical history. *Social History of Medicine* 5:183–206.

ROACH, W.H., JR. 1981. Access to medical records, Part 2: Liability for improper distribution of medical records. *Topics in Health Records Management* 2:41–48.

ROSENBERG, C.E. 1987. *The Care of Strangers: The Rise of America's Hospital System*. New York: Basic Books.

SHEPPARD, J., AND A. NICOL. 1985. Why keep hospital records? *British Medical Journal* 290:263–64.

TEMKIN, O. 1977. *The Double Face of Janus*. Baltimore: Johns Hopkins University Press.

WARNER, J.H. 1985. *The Therapeutic Perspective.* Cambridge: Harvard University Press.

WATERS, K.A., AND G.F. MURPHY. 1979. *Medical Records in Health Information*. Germantown, Md.: Aspen Systems.

WEED, L.L. 1969. *Medical Records, Medical Education, and Patient Care*. Cleveland: Press of Case Western Reserve University.

WELLCOME UNIT FOR THE HISTORY OF MEDICINE. 1979. *The Preservation of Medical and Public Health Records*. Research Publication no. 1. Oxford: Wellcome Unit for the History of Medicine.

———. 1980. *Medical Records Newsletter,* ed. L. Jordanova. Research Publication no. 4. Oxford: Wellcome Unit for the History of Medicine.

4

Collecting Scientific Data with Ongoing Value for Research and Teaching

Jane Williams

WHEREAS PATIENT RECORDS and scientific research data share many characteristics in terms of format, content, and medium, these two types of documentation differ significantly in that they are created for distinctly different purposes under different sets of circumstances, guidelines, and regulations. Patient records are created to verify processes of diagnosis and treatment. Research records are generated to verify processes of scientific experimentation and observation. Patient records, especially in hospitals affiliated with academic health centers, are usually created with the intention that they may also be used for study in the health and related sciences.

The health sciences include a broad range of clinical and applied science disciplines that crosscut many professions, including medicine, nursing, dentistry, public health, and the ancillary health occupations. The biological sciences and life sciences span the basic science disciplines that study living organisms and their systems. Whereas the health sciences revolve around the diagnostic, therapeutic, and socioeconomic aspects of health care delivery, the biological sciences and life sciences focus on the study of biological, biophysical, and biochemical phenomena. For a more definitive discussion of discipinary distinctions in the health sciences and the life and biological sciences, see the chapter by Paul Anderson in Joan Krizack's *Documentation Planning for the U.S. Health Care System* (Krizack 1994).

A key difference between patient records and the records from studies in the health and related sciences involves controls. Whereas regulatory controls have standardized the design of the patient record, regulatory agencies have been unable to reach consensus on standards for research records. Because the structure of research records tends to be discipline specific, a high degree of standardization is neither possible, nor desirable. Most research records are generated in controlled laboratory settings, while patient records are created in a situational mode that must accommodate the immediacy of the patient's condition.

At academic health centers, patient records and scientific research data are used interactively to further functions of health care delivery, teaching, and research. Many scientists in the health fields rely on access to patient records to gather baseline information for prospective studies. Some research findings in the basic sciences may have immediate clinical applications that can be tested in clinical trials with a select group of patients. On the other hand, a biological marker found in a selection of patient records may have special implications for research in the basic sciences.

Archivists at institutions in the health fields must balance priorities for the acquisition of patient and research records. Whereas it is possible to develop general schemes for the sampling of patient records because their in-

formational components are standardized, a common rational approach cannot be developed for sampling scientific records because of the lack of standardization in their design. However, by studying discipline-specific methodologies for generating research data, individual sampling approaches may be developed for certain areas of science. Appraisal procedures for scientific data should focus on the role of the data in verifying research findings. Thus, the criteria and standards for verifying research findings should be incorporated in the appraisal of scientific records.[1]

Although some archivists and historians may question whether or not the acquisition activities of archival programs should include the area of research data, pressures do, however, exist at institutions in the health fields for archival repositories to accept some samples of research data on a regular basis. As institutional administrators at the Johns Hopkins Medical Institutions have had to deal with the scientific, historical, and regulatory issues that pertain to the retention of research data, they have requested that selections of research data that may be used for ongoing studies and as pedagogical examples for teaching be deposited in the institutional archives.

Because these selections of research data documented significant research initiatives at the Medical Institutions and also had far-reaching importance in the health fields, the archives staff felt a compelling responsibility to accession these materials. While these samples of research data have presented challenges in terms of processing and preservation, they also afford new opportunities for research to investigators from a number of different disciplines. As sociologists, anthropologists,

1. The Center for the History of Physics at the American Institute of Physics (AIP) has taken a leadership role in appraising research records. Archivists at AIP have written appraisal guidelines that are applied at other institutions in the field of high-energy physics (e.g., the Stanford Linear Accelerator Center). While some of the issues surrounding research records in the health fields are different than those associated with physics, AIP's program nonetheless stands as an excellent model for appraising the records of scientific research. For further discussion, see Warnow-Blewett 1987, 1989, and 1992.

historians, and other types of social scientists engage in the study of scientific processes, they must examine research methodologies as well as actual samples of data.[2]

Investigators in the health and related sciences may use samples of these data to study the origins of basic concepts in their fields and to reanalyze these data in view of new questions and new knowledge. Educators in the health and related sciences find that these samples of research data serve as excellent teaching tools to demonstrate the evolution of research methodologies and experimental design. The acquisition of research data documents key institutional functions and at the same time stimulates new areas of study.

Because of variations in research methodologies and differences in how data are generated and used, it is impossible to make standardized, broad-sweeping acquisition guidelines that apply to the full spectrum of research data in the health fields. Whereas professional associations for some scientific disciplines have begun to develop data retention guidelines for purposes of defending research findings, institutions will not be able to develop a body of inclusive policy for data retention until the disciplines themselves issue more definite guidelines. The criteria and standards that the individual disciplines provide to guide the retention of research data for the purpose of verifying research findings should in turn be adapted by archivists in the appraisal of scientific research data. For an overview of the role of professional organizations in the health sciences and biological and life sciences, see James Carson's chapter on voluntary and professional organizations in the U.S. health care system in Krizack 1994.

While archival programs cannot be expected to assume the functions of a data center for their institutions, they do, nevertheless, have a responsible role to play in the identification and preservation of key research data at their institutions. On an institutional level they should work with administrators and scientists to develop policies and strategies for the selection and preservation of significant

data sets. At this level they should play an activist role in seeing that some selections of data are placed in data centers or laboratories where they will be utilized in ongoing studies. At the repository level, they should make provisions in their programs for the acquisition, processing, and management of samples of research data and also address issues of access and use. In developing documentation plans they must strive to balance the selection of research data with the acquisition priorities for the archival programs. The acquisition of research data is just one of the many options in the development of archival holdings.

This chapter does not intend to suggest that archives in the health sciences depart from their traditional functions to become centers for the exclusive collection of institutional research data. The aim is to encourage archival repositories to enlarge the intellectual scope of their mission by documenting the research activities of their institutions. A main purpose is to advocate the selection of data on the basis of its integrity for reanalysis and verification of research findings. By allowing the research methodologies of the relevant scientific disciplines to guide their standards and criteria for selection, archivists will be able to build a body of intellectually coherent data that may be manipulated in the process of reanalysis. A main objective is to encourage archivists to select samples of data that are representative of the scientific activities at their institutions.

ARCHIVAL ISSUES IN THE ACQUISITION OF SCIENTIFIC RECORDS

Whereas archival appraisal of scientific records has focused largely on records that document significant discoveries and major events in the research community, other issues have emerged in the appraisal of research records. In recent years scientists as well as health policy specialists, historians, anthropologists, and other scholars have turned their attention to

2. The historian F.L. Holmes has utilized laboratory notebooks for the study of research processes (Holmes 1990).

the potential reuses of research data in applications to new questions and new areas of study. Because many of the research methodologies in the health and related sciences are inductive and rely upon the collection and analysis of large sets of data, there is a superabundance of research data from both the present and the past at institutions throughout the health fields. The investigators who collected these data, as well as the research institutions and funding agencies that supported their collection, are sometimes reluctant to dispose of these materials after the expiration of regulatory retention requirements. They often hold hopes of gaining more returns from their original intellectual and financial investment.

Over the years the duplication of research efforts has inevitably led to redundancies in data collection. Because some collections of research data do contain materials that may be utilized in ongoing studies, they may be regarded as an untapped resource of potentially recyclable data. With recent funding constraints and calls for reforms in research practices in the health fields, investigators are compelled not only to cut costs but also to make more prudent and creative use of existing resources. While these collections of data may constitute a viable research resource for some ongoing studies in the health sciences, they may also serve as a primary resource for studies in other fields, such as the humanities and the social sciences.

Concerns have focused on the fate of these data collections after their immediate primary use, especially when research projects conclude and principal investigators retire or die. As archivists are drawn into the effort to preserve viable samples of research data, they face a number of major challenges. They must learn not only how to appraise and select pertinent samples of research data but also how to make these samples of data accessible for different forms of research.

Archivists must concentrate on strategies for documenting the scientific activity of institutions in the health fields. They will have

to address issues about the underutilization and loss of data resources at their institutions. As archivists consider the potential reuses of scientific data for ongoing studies in the health sciences and other fields, they must develop criteria and standards for assessing the quality and viability of these materials for research purposes. Although archivists who are responsible for the records of the health sciences should continue to acquire records that document key discoveries and major historic events, they must also begin to address the new issues associated with the selection and management of data samples that are to be reused for studies by investigators from a number of different fields.

Types of Biomedical Research Data

Data in the field of biomedical research include both *observational data* (data collected through observation of natural phenomena) and *experimental data* (data collected through experimentation). Experimental data are by definition not unique, because experiments must be repeatable. Whereas the need to preserve unique observational data—for example, in longitudinal and epidemiological studies—is well established, the case for preserving repeatable experimental data is less clear-cut.

Observational data may include individual case studies as well as large surveys of special patient populations and communities; most experimental data represent the results of laboratory research. However, some types of clinical laboratory data—for instance, blood test and urinalysis results—fall somewhere between the categories of observational and experimental data. Many research records in the health sciences contain a combination of observational and experimental data. The data from clinical trials, patient case studies, and epidemiological, biostatistical, longitudinal, latitudinal, and quality assurance studies are examples of the types of data that may have potential value for reuse in related or other forms of research.

The types of data in the health sciences that are most viable for reuse are as follows (adapted from Cordray, Pion, and Boruch 1990):

- The data produced in basic biomedical research, which include the digital or graphic output of laboratory instruments; notebooks containing experimental data; histological samples; and biochemical and other assays
- Clinical research data, which are similar to those generated in basic biomedical research and may also include medical records and diagnostic tests
- Behavioral research data, which may include tests, questionnaires, investigator-developed checklists, structured behavioral assessments, and unstructured interviews
- Epidemiological data, which are similar to those produced by basic biomedical studies and by behavioral studies and may include laboratory tests, diagnostic media, and clinical observations, as well as structured surveys

Data Sharing and the Ethos of Science

Scientific research is a collective activity, the products of which are assumed to be the common property of the scientific community. This idea is embodied in the "ethos of science," which has been expounded by the sociologist of science Robert Merton (Merton 1973, 268). According to Merton, four unwritten but socially articulated "institutional imperatives" or "norms of science" (Merton 1973, 270) govern the behavior of scientists and, moreover, are essential to scientific methodology:

- Universalism: the concept that the validity of scientific knowledge should transcend the divisions of race, nationality, religion, and class
- Communism: the concept that the products of science should belong not to the individual researcher but to the community as a whole

- Disinterestedness: the concept that science should not be influenced by the political, religious, or personal beliefs of its practitioners
- Organized skepticism: the concept that science should involve a temporary suspension of judgment and detached scrutiny of beliefs in terms of logical criteria (Merton 1973)

Indeed, it has been argued that openness to criticism is essential to the proper functioning of the scientific method. It follows that it is only through scrutiny, testing, and replication of research findings that scientific knowledge may be validated (Popper 1959).

In this context, the sharing of historical or contemporary research data might be assumed to be in keeping with normal scientific practice, and disputes over ownership and disclosure would be the exception. The scientific community and the knowledge it generates are, however, subject to the same social and economic forces that characterize modern industrial societies. Hence, research performed in a commercial environment will be subject to proprietary restrictions, and competition for peer recognition and promotion within the academic sector may influence a researcher's attitude to sharing data with potential rivals.

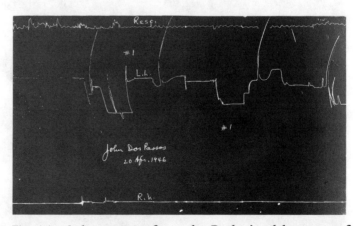

Fig. 4.1 **A kymogram from the Pavlovian laboratory of Horsley Gantt.** During the twentieth century machine-generated data became prevalent in the laboratories of bench scientists. *Source: Alan Mason Chesney Medical Archives, the Johns Hopkins Medical Institutions.*

Although the real-life situations in which scientists work are complicated by such considerations, open inquiry continues to be upheld as a fundamental value of science, and the sharing of knowledge is still imperative to scientific progress (Fienberg, Martin, and Straf 1985). The justification for sharing data is particularly strong in the case of publicly funded research because it may be argued that the results of such research should be used for the benefit of society. Accordingly, it may follow that data from publicly funded research should be made available for reuse, the only exceptions being information harmful to human subjects or to national security (Ceci and Walker 1983). Such sharing of data may also maximize the value obtained from a single piece of research and thus result in more effective and economical use of public funds. In the United States, this argument is particularly pertinent to the field of biomedical research, where a large proportion of research is funded by the taxpayer.

IMPLICATIONS FOR PROMOTING THE SHARING OF SCIENTIFIC DATA

The Rise of Scientific Research

Science has never before been so pervasive nor so integral to economic life as it is today. Since the end of World War II, support for scientific research has grown at a phenomenal rate, and it is now a significant item of national expenditure. Between 1970 and 1986 the total U.S. expenditure on research and development increased from $62 billion to $102 billion (Na-

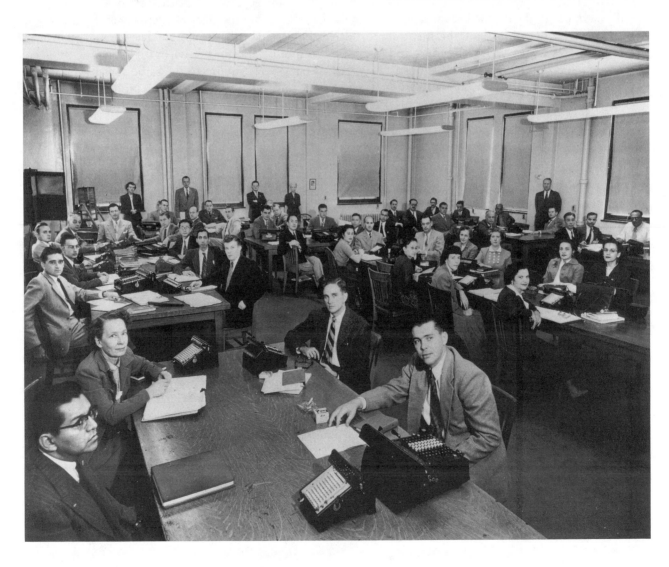

tional Science Foundation 1987). This rise in government spending represents not only an increase in the amount of research supported but also an increase in the cost of performing research as the tools used become more sophisticated.

On a longer time scale, the steady growth of scientific activity during the last three centuries has been accompanied by a commensurate increase in means of scientific communication. The escalation of scientific publishing has been particularly significant. In both books and journals, scientists have competed for precedence. The historian Derek de Solla Price has pointed out that the number of scientific journals published increased from one in 1665 (the *Philosophical Transactions of the Royal Society of London*) to about one hundred thousand in the early 1960s. He commented that the number of journals has grown exponentially, doubling about every fifteen years (Price 1961, 96). Price also used the number of papers published in a particular field (as recorded in *Physics Abstracts*) and the number of people employed in a science-based industry (electrical engineering) as indexes to trace the growth in scientific activity. All showed the same pattern of exponential growth (Price 1961, 101–3).

Since Price's studies, scientific publishing has continued to grow at an exponential rate and is currently undergoing a major shift in medium. Whereas printing presses have been the main vehicles of scientific communication for the past three centuries, computers have now entered the arena of scientific communication and are beginning to transform both journal and book publication. Reference books such as *Mendelian Inheritance in Man* (published electronically as GDB/OMIM) are

published in electronic formats so that they may be more easily and more rapidly updated on a regular—sometimes daily—basis. Scientific abstracts and citation indexes are also being computerized to facilitate more rapid collection and dissemination of scientific information. [3]

The interactive nature of research and scientific publishing has held and continues to hold special implications for archivists who are involved in the appraisal and selection of research data. [4] Because the editorial peer review processes that publishers employ do inevitably involve some biases and may result in skewed decisions, the published record is not necessarily the most thorough or accurate record of scientific activities. For instance, the results of some significant studies may not have been published because of objections to either the principal investigator or the topic of the studies. Personal and political biases affect scientific publishing, as do trends and popular fashions in research topics. Whereas archivists must concentrate on preserving examples of data from major studies that have been published, they, at the same time, should not overlook the data from key studies that have not been published.

Thus, the publishing status of data is another issue to be considered in archival appraisal. Recent requirements in scientific publishing, to review the data upon which articles are based, also have archival implications. In order to publish, scientists will be compelled to retain their primary research data for longer periods of time. [5] Because of recent incidents

---

Fig. 4.2 **Biometrics laboratory, circa 1935.** The introduction of new technology and quantitative methodologies for research in biometrics, biostatistics, and epidemiology have transformed the recording, collection, and use of documentation in these fields. *Source: Alan Mason Chesney Medical Archives, the Johns Hopkins Medical Institutions.*

3. Currently more than forty medical journals are available in electronic format, as are many scientific and technical journals. About three dozen journals in various disciplines exist only as electronic journals (Michelson and Rothenberg 1992, 273, 274).

4. In discussions with Nancy McCall and Lisa Mix about the documentation of scientific activity in the health fields, Harry Marks, of the Johns Hopkins University Institute of the History of Medicine, urged that they not overlook the role of publishing in their study. Marks is particularly concerned that the archives of scientific journals be preserved and made accessible for research, so that the impact of publishing decisions may be better understood.

5. In the past, both publishers and the scientists who submitted manuscripts to them operated on an honor system.

of scientific fraud and the growing complexity of scientific data in the health fields, publishers have had to hire statisticians and data auditors to review data from manuscripts that are under consideration for publication. In some instances journals may also include excerpts of data in the publication of manuscripts to augment the textual account because some studies cannot be fully understood by verbal descriptions alone.

Because both individual and institutional prestige is achieved through successes in grantsmanship and publishing, the research community in the health sciences is forced to comply with the rise of data-retention requirements from granting agencies and publishers. As the data from research projects accumulate at institutions in the health fields and increase at an exponential rate with the overall expansion of research activities, institutions are forced to review their responsibilities for the retention of these data.[6] Because of the volume and complexity of the data and variation in retention requirements, it is impossible for institutions, especially large academic health centers, to manage the retention of data effectively in any single formalized approach. In some institutions, such as the Johns Hopkins University School of Medicine, institution-wide policies have been adopted to promote the responsible collection, management, and retention of research data. Whereas the objectives of the Johns Hopkins policies are broad-sweeping on an institutional level, the central administration has placed responsibility for the physical storage and management of the data on the individual departments.

To document scientific activity at institutions in the health fields, archivists must engage in not one strategy but a combination of different strategies. In confronting the surfeit of research documentation at their institutions, they must recognize that they face a variety of options for selection. Their greatest challenge is to prioritize these options in a clearly designated documentation plan. A major goal of the documentation plan should be to balance the selection of data from representative scientific activities with the selection of data from key areas of specialization. Criteria and standards should be set to ensure the selection of documentation that is physically, intellectually, and technically viable for use in various forms of research.

Whereas the issues that have attended the rapid expansion in scientific research are manifold, essentially three can be singled out as having particular relevance to the preservation of scientific data:

- Data may be reused as source material for new or related studies in the same scientific field.
- Data may be reused as source material for studies in other scientific fields.
- Data may be reused as source material for studies that examine the role of data in the scientific research process. Such studies include data analyses in fields that study scientific research methodologies (history, sociology, anthropology, ethnography, etc.), and verifications of research findings and data audits in investigations of research fraud.

Reuse of Scientific Data in New or Related Studies

The large-scale support for research since 1945 has resulted in the accumulation of vast quantities of scientific data. Some of these data have been published in the literature, but

---

Publishers relied largely on the logic and the persuasion of the scientists' arguments, on peer review, and on the professional integrity of the investigators. Seldom did they require audits of primary data.

6. Archivists who are responsible for documenting the scientific activities of their institutions are also faced with a dilemma about the appraisal of research protocols for projects that granting agencies did not fund. Because funding decisions, like publishing decisions, may be affected by personal biases as well as by trends in research topics, archivists should consider the place of rejected research protocols when developing institutional acquisition plans. Retaining documentation from successful endeavors (e.g., funded projects) and disposing of documentation from unsuccessful endeavors (e.g., projects rejected for funding) would not provide an accurate view of scientific activity at their institutions.

the remainder have never been systematically appraised for their potential value to other researchers and thus may be considered an important unexploited resource (Elliott 1983; Haas, Samuels, and Simmons 1985; Sieber 1991).

The escalating cost of performing scientific research also has implications for the preservation of research data. The desire to avoid unnecessary duplication and maximize the value obtained from each research project has provided the motivation for professional organizations and funding agencies to examine the potential for data sharing.[7]

Traditionally the results of research are shared through publication in recognized journals in an appropriate field, yet only a small fraction of research data is published in the literature. The formidable problems created by the vast amounts of unpublished data produced in the course of scientific research have been described in a report (Elliott 1983) published by the Joint Committee on Archives of Science and Technology (JCAST). (The recommendations of the JCAST report are discussed more fully in chapter 7.) Sieber's important work *Sharing Social Science Data* (1991) presents a model for reusing data in the social sciences. This model may also be adapted for numerous disciplines (e.g., epidemiology) that collect and study observational data in the health sciences. The Sieber text presents examples of various data-sharing approaches in the population sciences, anthropology, and the social sciences. The elements of data sharing are discussed, including guidelines for developing and managing a social science data archive, and the use of shared data sets in the teaching of statistics.

Data that have been retained by the original investigator or deposited in a data bank may be of value to researchers in the same field or a related one, or to investigators working in areas far removed from the original research topic. Two of the possible uses of research data are reanalysis and secondary research. An investigator conducting a reanalysis studies the same problem as the original investigator

did, and may or may not use the same data. When the reanalysis uses independently collected data to study the same problem, it is called a replication; when the same data are used in the reanalysis, it is a verification. Secondary research may be defined as research that uses existing data but has objectives that differ from those of the original investigation. In some areas the use of existing data is fundamental to the research process; for example, epidemiological research is often based on several data sets collected over a long time period (Fienberg, Martin, and Straf 1985).

Reanalysis of Scientific Data to Study Processes of Research

Studying Scientific Research Methodologies Some of the most recent works in the history and sociology of science and technology have focused on the social construction of science and technology and have provided several theories about the crucial role of instrumentation, measurement techniques, and recording methods in the generation of scientific knowledge (Mackenzie and Wajcman 1985; Latour and Woolgar 1986; Bijker, Hughes, and Pinch 1989), notably that the instruments (apparatus and other resources) used in the laboratory embody prior social selections (Knorr-Cetina 1981). This view suggests that the adoption of a particular technology in scientific practice can be influential in defining the nature of the phenomena it is used to observe (Woolgar 1991a). Arguments in the anthropological literature similarly in-

7. In April 1990, the Department of Health and Human Services (DHHS), the U.S. Public Health Service (PHS), and the Office of the Assistant Secretary for Health (OASH) sponsored the workshop Data Management in Biomedical Research. This special-invitation workshop included a broad cross-section of professionals from the biomedical research community, ranging from deans of medical schools, bench scientists, and social scientists to officials from federal agencies, attorneys, entrepreneurs in biotechnology, journalists, and archivists. The topics included data ownership, data retention, and data sharing. The participants were polarized on nearly every topic, and the consensus was that the topics warranted further discussion. The report of the workshop Data Management in Biomedical Research is available through the Department of Health and Human Services.

dicate that different ways of representing and classifying knowledge have profound effects on what counts as adequate knowledge (Goody 1977).

The influence of anthropological and ethnographic techniques, especially participant observation, on the recent literature of the history and sociology of science has been enormous. The justification for this approach is that it allows the researcher to examine decisions in the laboratory as they are being made, before recollections are affected by rational reconstruction. Developed in recent years for the in situ study of the scientific research process (Latour and Woolgar 1986; Lynch 1985; Traweek 1988), participant observation techniques have now been extended to technology, with particular reference to information technology (Woolgar 1991b). Participant observation requires that the investigators become part of the situation they observe; by doing so they are able to develop a heightened appreciation of the technical problems and other difficulties encountered by the other participants. This method of observation complements broader survey approaches by focusing in detail (Hammersley and Atkinson 1983) on a single research site. In its application to technical and scientific settings, participant observation entails intensive and sustained monitoring of how a research design evolves and is carried out. It involves systematically taking field notes; collecting correspondence, reports, memoranda, and other relevant archival documents; making audio and video recordings; and transcribing these data, as well as both structured and unstructured interviews, for subsequent analysis.

Both before and during the participant observation, research typically involves collecting documents—usually external reports and discussions, and internal communications, texts, memoranda, and reports; and often raw scientific results. Of particular interest of late are the varying social functions fulfilled by different types of documents both within and beyond the research site or the particular dis-

cipline (e.g., the extent to which an electronic format is a viable substitute for hard copy, or the relationship between the visual design of a chart or graph and the statistical information it presents).

Data Audits and the Verification of Research Findings   At institutions in the health fields one of the primary reasons for the retention of scientific data is to be able to demonstrate the integrity of research processes. Several cases of alleged scientific fraud came to light in the 1980s and attracted considerable publicity. Such instances have alarmed the scientific community and have led to calls for formalized mechanisms to ensure that scientists adhere to accepted standards of conduct in their research. Of particular concern to scientists is the fact that public disclosures of fraud may undermine popular support for science and thus limit access to federal funding.

The scientific establishment has responded quickly to concerns about the integrity of scientific research. Organizations such as the National Academy of Sciences (1989) and the Association of American Medical Colleges (1990) have issued guidelines on responsible conduct in research, and funding agencies have made the award of future grants subject to conditions that certain protocols be observed in investigating cases of fraud or misconduct (U.S. Department of Health and Human Services 1989). The National Science Foundation (1989) issued a notice to presidents of colleges and universities that reaffirms its commitment to open, rapid dissemination of research performed under its sponsorship, and to open communication in science. The National Institutes of Health, amid some controversy, set up an Office of Scientific Integrity, and there has also been a move for federal legislation against scientific fraud, although this proposal has not yet been implemented (Culliton 1988a). Because the adequacy of laboratory records is often a central issue in cases of alleged fraud, laboratory notebooks have become the focus of the guidelines on responsible conduct in research that have been introduced by several universities and medical schools (Cordray, Pion, and Boruch 1990).

The subject of data preservation has become bound up with the need to demonstrate the integrity of research processes, although not without producing considerable dissension within the scientific community. Because of the use of research data in fraud investigations and research audits, it is important to distinguish between research data retained for their potential value in future research and those retained for legal reasons or audit purposes.

PROSPECTS FOR DATA SHARING IN THE HEALTH, LIFE, AND BIOLOGICAL SCIENCES

The informal sharing of research and clinical data has traditionally been a common practice in medicine, and physicians have routinely discussed clinical observations and research results with their colleagues. Pressures within the researcher's work environment, however, may create barriers to data sharing. The question of how to encourage and formalize data sharing is therefore receiving considerable attention in the health sciences (Fienberg, Martin, and Straf 1985; U.S. Department of Health and Human Services 1990).

Benefits to Be Promoted

The National Research Council's Committee on National Statistics published a report, *Sharing Research Data* (Fienberg, Martin, and Straf 1985), which describes the ways in which data sharing may benefit research. These include both financial benefits for funding agencies and an improvement in the quality of the research performed. Although this report was concerned primarily with the social and behavioral sciences, its analysis clearly applies equally well to most other scientific research.

The benefits of data sharing that are identified in the report may be summarized as follows:

- Allowing one's peers to test the validity of one's conclusions is an important

mechanism for maintaining the quality of scientific research. Without such openness, research is vulnerable to undetected error or even to deliberate misrepresentation or falsification of results.
- Reexamination of data, either by the original investigator or by an independent researcher, may lead to new interpretations of existing data or to completely new lines of research.
- Comparing different data sets from independent studies may test the generality of an individual's findings. In addition, linking data from several sources may reveal phenomena that might otherwise go undetected.
- The examination of researchers' data and research methodology by other researchers often leads to suggestions for improvement of the experimental procedures or design.
- Data sharing promotes the efficient use of resources by ensuring that the maximum use is made of research data.
- Pooling existing data sets creates useful resources for secondary research by other scientists and may provide information sources of considerable value to professionals involved in policy decisions.

The existence of well-documented data sets may also be a valuable resource for research training. Such data sets may be used to demonstrate research methodology and experimental design, and can also be used in worked examples and exercises in applying analytic techniques (Sieber 1990).

Impediments That Exist

Although it is clear that data sharing is beneficial to science, such openness is not always in the interest of the investigator who generated the data. The scientific reward system as it exists gives little credit to researchers who share their data or establish data banks as shared resources. It is, therefore, not surprising that researchers are reluctant to spend valuable time making data available for use by others. Moreover, obstacles such as cost to the original investigator and technical considerations of compatibility further inhibit data sharing.

Inherent Costs   Sharing research data entails performing a considerable amount of additional labor to establish a useful and workable context for those data. This effort includes providing relevant documentation for the data, publicizing the data's existence, providing training in its use, and answering questions from users. The costs of these activities are not usually provided for in research grants, and they therefore fall to the investigator. The use of another researcher's data also involves costs to the secondary researcher. Time and effort must be expended in becoming familiar with the data and sometimes in reorganizing them and converting them to another database system.

Technical Obstacles   Accessibility is an important consideration in data sharing, one that depends on the storage medium. Social scientists and demographers are increasingly facing the problem of having data stored in media that have become obsolete. Whereas the results of research performed before the 1950s were recorded in notebooks or as photographic images, recent research is often recorded in machine-readable media such as computer punch cards, magnetic tapes, magnetic disks, and videotapes.

Incompatibility between different kinds of computer hardware and software continues to present a real barrier to more widespread sharing of data. Recent advances in the technology of data storage and retrieval may help in the "retrofitting" of data, but no simple "technological fix" is available to render old data reusable. A more fruitful approach is to design shared-access data sets prospectively rather than retrospectively.

Investigators' Reluctance   Like the costs of sharing data, investigators' concerns about the consequences of making their data available to others are a powerful disincentive to sharing. Many researchers feel that such dis-

closure could invite criticism—either warranted or unwarranted—of their work, and that they could be forced to spend valuable time rebutting this criticism. Furthermore, revealing data before the principal investigator has had a chance to analyze them fully may allow credit for the research to be preempted by other researchers, who would have a chance to get their own analyses into print first.

Information Involving Human Subjects Under the Privacy Act of 1974, individuals have the right of access to any information concerning themselves that is held by the federal government, and the disclosure of such information to third parties may occur only with the explicit consent of the individual involved. Hence, if records are individually identifiable, there are restrictions on their disclosure. Methods for assuring privacy—for example, the removal of personal identifiers —may be used to overcome concerns about confidentiality, but this approach can prove to be time consuming and costly (Cordray, Pion, and Boruch 1990).

These obstacles are by no means trivial, and they will have to be addressed if data sharing is to become more widespread. In some cases the obstacles may be overcome by technical solutions or by designing experiments so as to allow for data sharing. In other cases, such as when investigators are concerned about sharing data, the obstacles may be addressed only by changing the environment in which the investigators work (for example, by funding agencies' making grants conditional on data being made freely available) and by covering the costs associated with sharing data.

FOSTERING ALTERNATIVE RESEARCH USES
FOR SCIENTIFIC DATA

Until recently, archivists have been involved only in a limited way with discrete selections of inactive research data, not with the management of collections of active data. The prevalence of recently retired collections of data that still have long life spans for active research, and the increasingly high profile of data sharing in research and educational institutions, means that archivists will need to become familiar with the issues involved in preserving and accessing data for ongoing and active use in scientific research. In considering the role of archives in data preservation, it is helpful to distinguish between data banks or scientific data centers, which are concerned with the storage of active research data, and archives of historical scientific data. A fundamental difference between data centers and research archives is in their basic mission. Whereas data centers are designed to collect specific kinds of data for specifically designated functions, archives have more varied acquisition policies and must serve a broader range of research needs. The criteria and standards for archival acquisitions are set at the institutional level; the criteria and standards of data centers are usually set by the professions and their various validating activities. Data centers are required to enforce rigid standards set by professional associations regarding the quality of data they will accept, and normally have established procedures for the evaluation of data that are subject to collection. The researchers who utilize data banks are generally professionals who are highly specialized in the particular subject area of the data that are stored.

It is worth exploring the ways in which archivists may play a larger role at their institutions in the identification, preservation, and management of collections of retired data that are still viable for some forms of active use. Some of the issues that need to be addressed if archivists are to broaden their traditional role are outlined below. They are illustrated by reference to the Curt Richter Papers at the Johns Hopkins University School of Medicine, a collection of detailed documentation maintained by this well-known investigator during the course of his research in the psychobiology laboratory at Johns Hopkins from 1919 to 1988.

The volume, as well as the scientific and technical complexity of contemporary bio-

medical research make the appraisal of biomedical research records by archivists a particularly difficult task. Moreover, the need to evaluate documentation varies according to the potential use of the research data, further complicating decisions on retention. Each case is unique, and a selection strategy is needed to take into account the specific requirements of each situation. Consequently, archivists need to approach the appraisal of scientific data with an open mind and to think creatively about the various needs of potential users.

To assess the overall importance and potential research value of scientific data, it is necessary to consult with the peers of the scientist who created the data, as well as with a broad spectrum of other experts, including scientists from related fields, historians of science, and archivists. When data are acquired after a scientist's death, that individual's peers may be identified from his or her papers or from citation indexes. In the case of Curt Richter, the diversity of Richter's research activities made it necessary to divide his work into major research areas and then to consult specialists in each area. Three complementary means of consultation were used to elicit advice: questionnaires, direct interviewing, and review by an expert panel.[8]

The most significant and important results of research are, in general, disseminated

---

8. In 1989, the staff of the Alan M. Chesney Archives inventoried and moved the contents of Curt Richter's laboratory (including over sixty years of data, professional papers, and laboratory equipment) to off-site storage space. The staff then began a study to assess the significance of the material. I conducted telephone interviews and sent questionnaires to scientists in Richter's fields of research. In 1990, I gave a presentation on Richter's research at a meeting of the Society for the Study of Ingestive Behavior. McCall, Mix, and I presented examples of Richter's data at the 1990 meetings of the Eastern Psychological Association and the American Association of the History of Medicine, inviting members of these organizations to examine and comment upon the records. It should be noted that the scientists took a greater interest in Richter's research records than did the historians. Whereas a number of archivists and historians recommended that Richter's laboratory data be microfilmed for purposes of preservation, the scientists were opposed to microfilming. Instead, they urged that the data be converted to a computer format so that they would have the ability to manipulate the data.

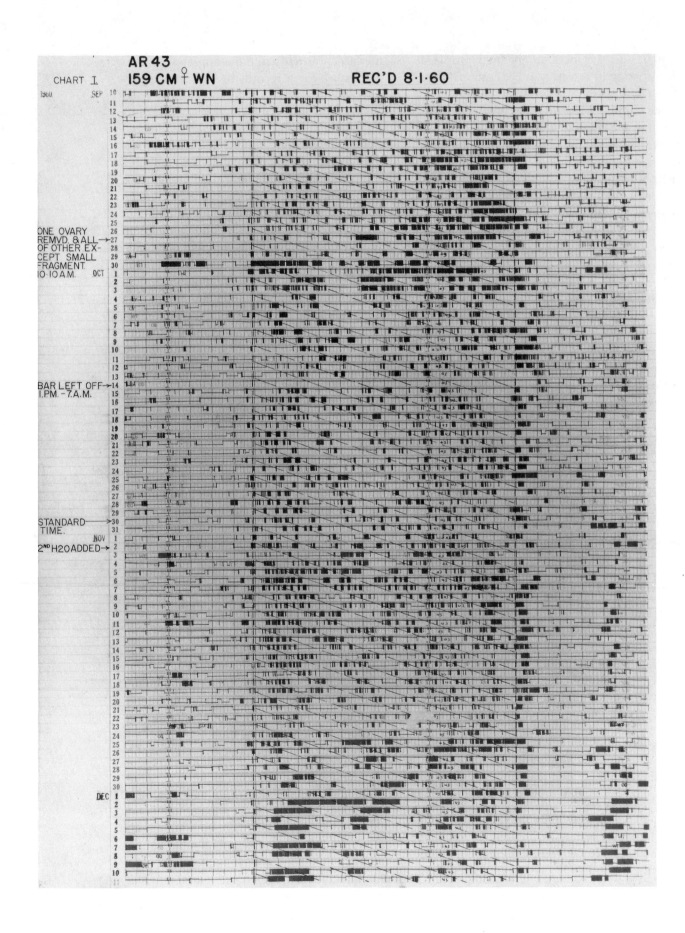

through the published scientific literature. However, information and data are published in a highly selective manner, and the results of unsuccessful experiments, or results deemed to be uninteresting, are generally not published. Such information may, however, subsequently prove to be of interest either to the original researcher or to others viewing the data from a different perspective. For example, researchers familiar with Richter's work felt that his papers might contain unpublished material that, in light of subsequent research, would be of value to contemporary investigators.

Archives have traditionally retained documents either in the original format and medium (usually paper) or in microform. However, new storage and retrieval technologies such as videodisks and computer-based retrieval systems may now be used to address problems of storage, preservation, and access. Because of the large number of records in the Richter papers, several preservation options using machine-readable media are being considered.

In appraising scientific research data, it is important to bear in mind the need for comprehensive documentation (Haas, Samuels, and Simmons 1985). Although the documentation requirements are specific to each particular case, some general conclusions may be drawn:

- Primary data form an essential element of a scientific database, since they are the raw material that is obtained by the research and is the subject of subsequent analyses.
- A full account of the experimental design and methodology is important to understanding and interpreting the data. Although this information may be provided in publications, published accounts

rarely contain sufficient detail to allow other scientists to replicate an experiment.

- In addition to the primary data, supplementary information concerning the experimental conditions and external factors that might have affected the results is also important, since this information may influence the interpretation of the data.
- The researcher's inferences from and interpretations of experimental data are also important for understanding the research.

The need for comprehensive documentation of research data will inevitably conflict with the practicalities and economics of the archival process, which dictate that a high degree of selectivity be used in decisions on preservation.[9] A balance must therefore be achieved by assessing the costs and the benefits of retention. If excessive costs are involved in making data available, the value of the data might not be great enough to justify the price of preservation.[10] It is of course difficult to assess the potential worth of data in many cases, and it is an inevitable fact of appraisal that the value of the material may become apparent only in retrospect.

CONCLUSION

Although the challenge of managing published material has been alleviated to some extent by the introduction of new information

Fig. 4.3 **An Esterline-angus chart from the psychobiology laboratory of Curt Richter.** *Source: Alan Mason Chesney Medical Archives, the Johns Hopkins Medical Institutions.*

9. In 1990, the staff of the Alan M. Chesney Archives consulted with Sociometrics, a California-based firm that specializes in the retrofitting of research data. Sociometrics recommended that, in deciding which data sets should be converted to machine-readable form, the archives should identify the types of records that would be most useful to researchers and most adaptable to conversion (e.g., logbooks, plotted graphs of daily observations), and should focus on data from key experiments (as determined through consultation with scientists). Data sets from these key experiments may then be converted first, and other data sets could subsequently be converted as resources became available. Priorities would then be determined by the demand for the material.

10. Many research data that are generated and stored in laboratory settings are contaminated with hazardous substances

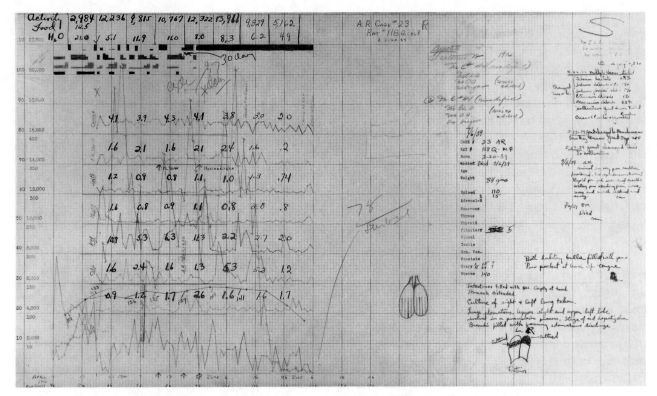

Fig. 4.4   **An activity chart from the psychobiology laboratory of Curt Richter.** Annotations on charts carry important details that should be considered in the appraisal of laboratory records. *Source: Alan Mason Chesney Medical Archives, the Johns Hopkins Medical Institutions.*

technologies, the problem of adequately cataloging the vast quantities of unpublished research data remains. The reasons for preserving such data are threefold. First, they have potential value for both current and future scientific research. While the usefulness of large data centers set up by the research community is already recognized, the data collected by individual scientists are also of potential value for further research: these data may be used either for secondary research or for reanalysis of the original research, and such reexamination of the data may lead to new interpretations of the results or even to completely new lines of research. Second, in addition to the intellectual and research benefits of preserving data, there is also the potential economic benefit of maximizing the value obtained from research expenditures. The possibility of this benefit is particularly significant when a research project involved a large investment of money,

time, and effort. Third, much of the impetus for examining the question of retaining research data has come from current concern about allegations of misconduct or fraud in science.

In the context of these developments, considerable attention has been given to the possible role of data sharing in promoting responsible conduct in research and in making effective and economical use of research resources. Although data sharing is a generally accepted norm of science and is common practice for many researchers, there are significant obstacles to its more widespread adoption. These barriers include the financial costs

---

from the laboratory environment. In the instance of the Richter papers, the presence of lead paint dust poses many problems and potential costs. To justify the expenditure of funds, the intrinsic value of these materials must be weighed against the costs of preservation and decontamination.

of making data accessible, problems of incompatible technologies, and the need to protect individual privacy in the case of clinical and human-subject data. Further obstacles to sharing arise from investigators' fears of attracting criticism of their work, and their suspicion that free access to their results might allow other researchers to publish analyses of those results before the original study could be completed.

To surmount these barriers, professional and scientific organizations have attempted to promote the sharing of data by introducing guidelines on openness and responsible conduct in research. However, more systematic data sharing is prevented by the lack of any institutional structures designed to facilitate such sharing. In some areas the establishment of data centers for active data has begun to address this problem. This chapter is not suggesting that archival programs take on the large-scale functions of a data center, but rather that archival programs follow the data center model in acquiring relevant scientific data and making that data available to a wide range of users. Archivists must begin to enlist the help of the scientific community in the appraisal and processing of historical research records. It is important to ensure that decisions concerning the selection, preservation, and management of data are sound and that the data will be of genuine value to the research community and made widely accessible for their use. These goals may be achieved only by involving that community and engaging their commitment and support.

ACKNOWLEDGMENTS

The author and editors are grateful to the following individuals for their contributions to the content of this chapter: David Blake, Rosemary Chalk, Barbara Craig, Deborah Day, Clark Elliott, Joan Krizack, Joan Sieber, and Joan Warnow-Blewett.

BIBLIOGRAPHY

ALLEN, F.H., O. KENNARD, AND R. TAYLOR. 1983. Systematic analysis of structural data as a research technique in organic chemistry. *Accounts of Chemical Research* 16:146–53.

ALTMAN, L.K., AND L. MELCHER. 1983. Fraud in science. *British Medical Journal* 286:2003–6.

ANGELL, M., AND A.S. RELMAN. 1988. Fraud in biomedical research. *New England Journal of Medicine* 318:1462–63.

ASSOCIATION OF AMERICAN MEDICAL COLLEGES. 1990. *Framework for Institutional Policies and Procedures to Deal with Misconduct in Research*. Washington, D.C.: Association of American Medical Colleges.

BARNES, B. 1974. *Scientific Knowledge and Sociological Theory*. London: Routledge and Kegan Paul.

BIJKER, W.E., T.P. HUGHES, AND T. PINCH, EDS. 1989. *The Social Construction of Technological Systems*. Cambridge: MIT Press.

CECI, S.J., AND E. WALKER. 1983. Private archives and public needs. *American Psychologist* 38:414–23.

CECIL, J.S., AND R.F. BORUCH. 1988. Compelled disclosure of research data. *Law and Human Behavior* 12:181–89.

CORDRAY, D.S., G.M. PION, AND R.F. BORUCH. 1990. Sharing research data: With whom, when, and how much? In *Proceedings of the Workshop on Data Management in Biomedical Research*, pp. 39–85. Washington, D.C.: U.S. Department of Health and Human Services.

CULLITON, B.J. 1988a. Bill would set fraud guidelines for scientific publications. *Science* 242:187.

———. 1988b. A bitter battle over error. *Science* 240:1720–23.

———. 1988c. A bitter battle over error. *Science* 241:18–21.

———. 1988d. Scientists confront misconduct. *Science* 241:1748–49.

ELLIOTT, C.A., ED. 1983. *Understanding Progress as Process: Documentation of the History of Post-War Science and Technology in the United States*. Final report of the Joint Committee on Archives of Science and Technology. Chicago: Society of American Archivists.

FIENBERG, S.E., M.E. MARTIN, AND M.L. STRAF, EDS. COMMITTEE ON NATIONAL STATISTICS, NATIONAL RESEARCH COUNCIL. 1985. *Sharing Research Data*. Washington, D.C.: National Academy Press.

GOODY, J. 1977. *The Domestication of the Savage Mind*. Cambridge: Cambridge University Press.

HAAS, J.K., H.W. SAMUELS, AND B.T. SIMMONS. 1985. *Appraising the Records of Modern Science and Technology: A Guide.* Cambridge: MIT Press.

HAMMERSLEY, M., AND P. ATKINSON. 1983. *Ethnography: Principles in Practice.* London: Tavistock.

HOLMES, F.L. 1990. Laboratory notebooks: Can the daily record illuminate the broader picture? *Proceedings of the American Philosophical Society* 134:349–66.

INTERNATIONAL UNION OF CRYSTALLOGRAPHY, COMMISSION ON BIOLOGICAL MACROMOLECULES. 1989. *Acta Crystallographica* A45:658.

KNORR-CETINA, K.D. 1981. *The Manufacture of Knowledge.* Oxford: Pergamon.

KRIZACK, J.D., ED. 1994. *Documentation Planning for the U.S. Health Care System.* Baltimore: Johns Hopkins University Press.

LATOUR, B., AND S. WOOLGAR. 1986. *Laboratory Life: The Construction of Scientific Facts.* Princeton: Princeton University Press.

LYNCH, M. 1985. *Art and Artefact in Laboratory Science.* Cambridge: Cambridge University Press.

MACKENZIE, D., AND J. WAJCMAN, EDS. 1985. *The Social Shaping of Technology.* Milton Keynes, England: Open University Press.

MERTON, R.K. [1942.] 1973. The normative structure of science. In *The Sociology of Science,* ed. N. Storer, pp. 267–78. Reprint, Chicago: University of Chicago Press.

MICHELSON, A., AND J. ROTHENBERG. 1992. Scholarly communication and information technology: Exploring the impact of changes in the research process on archives. *American Archivist* 55:236–315.

NATIONAL ACADEMY OF SCIENCES. 1989. On being a scientist. *Proceedings of the National Academy of Sciences* 86:9053–74.

NATIONAL INSTITUTES OF HEALTH, INSTITUTE OF MEDICINE. 1989. *The Responsible Conduct of Research in the Health Sciences.* Washington, D.C.: National Academy Press.

NATIONAL SCIENCE FOUNDATION. 1987. *Science and Engineering Indicators.* Washington, D.C.: National Science Foundation.

———. 1989. Important notice to presidents of colleges and universities and heads of other National Science Foundation grantee organizations. Notice no. 106. April 17, 1989.

NELKIN, D. 1984. *Science as Intellectual Property: Who Controls Research?* New York: Macmillan.

POPPER, K.R. 1959. *The Logic of Scientific Discovery.* New York: Harper & Row and Basic Books.

PRICE, D.J. DE SOLLA. 1961. *Science since Babylon.* New Haven: Yale University Press.

SIEBER, J.E. 1990. Investigators' concerns about data sharing. In *Proceedings of the Workshop on Data Management in Biomedical Research.* Washington, D.C.: U.S. Department of Health and Human Services.

———, ED. 1991. *Sharing Social Science Data.* Newbury Park, Calif.: Sage.

TRAWEEK, S. 1988. *Beam Times and Life Times: The World of High Energy Physicists.* Cambridge: Harvard University Press.

U.S. DEPARTMENT OF HEALTH AND HUMAN SERVICES. 1989. Responsibilities of awardees and applicant institutions for dealing with reporting possible misconduct in science. *Federal Register* 54 (151): 32446–51.

———. 1990. *Proceedings of the Workshop on Data Management in Biomedical Research.* Washington, D.C.: U.S. Department of Health and Human Services.

WARNOW-BLEWETT, J.N. 1987. Saving the records of science and technology: The role of a discipline history center. *Science and Technology Libraries* 7 (3): 29–40.

———. 1989. The role of a discipline history center, part II: Promoting archives and research in science and technology. *Science and Technology Libraries* 9 (4): 85–104.

———. 1992. Documenting recent science: Progress and needs. *Osiris,* 2d ser., 7:267–98.

WOOLGAR, S. 1991a. Beyond the citation debate: Towards a sociology of measurement technologies and their use in science policy. *Science and Public Policy* 18:319–26.

———. 1991b. Configuring the user: The case of usability trials. In *A Sociology of Monsters: Essays on Power, Technology, and Domination,* ed. J. Law, pp. 57–99. London: Routledge.

5

Computerization and a New Era for Archives

Nina W. Matheson

BECAUSE MUCH DOCUMENTATION that is being generated in the primary functions and administrative activities of health care delivery, education, and research is in computerized formats, archivists must face and come to terms with the electronic information environments of their institutions. They have to recognize the scope of their new roles in this era of electronic information and assume greater responsibility for the archival selection, preservation, and management of institutional documentation in computerized formats. In so doing they will have to develop effective strategies for dealing with the physical and technical fragilities of electronically stored data and information. Their leadership in establishing criteria and setting standards for electronically stored records is critical to the survival of key institutional documentation.

This chapter assesses the evolution of computing applications in the health fields. It is intended to provide an overview of the development of computerization in settings for health care delivery, education, and research, and serve as a guide to current computer applications in these settings. Archivists as well as educators, clinicians, and researchers must keep abreast of generational shifts in computerization, because in their work they may encounter computerized documentation from bygone eras. Archivists at institutions in the health fields need to become more involved in computerization issues at their institutions as well as at their repositories.

The problems associated with the preservation of computerized documentation involve nearly as many complex philosophic issues as matters of technology. When there is more consensus about the types of data and information that need to be saved to preserve the knowledge base of the health fields, there should then be greater incentive to press for the appropriate technical solutions. Therefore, a goal of this book is to stimulate thought about the ongoing data and information needs of health care delivery, research, and education. To work toward technical solutions, the users of data and information systems in the health fields must interact with both hardware and software specialists in the computer industries to develop safeguards for the preservation, access, and use of data and information in electronic media.

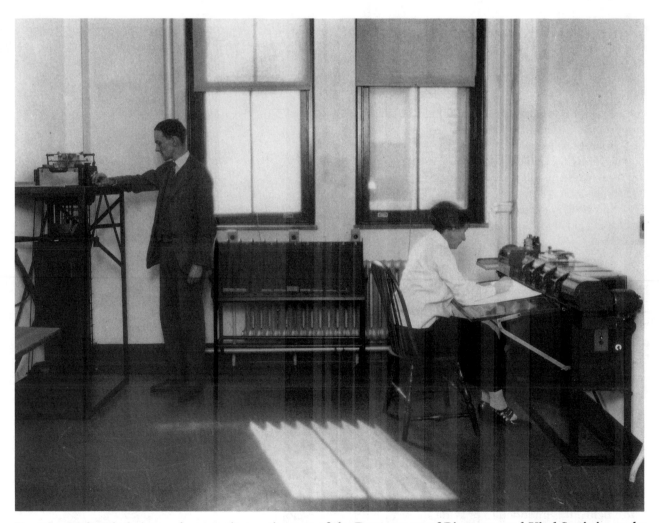

Fig. 5.1 **Early tabulating and computing equipment of the Department of Biometry and Vital Statistics at the Johns Hopkins University School of Hygiene and Public Health.** *Source: Alan Mason Chesney Medical Archives, the Johns Hopkins Medical Institutions.*

AN OVERVIEW OF COMPUTERIZATION
IN THE HEALTH FIELDS

Since their commercial introduction in 1947 with UNIVAC I, three generations of computers have come and gone. The modern world cannot function without computers and the associated telecommunications technologies. Computers are now involved in the manufacture of most products; they even manufacture the key components necessary to assemble themselves. As they near the end of their fourth generation, high-speed, parallel supercomputers are about to shrink to the size of a desktop microcomputer workstation. However, while astrophysicists use computers to study phenomena too remote to be humanly perceived without their aid, and biophysicists use them to model submolecular structures, the use of computers to improve the educational process and the management and delivery of health care is still at an early stage.

The application of computer technologies in academic health centers began in the late 1950s. During the past ten years, computers have become so integral to science and medicine that there is no question of turning back or slowing down, but their applications are still unevenly developed. Computer systems underpin the administration of hospitals and health centers, they monitor and manage patient care, they have revolutionized biomedical research, they are inexorably changing the process of health sciences education, and they have changed how health knowledge is accessed and displayed.[1]

The history of health care computing is well documented in a number of recent sources (Ball and Hannah 1984; Blum 1986; Blum and Duncan 1990; Enterline, Lenhard, and Blum 1989; Schwartz, Patil, and Szolovits 1987). While the December 1986 special issue of the *Western Journal of Medicine* is still useful, the book by Shortliffe et al. (1990) provides the best overview of the current status of health care computing. Other health professions, such as nursing (Ball 1988) and dentistry (Salley, Zimmerman, and Ball 1990),

have developed informatics strategies for managing information in their special domains. Austin (1988) treated hospital information systems thoroughly in his standard textbook; Adlassnig (1991) provided a perspective on the European scene.

In assessing developments in medical informatics, Bruce Blum has said,

> Much of what has happened in medical informatics has centered around patient care and education. The digital records of images and the attempts to automate the medical record have been concerned with data and information regarding specific patients. Simulations used in education and testing are more general, but they limit themselves to the accurate presentation of medical knowledge and the evaluation of the student's understanding of that knowledge. More typical library functions, for example MEDLINE, attempt to provide targeted access to desired knowledge; where (as in some IAIMS settings) the bibliographic access is available in the clinical setting (e.g., at an HIS terminal), this knowledge is used to support decision making for individual patients (or students in clinical training).
>
> Having said this, I recognize several overlapping issues: patient care in which the data for each patient should be available for the life of the patient; medical research in which access to the data of individual (and informed) patients should be available for an indefinite period; medical education in which real (e.g., clinical exemplars) and structured (e.g., simulated) data should be made available in a specialized environment; bibliographic resources in which the resource or its surrogate must be available with reasonable performance; and historical analysis in which (among other things) data policy decisions must be retained and organized for subsequent use. (Blum 1993).

---

1. Part III of the National Records Survey of Academic Medical Centers (conducted in 1987 as part of the Johns Hopkins Medical Institutions Records Project) dealt with computer issues. The following observations may be made from the survey data: Almost half (45%) of the hospitals surveyed installed their major computer systems in the 1980s; among systems installed earlier, financial and accounting systems were more prevalent than clinical systems. Fifty-nine of the seventy-eight respondents reported that computers were used on inpatient floors, while sixty-four respondents reported using computers in outpatient clinics; the four most prominent types of information reported as "routinely available" on these computers were patient demographics, patient identification information, billing data, and laboratory values. At the time of the survey,

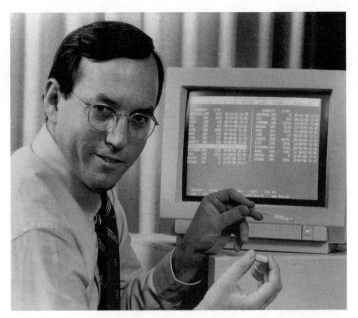

Fig. 5.2 **The ingestible thermal monitoring system, which measures body "core" temperature.** This system has applications as a diagnostic tool for infertility, exercise physiology, and obesity monitoring. It is one of the many new clinical applications that have been introduced through computerization. *Source: Alan Mason Chesney Medical Archives, the Johns Hopkins Medical Institutions; photograph by Rob Smith.*

The discussion in this chapter is guided by Blum's (1984) grouping of medical computing applications according to three classifications: data, information, and knowledge. Data are uninterpreted elements, such as numbers, names, or test results; information is an assemblage of data that conveys meaning and has value over time; and knowledge is derived from the relationship between data and information. Medical computer systems increase in complexity and sophistication as they expand to handle these.

The importance of computational support for data analysis and image processing in biomedical research is undisputed. For example, human gene mapping would be impossible without data management. New research areas, such as the mapping of the brain, have extraordinary implications for clinical medicine (Pechura and Martin 1991). Computers augment medical education in new ways, through case simulations and through alternative representations of familiar information,

such as the "electronic cadaver." Computational visualization of internal human structures is very new but is already having an effect on such specialties as neurosurgery and orthopedic surgery. In the next decade computers are likely to become as basic to medicine and science as the stethoscope and the microscope are now. As early as 1983, a survey conducted at the Duke University School of Medicine indicated that, of the one hundred members (88%) of the first-year class who responded, more than two-thirds had prior experience with computers, 45 percent had programmed computers, 20 percent had used standard computer programs such as statistical packages, and 22 percent owned or had access to home computers (Saltz, Saltz, and Rabkin 1985). Today some schools, such as Case Western Reserve, issue laptop computers to incoming freshmen.

Harold Lehmann, director of the Office of Medical Informatics Education at the Johns Hopkins University School of Medicine, has summarized the responses of three medical school classes at Johns Hopkins to questions about their ownership of, experience with, and expectations of computers: Eighty-eight percent of the entering class (the class of 1997) responded; 82 percent of the class of 1996 replied at the end of their first year; and 73 percent of the class of 1995 replied to a mailing. The results show ownership of computers in the first- and second-year classes (61% and 59%) to be about the same, but much greater than in the third-year class (43%). In terms of computer experience, the first-year class seems far ahead of the other classes in data analyses and literature searching. Approximately 75 percent of the first-year class perform data analysis, in contrast to 40 percent of the second-year class and 50 percent of the third-year class. The greatest disparity in experience is in literature searching, in which about 70

computers were used more often for administrative applications than for clinical applications, but clinical use appeared to be increasing.

percent of the first- and second-year classes have experience, in contrast to 20 percent of the third-year class (Lehmann 1993).

Resistance to computerization among health care professionals is diminishing rapidly.[2] Systems are improving in sophistication and reliability, experience with computers is more widespread, and the capabilities of computers are better understood. Certain office automation functions such as word processing programs and billing and accounting systems have become ubiquitous. Still, the use of computers in health care management falls far short of realizing the visionary dreams of the early pioneers. In 1970, for example, Schwartz predicted that by the year 2000 computers would be able to act as powerful extensions of the physician's intellect (Schwartz 1970). He and other pioneers envisioned intel-

ligent systems that would not only be tools integral to the advancement of medical research, education, and health care but would also be partners in advancing those fields. The essence of these systems was living knowledge—knowledge that was immediate, growing, changing, and capable of being reinterpreted, interrelated, and recombined at will.

Certainly within reach is an environment in which a physician or health care worker, while examining a patient, can turn to a single device and use a nationwide computer network to retrieve and consult the individual's electronic medical record, obtain information from an expert diagnostic consulting system, and examine laboratory reports, as well as review drug-interaction databases and consult the most current literature on relevant topics. Individual components of this scenario exist but have not been assembled into a coherent, usable system. Progress toward more visionary goals, such as intelligent systems capable of learning from experience, will accelerate as new, more powerful generations of computer software and hardware emerge and as the field of health-related and medical informatics matures as an academic discipline.

This new vision has several implications for the long-term and archival management of electronic data and information. Information generally passes through at least three phases. For information in the first phase—current information necessary to the optimal daily operation of an enterprise—the electronic environment is essential. Once past this short-term phase, some information may have extended value as documentation or as evidence of practice and procedure. The demand for this information may be sporadic and unpredictable over a period that may range from ten years to one hundred years in

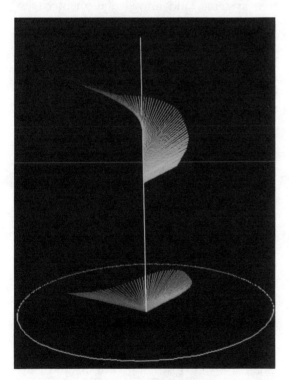

Fig. 5.3 **Computer simulation of thought processes in a monkey trained to move a lever counterclockwise to the 11 o'clock position when a light flashes at 2 o'clock.** Computerization is used in many new areas of basic research. *Source: Science 243 (January 1989): cover; photograph by Aposotolos Georgopoulos; copyright 1989 by AAAS.*

2. The breakdown in resistance is largely because of the emergence of a new generation of professionals with experience in using computers. Whereas this technology is still new to part of its user community, it is gradually being assimilated and more steadily accepted as professionals with computer sophistication enter the health fields.

length. Finally, there is information of permanent historical value, which requires archival (permanent) retention.[3]

Records managers and archivists must approach the electronic environment on two levels, keeping in mind both their need to manage information *about* the resources for which they are responsible, and their need to manage the accessibility and utility of the *content* of the materials they store and retain. They can take full advantage of computational methods to store and retrieve information about the records and documents for which they are responsible. In using computers as a management tool, records managers and archivists share the same problems in making the technologies perform at the most intelligent levels possible (Kesner 1984; Kesner 1988). It is in the realm of *content management* that the electronic media pose problems that are still unsolved (Michelson and Rothenberg 1992). So long as materials are human-readable, that is, on paper or its microform analog, the issues are the cost, efficiency, and durability of the storage media. The trade-offs between paper and microforms are well documented and well understood (Hendley 1983).

Until recently, attention has focused on the storage capacity (enormous) and the durability (disappointingly limited) of electronic formats such as magnetic media and optical disks (Geller 1983; Hedstrom 1984; Hendley 1985; Hendley 1987). Several new studies, however, have concluded that the retrieval technologies for machine-readable information are the critical and vulnerable variables (Mallinson 1986; National Archives and Records Administration 1986; Smithsonian Institution Libraries 1986; Michelson and Rothenberg 1992). The fundamental problem is the machine. The planned useful life of electronic devices is between ten and twenty years. All such devices have critical components that cannot be repaired and are not interchangeable among devices. The underlying reason is the tiny size of the components (Mallinson 1986).

The swift obsolescence of retrieval software and storage formats is no less a problem. (Lisa Mix explores these issues further in chapter 9 of this volume.) Tape and disk formats change every four or five years, along with the machines required to read them. They are not backwardly compatible. Whereas it is possible to regenerate information with every new format, and it is actually essential to rewrite tapes and disks within the same time periods, the constantly expanding volume of data makes this strategy economically and practically unfeasible.

This chapter will describe the features of key systems currently in use and will point to the complex security and archival issues that surround these applications. Both aspects will be discussed with respect to each of three types of systems: hospital and/or clinical information systems, bibliographic information systems, and knowledge-oriented systems. As noted earlier, the discussion is guided by Blum's (1984) grouping of medical computing applications according to three classifications: data, information, and knowledge.

HOSPITAL AND/OR CLINICAL INFORMATION SYSTEMS

Range of Applications

The first generation of hospital data-processing systems concentrated on the financial management of patient billing and collections. This business application still predominates, although systems have become more sophisticated as a result of the increasing complexity of hospital financing and the need for information in strategic program planning (Grams et al. 1985).

Early auxiliary systems included admissions and/or registration systems and automated clinical laboratory systems. Order-

---

3. In considering archival retention, the implications of networking should not be overlooked. Archives may end up with a distributed responsibility for the long-term retention of different collections that can be integrated within the network.

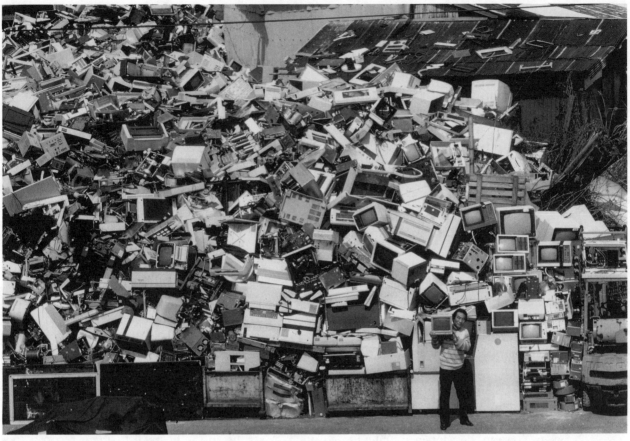

Fig. 5.4 **A computer graveyard in Japan.** This scene is an indication of the rapid obsolescence of computer hardware. *This photograph appeared previously in the* New York Times Magazine, *25 June 1989. Source: Gamma Liaison, by permission; photograph by Mitsuhiro Wada.*

entry systems for nursing stations emerged in the mid-1970s. More recent are pharmacy systems and radiology systems that capture physiological data through diagnostic tools such as electrocardiograms, and diagnostic imaging techniques such as computerized tomography scanners (CT) and nuclear magnetic resonance (NMR) spectroscopy. Typically, these systems are stand-alone systems meant to serve only one specific function. They are not integrated, nor are they even linked to one another, and remote access through electronic networks is relatively rare. They tend to be data-capturing systems with limited reporting capabilities. They are management systems, not care systems. The distinction between these two conceptual orientations, toward data and toward information,

is growing more and more critical to the design of the next generation of systems.

In his description of the systems in use at the Beth Israel Hospital and the Brigham and Women's Hospital, Slack (1989) presented the argument that financial computing is most effectively and efficiently managed as a byproduct of clinical computing. Using clinical computing systems, staff members at these hospitals may ascertain the results of a patient's laboratory tests; view diagnostic reports from clinical departments; obtain a detailed account of the patient's history, including hospitalizations, surgical operations, blood transfusions, and ambulatory visits; scan a record of prescriptions filled in the outpatient pharmacy; request the patient's chart; notify other staff members of an unscheduled conference; and locate relevant references in the biomedical literature using the MEDLINE database (Slack 1989).[4] Other programs are under development in virology and blood banking, and a program to provide physicians with consultations will be available in the near future. This system is far from being fully electronic. The medical record, for example, is still a paper record. At this stage, the system is more oriented toward the retrieval and display of information. The ability to manipulate data and reorganize it for other purposes appears to be limited, and the issue of long-term storage of information remains to be addressed.

This type of integrated system is the exception rather than the rule, in part because of the high cost of either developing or purchasing such a system. Other systems reflect the particular priorities in an environment, the developer's professional orientation toward those priorities, and the resources available. Some of the best-known hospital and/or clinical information systems include the Technicon Medical Information System; the IBM Patient Care System, developed at Duke University; and the HELP System, developed at the Latter Day Saints Hospital in Salt Lake City, Utah, and now marketed by Control Data Corporation (Blum 1984).

Records Management and Archival Issues

The medical record is at the heart of patient care activities, serving as a record of current treatment, an archival record for further treatment, an evaluation tool for audit and utilization reviews, and a database for research studies. Yet in its current hard-copy state the medical record is universally recognized as a hopelessly inadequate medium. When it can be manually located at the time of the physician-patient encounter (which is the case only 70–75% of the time [Cerne 1988]) it is usually incomplete and frequently misleading (Burnum 1989). It would therefore appear to be a prime candidate for computerization (Dick and Steen 1991).[5] Thus far, however,

computers have been used primarily to assist in managing the paper records—assigning unique numbers, tracking the paper records' location, assisting in coding, and so forth. Digital representation of the record itself has involved legal problems as well as technical ones. The legal problem is that electronic records are subject to alteration and degradation in ways that paper records are not. The technical problems relate to the highly complex nature of the information and the difficulty of capturing data effectively and efficiently with current technologies.

Whereas practices for managing active medical records are highly variable, microfilm is the retention medium of choice for inactive records in a majority of institutions. The use of microfilm has been advocated largely by administrators whose primary interest is to reduce the physical volume of paper-based records in storage, to maintain more physical control of the component parts of the unit record by linking the documents photographically in microfilm reels, and to limit use of the patient record to a controlled setting in the hospital's patient records division where equipment is maintained to access and to read the miniaturized image of the record. Users, however, have been generally quite displeased by the limitations that microfilming places on both access to and use of clinical data and information. The means of linear access impede quick retrieval of data and information. Because documents and component parts are frequently photographed out of sequence, search time is burdensome. Often the photographic image is itself distorted or of such poor quality that the data and information cannot be interpreted. And finally, the reading equipment is awkward, difficult to operate, and not easily accessible to the clinicians on the wards.

---

4. "Note that the idea of bringing MEDLINE to the record is one of knowledge integration—bringing what is needed to the user in a coordinated way" (Blum 1993).

5. The advantage of automating patient records is that they may be accessed from anywhere and that the user may read all or part of the record.

Typically, hospitals microfilm their paper records, which are then stored in remote locations. Both the conversion to microfilm and the retrieval from microfilm are labor-intensive processes. Some records administrators have adopted the solution of optical disk storage with enthusiasm, despite the recognized technical limitations of this medium. The space-saving and dollar-saving arguments for optical disk storage are compelling: the equivalent of roughly eighty file cabinets' worth of paper records can be stored on a twelve-inch disk. By converting to an optical disk system, one medical center was able to eliminate some ten thousand square feet of storage space: Henry Ford Hospital estimated its annual savings at $427,880, of which 44 percent represents salary savings and increased user productivity (*Hospitals* 1986). Peter Waegemann, executive director of the Institute for Medical Record Economics, in Boston, estimated that conversion to optical disk storage would save the medical industry $80 billion (Cerne 1988).

The problems associated with retaining and archiving clinical information databases (except for those containing radiological data) have not been addressed at any detectable level in the literature. Retention and storage practices vary depending on the size and transaction levels of the system, as well as on the experiences that the individual responsible for the systems has had with requests for inactive datasets. In the Laboratory Medicine Division of the Johns Hopkins Hospital, for example, some pathology data are kept on-line in perpetuity, whereas other patient-specific data, such as blood counts, are purged from the on-line file and stored on microfiche a few weeks after a patient encounter. The Hopkins Oncology Center has a clinical information system in which a half-million patient days of clinical data on fifty thousand patients are retained on-line without archiving (Enterline, Lenhard, and Blum 1989). In the Cardiology Research Division at Johns Hopkins, the volume of data is low enough that all data are actively maintained on disk and routinely backed up on magnetic tapes. In this division the systems have gone through three generations of hardware and software development. Since the migration has all been within one vendor's hardware and operating systems, there has been little difficulty in transferring data, and the division has been able to satisfy every researcher's request for data from older files.

In most clinical settings radiologists have by far the most sophisticated and extensive experience with digitized data. CT scans and NMR imaging procedures have revolutionized radiology as a profession and have transformed other specialties such as surgery, because the digitized data can be used to produce multidimensional images capable of disarticulation as well as 360-degree rotation around any desired axis. It is estimated that 20 percent of all radiological images are now in digital format (Fischer 1988). The volume of data generated is enormous: in 1988, the examination of 115 patients in a 540-bed hospital resulted in 1.05 gigabytes of digital data per day (Templeton, Cox, and Dwyer 1988). The concerns regarding picture archiving of computerized images center around the need to compress the data for storage without causing degradation of the images. Templeton, Cox, and Dwyer (1988) envisioned a three-tiered system to meet immediate needs: networks would permit the transfer of images from point to point for current use in health care delivery. These networks would also provide access to optical disk jukeboxes capable of storing up to 150 fourteen-inch disks, or 1,020 gigabytes of data, which would be used for intermediate storage. Optical tapes would be used for storage periods of five to seven years (Templeton, Cox, and Dwyer 1988).

Information systems to support ambulatory care are designed to meet a different set of requirements. They typically include the following components: a medical records system, a financial system, an appointment system, and a management reports system. Some of the best known include COSTAR, one of the oldest, most complete, and most widely used systems; the Regenstrief Medical Record System, which emphasizes a reminder system; and The Medical Record (TMR), developed by the Duke University Department of Community Health Sciences with the goal of replacing the paper-based medical record (Blum 1986).

INFORMATION SYSTEMS FOR MEDICAL LITERATURE

Bibliographic Databases

By 1985, more than twenty-eight hundred databases were available on-line to the public; more than eight hundred of these were in the biological sciences (Williams 1985). The major developers and their on-line databases are the National Library of Medicine (MEDLINE and TOXLINE); Excerpta Medica (EMBASE); Biosciences Information Service (BIOSIS); the Chemical Abstracts Service (CAS); and the Institute for Scientific Information (*Science Citation Index* and *Current Contents*). These institutions provide direct access to their on-line services but also sell their files to third-party vendors and to libraries. Libraries have been developing local search and retrieval systems for subsets of these databases, or contracting for unlimited use of the databases. These contracts permit barrier-free (i.e., cost-free) access to the databases by all authorized users at the libraries' parent institutions. As a money-saving strategy, this approach may be feasible for some academic health centers. The rationale for the creation of local subsets of databases stems from the primary function of all libraries, which is to provide the information resources needed by faculty members and students as equitably as possible within the resources of the institution. Certainly, if libraries buy books and journals, they should also provide the means by which individuals can access and utilize the information in those resources.

The focus of computer usage in medical libraries is shifting from the control, processing, and management of library records to the management and distribution of bibliograph-ic and full-text database information on the premises through local networks. In a survey conducted in 1987, the Association of Academic Health Sciences Library Directors found that more than 50 percent of academic health sciences libraries provided on-line access to electronic book catalogs. At least one-third provided such access by means of local area networks (LANs).

It is the goal of the National Library of Medicine to make MEDLINE quickly and easily available for bibliographic searching by all four hundred thousand U.S. health care professionals. Within the foreseeable future, users searching MEDLINE could strike one computer key to receive photocopies of desired articles from their local medical libraries (which would all be linked through a national biomedical communications network).

In addition to purely bibliographic databases, other kinds of on-line files have appeared. The Physicians Data Query (PDQ), produced by the National Cancer Institute, provides information on cancer treatment protocols as well as a directory of specialists and references to the literature. Vendors such as BRS provide access to the full texts of books and journals in addition to an array of bibliographic systems. The new technology is creating a global system for knowledge transmission that makes the locations of users and libraries irrelevant. The need to have the knowledge contained in books and journals displayed in ways that assist in day-to-day problem solving and decision making is the impetus behind the rapid development of knowledge-oriented, or "expert," systems.[6]

The preservation of the printed biomedical literature is currently receiving significant attention. The National Library of Medicine, which is the world's largest research library in a single scientific and professional field and is

---

6. "If one uses the data/information/knowledge breakdown, then knowledge is what we know, and it is represented as text (e.g., the library holdings and their surrogates), tables, simulations, and machine sensible forms that permit automated reference" (Blum 1993).

the "library of record" for the biomedical sciences literature, has spearheaded the development of a national preservation plan and has begun implementation with its own collection. It should be noted that these preservation steps are being taken because the threat to the continued existence of some materials can no longer be ignored. The problem, however, has been known for at least the past three decades.

It is quite likely that the preservation problems inherent in digital data will be similarly ignored until a drastic loss of data is experienced. However, existing electronic databases, while large, are in constant use, which guarantees their regeneration through each new technological upgrading. In addition, paper analogues exist for most files, so significant portions of the data need never be lost. The need for permanent inactive storage has not yet emerged as a significant issue.

Knowledge-oriented Systems

Expert systems consist of computational tools that capture and make available the knowledge of experts in a field. The first experimental systems emphasized encoding large quantities of specialized medical knowledge. The program MYCIN, for example, advised physicians on antimicrobial selection for patients with bacteremia or meningitis (Buchanan and Shortliffe 1984). PIP (Present Illness Program) generated hypotheses from data about patients with renal disorder (Pauker et al. 1976). INTERNIST-1 is a comprehensive consulting program focused on 570 diseases in internal medicine (Miller et al. 1986). CAS-NET provided help with disease states in ophthalmology and made recommendations regarding the management of patients with glaucoma (Weiss et al. 1978).

Research in medically oriented artificial intelligence continues to make progress in unraveling the complex problems underlying such areas as knowledge acquisition and model-based reasoning. These early expert systems continue to evolve slowly. QMR

(Quick Medical Reference) succeeded INTERNIST-1 and expanded the flexibility and interactiveness of the program. QMR aims not so much at providing expert advice as at assisting the user in analyzing and managing diagnostic information. It is microcomputer-based and therefore well within the reach of the office-based physician. ONCOCIN is an advanced expert system building on the MYCIN experiments. It assists physicians with decisions regarding treatment protocols and decisions on topics such as managing drug dosage, delaying treatment, aborting treatment cycles, and ordering special tests (Shortliffe 1986).

Other expert systems in specialized areas have emerged in recent years as microcomputers and programming have become more accessible and simpler to use. ICON is an expert critiquing system that provides advice about differential diagnosis in radiology. TOXPERT models product safety, toxicology, and regulatory decision processes. The Transfusion Advisor is a knowledge-based system for blood banks; it draws conclusions about twelve hemostatic disorders and critiques the appropriateness of the use of frozen plasma, cryoprecipitate, and platelets, the products most commonly used for the treatment of these disorders. OVERSEER monitors the treatment of psychiatric patients in real time, monitors the clinical database, and issues alerts when standard clinical practices are not followed or when laboratory results or other clinical indicators are abnormal. COMMES Nursing Consultant System provides decision-making support in nursing. MENTOR provides continuous monitoring of decision making on drug therapy for hospitalized patients.

Among the early computer-aided instruction systems were Ohio State University's PLATO system and the Massachusetts General Hospital programs. These programs were expensive and cumbersome not only to produce but also to use. More recent microcomputer-based programs that are interactive and packaged with images are increasingly valuable adjuncts to classroom instruction. Currently, the driving force for expanding the use of these programs is the National Board of Medical Examiners. Within the next few years the traditional paper and pencil exams will give way entirely to interactive computer-based examinations.

Despite nearly two decades of work, knowledge-oriented systems are still in an early stage of development. Few systems have emerged from the prototype stage into the fully operational stage, in part because of the continuing change in the technologies, but more fundamentally because the systems are extremely complex and as yet limited in scope and applications. Some serious technical problems have yet to be solved, such as handling multiple manifestations of disease over time in a single individual. A major difficulty is in integrating the expert systems with the information systems that can provide them with the basic data. The archival concerns are more in the area of documenting the historical development of these systems than in the preservation of the systems' content.

BENEFITS AND PITFALLS OF COMPUTATION

The benefits of computational methods in medicine are similar to those in any field. Computers make it possible to perform tasks previously done manually more quickly, accurately, consistently, and reliably. When coupled with communications networks, computers can allow us to surmount the limitations of time and geography. A given set of data can be accessed and used by authorized users from any point in a network system, at any time. Finally, computational tools allow new configurations of data and knowledge. Complex experiments that once required physical models can be simulated by using computational tools. Data captured for one purpose, such as CT or NMR imaging, can be used to construct "artificial realities." Computer-generated images of such features as the human hip can be represented three-dimensionally. A body can further be displayed in layers, so that the skin layer can be removed to display musculature, and so forth, until the skeletal level is reached. Applications to science and health care, which have only begun, offer exciting opportunities for new approaches to the representation of knowledge.

The problems associated with information technology have also barely begun to be explored. A complex set of information policy issues needs to be addressed at every level, from the local level to the national and international levels. In addition to security, these issues include control of access, confidentiality safeguards, legal ownership of and responsibility for the software and databases, assurance of quality control of the system components, fees and charges, and standardization of computer protocols and interfaces.

With the introduction of every new technology there is uncertainty about the long-term management of the materials recorded by means of that technology. Sometimes the enormous volume of electronic data can assure its lack of preservation. Like routine radiographic records, electronically recorded data can be too extensive for its retention to be economically feasible.

The mechanisms are lacking in most institutions to develop the kind of information policies that can address these long-term issues. It is possible that these archival concerns can be addressed within the framework of the Integrated Academic Information Management Systems (IAIMS). The IAIMS was initiated in 1983 by the National Library of Medicine as a means of catalyzing the development of a new computer-supported information management environment in academic health centers. The program is based on two studies undertaken by the Association of American Medical Colleges (Wilson et al. 1982; Matheson and Cooper 1982) and is aimed at stimulating institution-wide use of computer and communications technologies to enhance the effectiveness of the biomedical community.

The IAIMS was designed in the expectation that institutions would evolve through three phases. The first is a planning phase that is to set out the guiding institutional information policies for the strategic development of an electronic environment. The second is a pilot development phase in which computer and communications technologies are used to demonstrate the feasibility of particular approaches within the institution. The third is the implementation of an institutional infrastructure and the widespread adoption of computer applications in the everyday work environment. More than fifteen institutions have been funded for one or more of these phases. There is evidence that many more are following similar pathways outside this programmatic framework. The experiences of these institutions are well documented (Broering 1986; Matheson 1988; Lorenzi 1992) and illustrate the problems, pitfalls, and opportunities inherent in the information technologies. Long-term archival management and records management for this fragile electronic environment have not been addressed.

A rare opportunity now exists for archivists and records managers at academic health centers to become involved in institutional strategic planning at an early and formative stage. Kesner (1984 and 1988) has emphasized the need for archivists not only to involve themselves in the planning process but also to impose themselves. Michelson and Rothenberg (1992) advocate that the archival profession take an active role in the emerging information infrastructure, and they present strategies for creating this role. If archivists do not take an activist role, the danger to research-oriented historical studies is real, for neither information systems managers nor librarians may appreciate the necessity of building in preservation safeguards. To be effective participants in this volatile and changing technological environment, the archivist and the historian must not only become technically knowledgeable but must also reevaluate, if not reconceptualize, what is historically significant. Scholars have been known to take the position that to be serious about history means a commitment to saving everything.

Such a position is unrealistic even in the most narrowly defined areas. Limits must be set for the selection and preservation of electronic documentation.

CONCLUSION

Archivists, computer specialists, and health professionals will have to work together closely to establish criteria and standards for the preservation of electronic documentation. Because of the greater permanency of paper-based records, archivists and health professionals have been lax in defining the types of documentation that need to be preserved for future studies. Moreover, the curatorial professionals in the health fields—from librarians and archivists to records managers and manuscript curators—until recent years have concentrated largely on materials in relatively durable paper-based media. As a result, many of those practicing in the curatorial professions today have not been fully sensitized to the short-life-span implications of computerization.

The ephemeral and fragile nature of electronic storage and the rapid obsolescence of computer hardware and software mean that the data and information that are stored in libraries, archives, and records centers in electronic media are highly vulnerable and at risk of loss. The impermanence of computer-based media also means that key primary materials that have not yet been slated for archival preservation are in jeopardy. Both the limitations of electronic storage and the slim prospects for a sweeping technical fix for preservation in the immediate future demand that these curatorial professions begin to operate in a triage mode to ensure that critical published and primary source materials are salvaged and maintained for future use.

Curatorial professionals need a new intellectual framework in which to operate that will enable them to function more effectively in the new electronic environments that they now inhabit. No longer do they have the luxury of the incubation of time to assist their collecting choices. Whereas records managers and archivists have always relied upon the factor of time in the appraisal and selection of electronic records, they can no longer defer final disposition and retention decisions to a future period in which they will be better informed about the value of the records. They must now seize every opportunity to act in the present to select key primary materials in electronic media so that they may make provisions for their preservation through schedules of regular electronic refreshment.

The situation demands that those curatorial professionals (archivists, records managers, and manuscript curators) who are responsible for preserving rare or unique documentation that is in electronic storage develop more effective strategies for identifying and appraising strategic documentation in the health fields so that they may then proceed more expeditiously to take the appropriate actions for preservation. In turn, the appraisal activities of these curatorial professionals will have to become more keenly focused on the informational and evidential content of documentation.

ACKNOWLEDGMENTS

The author and editors are grateful to Bruce Blum and Frank Burke for their contributions to the content of this chapter.

BIBLIOGRAPHY

ADLASSNIG, K-P., ED. 1991. *Medical Informatics Europe, 1991*. Lecture Notes in Medical Informatics, vol. 45. Berlin: Springer-Verlag.

AUSTIN, C.J. 1988. *Information Systems for Health Services Administration*. Ann Arbor: Health Administration Press.

BALL, M.J., ED. 1988. *Nursing Informatics: Where Caring and Technology Meet*. New York: Springer-Verlag.

BALL, M.J., AND J.K. HANNAH. 1984. *Using Computers in Nursing*. Reston, Va.: Reston.

BLUM, B.I., ED. 1984. *Information Systems for Patient Care*. New York: Springer-Verlag.

———. 1986. *Clinical Information Systems*. New York: Springer-Verlag.

———. 1993. Personal communication.

BLUM, B.I., AND K.A. DUNCAN, EDS. 1990. *A History of Medical Informatics*. New York: ACM Press.

BROERING, N.C., ED. 1986. Symposium on integrated academic information management systems. *Bulletin of the Medical Library Association* 74:234–61.

BUCHANAN, B.G., AND E.H. SHORTLIFFE, EDS. 1984. *Rule-based Expert Systems: The MYCIN Experiments of the Stanford Heuristic Programming Project*. Reading, Mass.: Addison-Wesley.

BURNUM, J.F. 1989. The misinformation era: The fall of the medical record. *Annals of Internal Medicine* 110:482–84.

CERNE, F. 1988. Optical disk technology: Going paperless. *Hospitals* 62:94–95.

DICK, R.S., AND E.B. STEEN, EDS. 1991. *The Computer-based Patient Record: An Essential Technology of Health Care*. Washington, D.C.: National Academy Press.

ENTERLINE, J.P., R.E. LENHARD, AND B.I. BLUM, EDS. 1989. *A Clinical Information System for Oncology*. New York: Springer-Verlag.

FISCHER, H.W. 1988. Danger ahead? *Radiology* 169:267.

GELLER, S.B. 1983. *Care and Handling of Computer Magnetic Storage Media*. National Bureau of Standards Special Publication no. 500-101. Washington, D.C.: U.S. Government Printing Office.

GRAMS, R.R., G.C. PECK, J.K. MASSEY, AND J.J. AUSTIN. 1985. Review of hospital data processing in the United States, 1982–1984. *Journal of Medical Systems* 9:175–269.

HEDSTROM, M.L. 1984. *Archives and Manuscripts: Machine-readable Records*. Basic Manual Series. Chicago: Society of American Archivists.

HENDLEY, A.M. 1983. *The Archival Storage Potential of Microfilm, Magnetic Media, and Optical Data Discs: A Comparison Based on a Literature Review*. British National Bibliography Research Fund Report no. 10, NRCD Publication no. 19. Hertford, England: Hatfield Polytechnic, National Reprographic Centre for Documentation.

HENDLEY, T. 1985. *Videodiscs, Compact Discs, and Digital Optical Disk Systems: An Introduction to the Technologies and the Systems and Their Potential for Information Storage, Retrieval, and Dissemination*. Cimtech Publication no. 23. Hartfield, England: Hatfield Polytechnic, Cimtech, and National Centre for Information Media and Technology.

———. 1987. *CD-ROM and Optical Publishing Systems: An Assessment of the Impact of Optical Read Only Memory Systems on the Information Industry and a Comparison between Them and Tradi-

tional Paper, Microfilm, and On-Line Publishing Systems. Cimtech Publication no. 26; British National Bibliography Research Fund Report no. 25. Hartfield, England: Hatfield Polytechnic, Cimtech, and National Centre for Information Media and Technology.

HORNY, K. 1992. Digital technology: Implications for library planning. *Advances in Librarianship* 16:107–26.

Hospitals. 1986. Out of room for medical records: Try optical disks. 60:86–87.

KESNER, R.M. 1984. *Automation for Archivists and Records Managers: Planning and Implementation Strategies.* Chicago: American Library Association.

———. 1988. *Information Systems: A Strategic Approach to Planning and Implementation.* Chicago: American Library Association.

LEHMANN, H. 1993. Personal communication.

LINDBERG, D.A.B., AND C.R. KALINA. 1989. NLM and the preservation of the biomedical literature. *SEA Currents* 7:1–2, 8–9.

LORENZI, N.M., ED. 1992. Integrated academic information management system (IAIMS). *Bulletin of the Medical Library Association* 80:241–43.

MALLINSON, J.C. 1986. Preserving machine-readable archival records for the millennia. *Archivaria* 22:147–55.

MANDELL, S.F. 1987. Resistance to computerization. *Journal of Medical Systems* 11:311–18.

MATHESON, N.W., ED. 1988. Integrated academic information management systems (IAIMS) model development. *Bulletin of the Medical Library Association* 76:221–67.

MATHESON, N.W., AND J.A.D. COOPER. 1982. Academic information in the academic health sciences center: Roles for the library in information management. *Journal of Medical Education* 57:1–93.

MICHELSON, A., AND J. ROTHENBERG. 1992. Scholarly communication and information technology: Exploring the impact of changes in the research process on archives. *American Archivist* 55:236–315.

MILLER, R.A., M.A. MCNEIL, S.M. CHALLINOR, F.E. MASARIE, JR., AND J.D. MEYERS. 1986. The INTERNIST-1/Quick Medical Reference Project —status report. *Western Journal of Medicine* 145:816–22.

NATIONAL ARCHIVES AND RECORDS ADMINISTRATION, COMMITTEE ON PRESERVATION OF HISTORICAL RECORDS. 1986. *Preservation of Historical Records.* Washington: National Academy Press.

PAUKER, S.G., G.A. GORRY, J.P. KASSIRER, AND M.B. SCHWARTZ. 1976. Toward the simulation of clinical cognition: Taking a present illness by computer. *American Journal of Medicine* 60:981–95.

PECHURA, C.M., AND J.B. MARTIN, EDS. 1991. *Mapping the Brain and Its Functions: Integrating Enabling Technologies into Neuroscience Research.* Washington, D.C.: National Academy Press.

SALLEY, J.J., J.L. ZIMMERMAN, AND M.J. BALL, EDS. 1990. *Dental Informatics: Strategic Issues for the Dental Profession.* Lecture Notes in Medical Informatics, vol. 39. New York: Springer-Verlag.

SALTZ, C.C., J. SALTZ, AND M. RABKIN. 1985. Perceptions and knowledge of medical students regarding computer applications in medicine. *Journal of Medical Education* 60:726–28.

SCHWARTZ, W.B. 1970. Medicine and the computer: The promise and problems of change. *New England Journal of Medicine* 283:1257–64.

SCHWARTZ, W.B., R.S. PATIL, AND P. SZOLOVITS. 1987. Artificial intelligence in medicine: Where do we stand? *New England Journal of Medicine* 316:685–88.

SHORTLIFFE, E.H. 1986. Medical expert systems: Knowledge tools for physicians. *Western Journal of Medicine* 145:830–39.

SHORTLIFFE, E.H., L.E. PERREAULT, G. WIEDERHOLD, AND L.M. FAGAN. 1990. *Medical Informatics: Computer Applications in Health Care.* Reading, Mass.: Addison-Wesley.

SLACK, W.V. 1989. The soul of a new system: A modern parable. *Clinical Computing* 6:137–40.

SMITHSONIAN INSTITUTION LIBRARIES. 1986. Report of the Smithsonian Institution Libraries Optical Disk Working Group. Washington, D.C.: Smithsonian Institution.

TEMPLETON, A.W., G.G. COX, AND S.J. DWYER III. 1988. Digital image management network: Current status. *Radiology* 169:193–97.

WEISS, S.M., C.A. KULIKOWSKI, AND S. AMAREL. 1978. A mode-based method for computer-aided medical decision making. *Artificial Intelligence* 11:145–72.

WILLIAMS, M.E. 1985. Electronic databases. *Science* 228:445–46.

WILSON, M., AND P.J. TYDEMAN. 1982. *The Management of Information in Academic Medicine.* 2 vols. Washington, D.C.: Association of American Medical Colleges.

PART II

PREPARING ARCHIVAL PROGRAMS
FOR THE HEALTH FIELDS

THE INCREASE in the rate at which empirical evidence is being generated, and the changes in the nature of the media in which that evidence is embodied, present complex challenges to every type of curatorial program, from records management and archives to manuscript and museum collections. The essential problem is that each type of program operates under a separate set of curatorial conventions and takes a different approach to the management of content, format, and medium. (See Figure II.1 for a typology of curatorial programs.) As a result, these various curatorial jurisdictions have become increasingly balkanized. The lack of either unification or standardization in the management of empirical evidence that may be inherently related in terms of content, format, and medium impedes the study and use of these materials. Such barriers to common access ultimately undermine the fundamental purpose of these programs, which is to further the growth of knowledge.

The curatorial management of documentation from the health fields is particularly complicated. Although some programs for the curatorial management of this documentation may exist at institutions in the health fields, other programs may be found in institutions outside the health fields. See Figure II.2 for the institutional context of curatorial programs with documentation from the health fields.

In most institutions in the health fields, special offices or divisions have emerged that operate either formally or informally to collect empirical evidence from both contemporary and past activities of the institution. These may be departments of a library, or the office of an executive administrator, or specifically designated curatorial programs such as records management, archival, manuscript, and museum programs. The conceptual framework for these curatorial

Types of curatorial programs	Scope of curatorial jurisdiction
Records management	**Contemporary records**—recorded documentation (inscriptive, visual, aural) that is generated and used in contemporary institutional activities. This curatorial area includes documentation that must be maintained by an institution for administrative, legal, and regulatory purposes, as well as for ongoing use in such functional areas as health care delivery, research, and teaching. *Records management programs* usually serve as the main curatorial component for the administration of contemporary institutional records.
Archival	**Historical records**—recorded documentation (inscriptive, visual, aural) that was generated and used in institutional activities in a prior era. This curatorial area includes rare or unique documentation that may have ongoing and long-term use for an institution in an administrative, legal, or regulatory capacity, and may serve as source materials for teaching and research in fields including the health sciences, life and biological sciences, the humanities, and the social sciences. *Archival programs* usually function as the main curatorial component for the administration of historical institutional records.
Manuscripts	**Personal papers**—recorded documentation (inscriptive, visual, aural) generated by individuals in the course of personal and professional activities. This curatorial area includes rare or unique documentation that is used to study the life and work of individuals. This curatorial area is usually administered by *manuscript programs.* However, when a particular individual has a strong affiliation with an institution, the personal papers may be placed under the jurisdiction of that institution's *archival program.*
Library	**Publications**—recorded documentation (inscriptive, visual, aural) that is mass-produced and widely disseminated. Publications include not only printed journals and books, but also films, videos, sound recordings, and computerized data bases. *Libraries* are the primary repositories for the administration of published documentation.
Museum	**Material evidence**—physical samples of empirical evidence, including natural specimens, chemical samples, artifacts, etc. This curatorial area includes rare or unique materials that may be collected as free-standing examples, or to supplement recorded documentation. *Museums* serve as the principal repositories for the collection of material evidence. However, special collections divisions of *libraries* and *archival* and *manuscript programs* sometimes engage in the acquisition of material evidence to enhance their holdings of recorded documentation.

Fig. II.1 **A typology of the curatorial programs that collect and administer documentation from the health fields.**

programs evolves largely from long-standing practices in the classification of empirical evidence. Terms of ownership, legal status, and the format of the materials usually constitute the primary criteria for their classification. After materials are assessed and assorted, it is on the basis of these criteria that they are channeled into particular collecting programs. Materials are assorted first according to format. Recorded documentation (inscriptive, visual, and aural) is usually directed to records management, archival, and manuscripts programs, while examples of material evidence (specimens, chemicals, and artifacts) are placed

Range of institutions with curatorial programs

Institutions within the U. S. health care system	Institutions outside the U.S. health care system
Health care delivery facilities	General educational institutions
Professional schools	Learned societies
Research institutes	Free standing repositories
Health industries	archives
Government agencies	libraries
Private foundations	museums
Professional and voluntary associations	

Fig. II.2 **The institutional context of curatorial programs that collect documentation from the health fields.** Although documentation from the health fields may be found in different types of curatorial programs from a broad range of institutions, most of this documentation resides in programs that are based at institutions in the U.S. health care system.

in object or museum collections. Distinctions in the distribution of recorded documentation are largely determined by the ownership and legal status of the materials.

By law, empirical evidence is defined as both intellectual and physical property. As a result, separate rights of ownership are established for the intellectual and physical properties of these materials. Ownership is decided mainly on the basis of the circumstances under which the evidence was created. Judgments take into consideration who contributed the ideas and who actually produced the work, as well as who paid for it. The overall ownership of both the intellectual and the physical aspects of the evidence often entails a joint arrangement between different parties. One party may be deeded the intellectual rights to the evidence, whereas the other may be awarded physical ownership. Such split property arrangements often complicate maintenance of, access to, and use of empirical evidence.

At institutions where collections of empirical evidence are maintained for ongoing reference and research, the role of ownership is a key factor in determining the distribution of documentation into particular curatorial programs. Evidence produced under the authori-

ty of the parent institution and corporately owned in part or in full is usually placed under the aegis of archival programs and records management programs. Recently created institutional materials (contemporary records) are most often distributed to records management programs, whereas the older corporate materials of the institution (historical records) are placed in the archives. Documentation generated and owned by individuals (personal papers) is placed in collections of personal papers and manuscripts. The intellectual and physical property rights to collections created by individuals are as a rule deeded to the institutions that accept those collections for deposit.

The chief reason for differentiating on the basis of the age of the evidence is that regulations governing access and use are often time-dependent. Regulations concerning current evidence usually carry more restrictions than do those for older materials. As a result, contemporary materials are usually segregated from older materials. In theory and sometimes in practice, the records management program is intended to serve as the precursor for the archival program. As the contemporary materials in the records management program increase in age and outlive time-dependent restrictions, they are to be evaluated for their potential usefulness in the archival program. Depending upon the outcome of the assessment, they are either destroyed or transferred to the archival program or to another repository for reference and research use.

In the health fields, many complex arrangements now exist to deal with the ownership of corporate evidence. The prevalence of outside funding for research, and of third-party payments for health care, have caused a major shift in the basic patterns of ownership of intellectual property rights at institutions in the health fields. An institution may own only the physical manifestation of evidence, while second and third parties share possession of its intellectual property rights.

In recent years, the parties that finance research, education, and health care delivery have gained greater control in the area of intellectual property rights. The provision of funding has entitled them to ownership of the intellectual property that is produced through their support. However, the physical property rights to the documentation created are deeded primarily to the institutions that have received their support. As a result of this shift, institutions in the health fields are burdened not only with the physical management of these materials but also with administering access to the intellectual property in accordance with the stipulations of its owners.

The range of curatorial programs (records management, archives, manuscripts, and museums) found at institutions in the health fields face compelling problems regarding not only access to their holdings but also the profusion of different formats and new media among these materials. The interrelationship of intellectual content that exists among curatorial holdings in the health fields is now ensnared by technological and legal complexities that control intellectual information. This situation demands that attempts be made to improve technical compatibility and to facilitate greater communication among the different curatorial jurisdictions.

Although numerous types of curatorial programs may be found at institutions in the health fields, they fall into a variety of organizational patterns at these institutions. Their placement within the administrative hierarchy usually defines the scope and scale of their curatorial activities. See Figure II.3 for an overview of patterns in the organizational relationship of these curatorial programs. Whereas the administrative structure of curatorial programs may vary from one institution to another, the conditions that influence their modes of practice are essentially the same. See Figure II.4 for an overview of the conditions that affect curatorial practices in the health fields.

Because the curatorial professions practice legally driven and format-driven conventions, critical segments of documentation from one project or from related projects may be dispersed to each of the institution's assorted curatorial programs: records management, archives, manuscripts, and museum and object collections. The current project reports for a given study may be distributed to the records management program, whereas the research protocols that were designed ten years earlier may be deposited in the archives. Moreover, the personal papers of the faculty member who pioneered the study might be found in the manuscript collection, and prototypes for the scientific apparatus used in the study might appear in the museum or object collections.

Despite the need for greater unification among these different curatorial areas, they should still function as separate collecting entities. Special format characteristics such as size and medium make it necessary to house some types of material in different sets of physical accommodations. For instance, three-dimensional objects and collections of papers do not easily cohabit. Moreover, biological specimens and chemical samples present threats of migration through leaking and leaching, and because of these conditions they should be isolated from cellulose and polyvinyl media

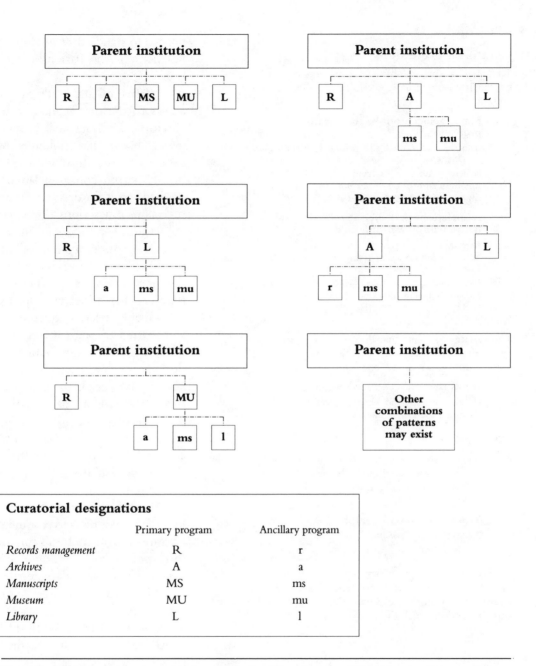

Curatorial designations

	Primary program	Ancillary program
Records management	R	r
Archives	A	a
Manuscripts	MS	ms
Museum	MU	mu
Library	L	l

Fig. II.3 **Patterns in the organizational relationship of curatorial programs.** Factors of precedence and subordination in organizational relationships affect the autonomy of curatorial activities. The placement of curatorial programs within the hierarchy of the parent institution usually defines the scope of primary and ancillary activities.

and should not be stored in close proximity to paper, film, magnetic tape, or computer disks.

The legal and regulatory environment presents other important reasons for maintaining three distinct curatorial programs for contemporary records, historical records, and personal papers. The scope of regulations and laws that pertain to the ownership and use of documentation in the health fields makes it administratively necessary to maintain distinctly separate curatorial programs.

Curatorial professions

The curatorial professions determine the conventions by which documentation is classified, organized, and utilized.

Major associations of the curatorial professions

Association of Records Managers and Administrators (ARMA)
Society of American Archivists (SAA)
American Association of Museums (AAM)
American Library Association (ALA)

Associations that specialize in documentation from the health fields

American Medical Records Association (AMRA)
Archivists and Librarians in the History of the Health Sciences (ALHHS)
Medical Library Association (MLA)
Medical Museums Association (MMA)

Intellectual disciplines

The specific discipline that documentation may represent provides criteria for the curatorial appraisal, description, and use in reference and research.

Fields that may be represented

Health professions and related sciences
Biological sciences and life sciences

Corporate sector

The regulations of the corporate sector in which a curatorial program is based guide the overall administration of its holdings and particularly affect terms of access and use.

Types of corporate sector

Public *(federal, state, local)*
Private *(for-profit, not-for-profit, religious)*

Fig. II.4 **Factors that control the development, management, and use of curatorial holdings from the health fields.**

Although curatorial programs for contemporary records, historical records, and personal papers must still function as separate collecting entities, the need for unifying the administration of these programs is increasing. The diffusion of related information into a variety of formats and media and eventual placement in different curatorial programs create complexities for access. The only uniform means of access to these materials is through content. A mechanism is, therefore, needed to standardize and link the descriptive practices of the various curatorial jurisdictions.

Systems of standardized and integrated access to the documentation in the various curatorial divisions will facilitate wider and greater use of these holdings. Making access easier and faster through a unified approach begins with a common language and standardized rules for description. Improving the precision of descriptive processes for each of the various curatorial divisions is a critical issue. Designation of points of linkage is another. When catalog entries fall short through either inaccuracy or insufficient information, they become misleading. In some instances, knowledge of certain documentation may be jeopardized through flawed catalog description. Because the description of documentation in the health fields requires a precise and highly specialized vocabulary, cataloging these materials is particularly demanding. The lack of uniform cataloging standards in archival, records management, manuscript, and museum practices for the description of documentation from the health fields only compounds the task.

One of the first steps toward unifying cataloging procedures is to coordinate the administration of an institution's curatorial programs (historical records, contemporary records, personal papers, and material evidence). In most institutions, these curatorial programs operate in varying degrees of formality as individual collecting units. Having evolved from different curatorial disciplines, they function with separate sets of practices for the management of documentation. Despite the obvious interrelationship between the documentation in archival and records management programs, they are often administratively isolated from one another. Personal papers are placed in manuscript programs which usually fall under the administration of libraries or archives. In general, records management programs are independent of library administration. Object collections are admin-

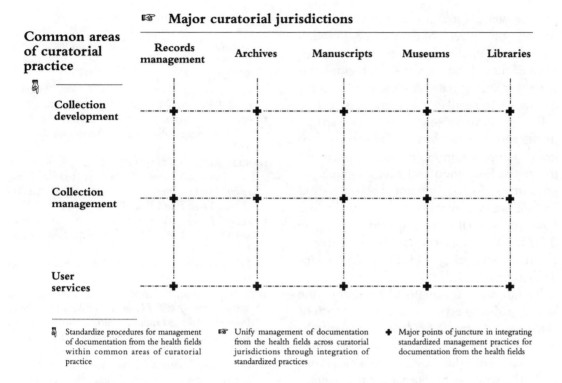

Fig. II.5 **Coordinating the management of documentation from the health fields within the various curatorial jurisdictions.** To promote a consolidated curatorial approach for documentation in the health fields, more standardization must be employed in common areas of curatorial practice.

istered either separately (as museum units) or as part of special collections units in archives or libraries.

Conventions for the management of contemporary institutional documentation employ principles of records management, whereas those used to manage an institution's older corporate materials follow archival principles. Principles of manuscript administration are employed in the case of personal papers, and museology principles are used in the management of material evidence such as specimens, chemicals, and artifacts. Although these four curatorial models vary in specific conventions of practice, they employ the same kinds of basic procedures, from appraisal and accessioning to processing and cataloging. However, much confusion arises because each of these curatorial models employs different descriptive terminology and variations in the styles for recording descriptive information. Differ-

ences in curatorial practice thus impede the ability to locate and use documentation with related content in different types of curatorial programs.

Because of the strong interrelationship of content that exists among the curatorial programs at institutions in the health fields, an effort should be made to provide better administrative and intellectual linkages among them. The expanding base and changing media of evidence in the health fields only heighten the need for a system of integrated access to the various curatorial programs. Administrative linkages as well as intellectual mechanisms must be put in place to facilitate access to these physically diverse but intellectually related holdings of documentation.

The objective of coordinating administrative and curatorial procedures for these programs is to foster cooperation in the overall development of holdings, as well as to improve systems for access and use. Although the integrity of each of the curatorial models should be maintained, new avenues of cooperation should be explored and employed wherever appropriate. A basic goal is to engender greater collaboration in areas such as collections development, collections management, and user services. If the various programs adopt a joint approach to collecting, the parent institution will have a unique opportunity to focus its curatorial objectives and to gain better control over the quantity and types of material to be acquired. See Figure II.5 for suggestions on how the practices of the major curatorial jurisdictions may be standardized and unified.

It is unrealistic for curatorial programs in the health fields to keep pace with the growth of evidence in the health fields merely by matching its volume in acquisitions. They must eventually limit the scale of their acquisitions to fit the scope of resources for the maintenance and use of these materials; collecting beyond their means is professionally irresponsible. If acquisitions cannot be processed and made available for use, their value is essentially diminished. When documentation was largely generated on paper, it could be stockpiled and processed at a later time as resources became available. However, many of the new media are so fragile and ephemeral that they cannot survive for long periods of time.

In this age of abundant evidence in short-lived media, new approaches to acquisition are necessary. To guarantee the long-term survival of holdings, both the selection and the processing of materials should be accelerated. Provisions for preservation must be introduced at a very early stage of the curatorial process. In addition, more focused collecting on a smaller scale should be undertaken to build better-quality holdings. Introducing joint administration among the collecting components can eventually reduce the collection of irrelevant and redundant materials. It also promises to streamline the management and use of holdings through greater standardization of policies and procedures.

BIBLIOGRAPHY

ADAMS, J.L. 1986. *Conceptual Blockbusting: A Guide to Better Ideas.* Reading, Mass.: Addison-Wesley.

BRADLEY, J., ED. 1983. *Hospital Library Management.* Chicago: Medical Library Association.

College and University Archives: Selected Readings. 1979. Chicago: Society of American Archivists.

DANIELS, M.F., AND T. WALCH, EDS. 1984. *A Modern Archives Reader: Basic Readings on Archival Theory and Practice.* Washington, D.C.: National Archives Trust Fund Board.

DARLING, L., ED., D. BISHOP AND L.A. COLAIANNI, ASSOC. EDS. 1982. *Handbook of Medical Library Practice.* Vol. 1, *Public Services in Health Science Libraries.* Chicago: Medical Library Association.

DARLING, L., ED., D. BISHOP AND L.A. COLAIANNI, ASSOC. EDS. 1988. *Handbook of Medical Library Practice.* Vol. 3, *Health Science Librarianship and Administration.* Chicago: Medical Library Association.

FLORANCE, V., AND N.W. MATHESON. 1993. The health sciences librarian as knowledge worker. *Library Trends* 42(1):196–223.

HACKMAN, L.J. 1988. *Strengthening New York's Historical Records Programs: A Self-Study Guide.* Albany: University of the State of New York.

NAISBITT, J., AND P. ABURDENE. 1986. *Re-inventing the Corporation: Transforming Your Job and Your Company for the New Information Society.* New York: Warner Books.

NATIONAL LIBRARY OF MEDICINE. 1986a. *Assisting Health Professions Education through Information Technology.* Report of Panel 5. Bethesda, Md.: U.S. Department of Health and Human Services.

———. 1986b. *Building and Organizing the Library's Collection.* Report of Panel 1. Bethesda, Md.: U.S. Department of Health and Human Services.

———. 1987. *Long Range Plan.* Report of the Board of Regents. Bethesda, Md.: U.S. Department of Health and Human Services.

PEACE, N.E., ED. 1984. *Archival Choices: Managing the Historical Record in an Age of Abundance.* Lexington, Mass.: D. C. Heath and Co.

SCHELLENBERG, T.R. [1956] 1975. *Modern Archives: Principles and Techniques.* Chicago: University of Chicago Press, Midway Reprints.

TOFFLER, A. 1990. *Powershift: Knowledge, Wealth, and Violence at the Edge of the Twenty-first Century.* New York: Bantam Books.

6

Reconceptualizing the Design
of Archival Programs

Nancy McCall

THE NEW INTELLECTUAL, PHYSICAL, and technical issues posed by late twentieth-century documentation in the health fields are providing unprecedented challenges to archival theory and practice. Archivists in these fields are forced to reexamine and redefine every aspect of program administration from collections development and collections management to user services. They must now strive to accommodate the quantity and complexity of late twentieth-century documentation. Today, issues associated with the physical, intellectual, and technical nature of the late twentieth-century documentation base call for the transformation of nearly every archival procedure, from accessioning, appraisal, processing, and preservation to modes of access and use.

Until recently, the holdings of archival repositories at institutions in the health fields were limited almost exclusively to historical administrative records in inscriptive format and paper-based media. Today, however, the holdings of a growing number of repositories have expanded to include a wider range of record types, from patient records to biomedical research records. This overall influx of records (ranging from administrative documents to clinical and biomedical research data) includes not only documentation in inscriptive format on paper but also documentation in other formats and media.

The inductive processes that guide scientific research, and decision making in health care delivery, account for the need to collect large quantities of data and information in many forms—not only recorded documentation but also material evidence such as specimens, biochemical compounds, and artifacts. Innovations in technology, meanwhile, have led to an expansion of formats and the introduction of new media, thus enlarging the documentation base in the health fields. Technology has also transformed the means of communication in these fields, thus facilitating more rapid exchange and dissemination of information. At the same time, these transformations in the generation and use of documentation have posed new challenges for archives in the health fields.

One issue that archivists must now face is the fragility of some new media in which contemporary biomedical evidence is stored. Many of these media (particularly ones that are electronically based) have special preserva-

tion requirements. Because they are machine-based and have relatively short life-spans, special precautions must be taken to ensure their continued usefulness.

A second issue raised by current documentation in the health fields is its built-in redundancy: the same evidence is commonly recorded in a number of different formats and media. For instance, a body of evidence surrounding a major action such as a diagnostic decision contains many overlapping pieces of evidence in different formats. Such diagnostic evidence includes both recorded documentation (e.g., written case histories and test reports, photographs, radiological images, and oral descriptions of gross pathological specimens) and related physical specimens from the patient. The need to verify processes of health care delivery directs the collection both of recorded evidence and of actual samples of the patient's tissue and fluids.

Another issue associated with twentieth-century records that must be addressed by an archival program is their multidimensionality: the data and information contained in these records have the potential to be used on a number of different levels for a wide variety of studies. Patient records or research records are frequently used for purposes other than the one for which they were primarily created. Therefore, archives in the health fields must begin to take steps to facilitate the secondary use of such data.

That documentation in the health fields has expanded in quantity and has become diverse in format and medium is of major concern to archival programs. The unprecedented amount of funding allocated to support the biomedical sciences since World War II has yielded a staggering quantity of biomedical research data. Meanwhile, the pressure exerted upon archives to accession scientific records is continuing to increase as principal investigators whose careers began at midcentury or earlier retire. They are leaving behind large quantities of data collected over long periods of time. Because much of the observational data collected over the past fifty years

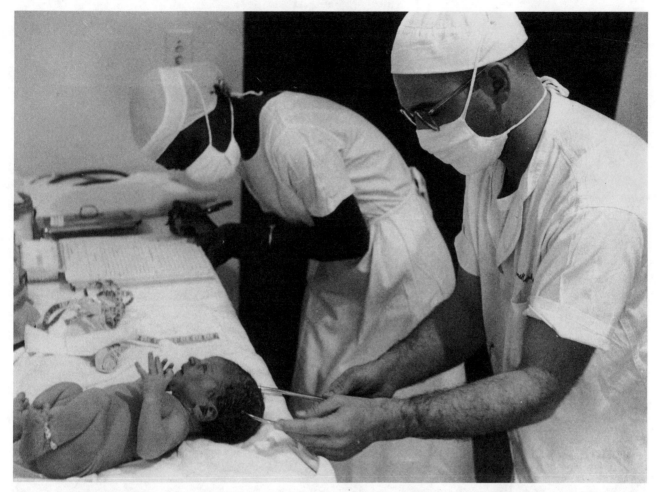

Fig. 6.1 **Observing and recording vital data.** "Observe, record, tabulate, communicate." This aphorism by William Osler aptly describes the role of documentation in the twentieth-century health fields. *Source: Alan Mason Chesney Medical Archives, the Johns Hopkins Medical Institutions.*

has not been fully studied or published, scientists and health policy experts are concerned that some of it may yet have value for ongoing research and teaching. Moreover, the level of funding, the extent of effort, and the range of talent allocated to the projects that have produced these data make granting agencies, recipient institutions, and principal investigators reluctant to consider large-scale destruction of these records and thus diminish the possibility of long-term returns from their original investments.

In addition to clinical and research documentation, archives are also required to retain many other types of documentation for evi-

dentiary purposes. Legal, regulatory, and administrative policies require a body of supporting documentation to verify corporate administrative processes and decision making. Although archival programs should guard against becoming a dumping ground for regulatory documentation, they must assume a responsible role in advising institutional authorities on managing this type of documentation.

Having to accession clinical and scientific records along with administrative records is transforming user service practices at archival repositories in the health fields. These repositories must now be prepared to facilitate sci-

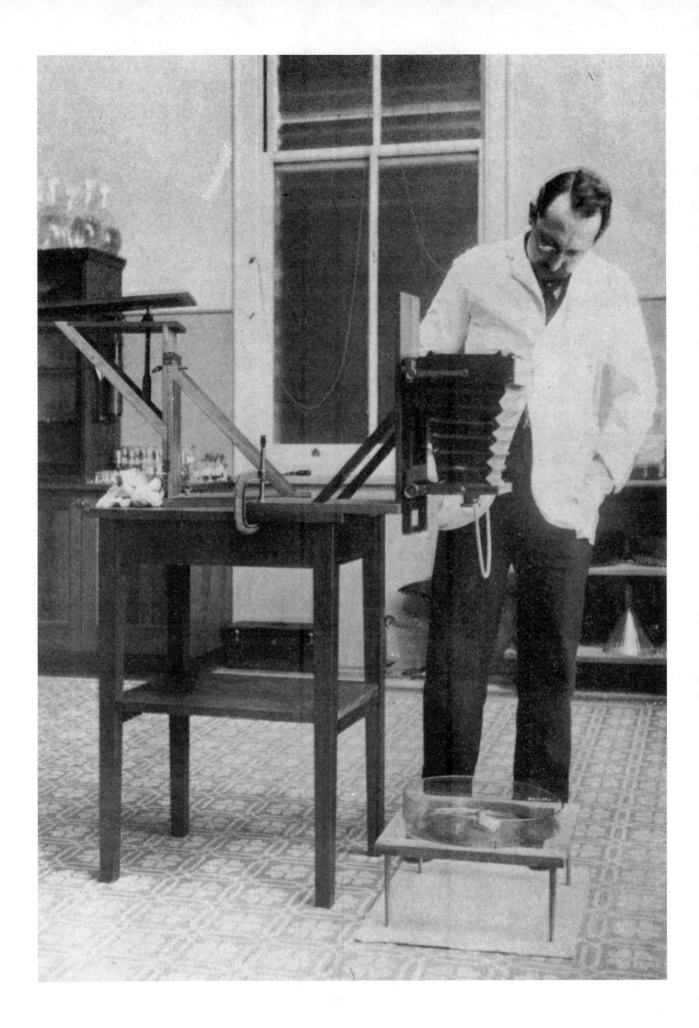

entific and clinical research in addition to research in history and the social sciences.

To meet the challenges posed by late twentieth-century documentation, archival and records management programs at institutions in the health fields must be prepared to consider new approaches to archival theory and practice. First, while continuing to fulfill their traditional functions as centers for institutional history, repositories must enlarge their intellectual horizons to accommodate the activities of scientific and clinical research. Second, they must expand their role as information clearinghouses for all types of institutional documentation, not just those records that are stored within the confines of their repositories; by providing basic information about other collections of documentation within the institution (e.g., patient records divisions and data centers), they will enhance wider research use of institutional documentation. And third, archives must collaborate with records management programs to promote the development of joint policies concerning the generation, maintenance, retention, and use of contemporary records at their institutions.

This chapter assesses the implications of the twentieth-century information revolution for archival and records management programs. A major goal is to encourage archival repositories in the health fields to find creative and responsible solutions to the challenges before them. It provides a theoretical framework as well as a practical approach.

The model that is presented advocates an evaluation of the intellectual, physical, and technical status of archival materials in order to deal with issues of redundancy and fragility. Focusing on the short life span of the media of documentation, this model recom-

mends acceleration of retention decisions so as to rescue valuable information in media that may be at risk. It concentrates on assessing the content of documentation so that the intellectual integrity may be safeguarded in preservation and processing activities. Through common language and standardized descriptive practices, the content of documentation is to be elucidated. Making the content of holdings known and accessible for reference and research is a key objective of the model.

RECONCEPTUALIZING ARCHIVAL THEORY AND PRACTICE TO ACCOMMODATE THE ACQUISITION, MANAGEMENT, AND USE OF TWENTIETH-CENTURY DOCUMENTATION

If an archival program is to support the mission of its parent institution, it will have to document the institution's administrative structure as well as its mandated functions such as teaching, research, and health care delivery. Archival programs in the health fields must in turn adapt their theoretical framework and traditional practices to meet the contemporary challenges of their institutions. Although their primary responsibility is still to acquire a core segment of evidence that documents their institutions adequately and appropriately, they must adopt more stringent standards in the selection of documentation to assure the development of holdings that are physically durable and strong in intellectual content. They will have to explore new and better ways of maintaining their holdings and of making them more easily accessible for reference and research use.

Because the inscriptive paper record no longer stands alone as the authoritative basis of documentation, archival theory and practice have to accommodate a broader range of materials in different formats and new media. The great diversity of recorded documentation and material evidence at institutions in the health fields demands new archival approaches to selection, preservation, management, and use.

A fundamental objective of archival programs at institutions in the health fields is to

Fig. 6.2 **Photographs of patients and specimens, a significant part of visual documentation in the health fields.** The intellectual and physical control of visual documentation presents many new challenges to archival management in the health fields. *Source: Alan Mason Chesney Medical Archives, the Johns Hopkins Medical Institutions.*

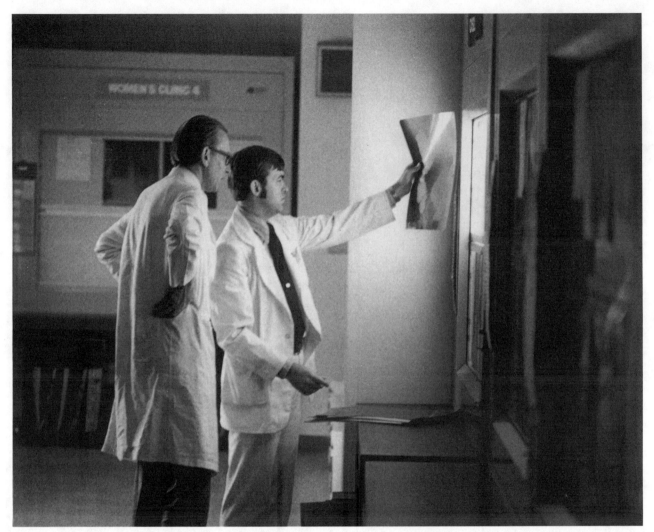

Fig. 6.3 **X rays and radiological images providing interior views of the body.** *Source: Alan Mason Chesney Medical Archives, the Johns Hopkins Medical Institutions.*

rein in a critical mass of core records that will be useful in activities of administration, teaching, and research. This goal may be achieved by targeting records that document institutional policy and organization, as well as records that document the mandated functions of these institutions—teaching, research, and health care delivery.

The archival model proposed in this chapter is an outgrowth of six guiding principles: (1) making documentation accessible for use should direct all aspects of archival practice

from acquisitions to collections management and user services; (2) standards for intellectual, technical, and physical quality should guide the selection of acquisitions; (3) administrative cooperation and unification of policies and procedures should be promoted within the related curatorial jurisdictions of the archival program and the institution; (4) archival programs should assume an activist role in issues pertaining to contemporary institutional documentation; (5) standardized descriptive procedures should be employed within the different curatorial jurisdictions of the archival program and the institution in which it is based; and (6) computerization should be employed to improve the management, accessibility, and use of archival holdings.

Adopting a Use-oriented Approach

Studies of the academic health community indicate the need for archival programs that will address the issues of contemporary documentation. Of particular concern is how this documentation may be used to further various forms of research—historical, scientific, and clinical.[1] In response to these concerns, we present a use-oriented model for archival programs in the health fields. The objective of this model is to help archives develop programs that fit the context of their parent institutions and the scale of their resources; to build select and strong holdings; and to strengthen their organization and management so that their holdings will be more easily accessible for use. This approach recommends that the inherent usefulness of materials for administrative, research, and educational purposes guide all acquisition activities, and that strategies for making holdings more easily accessible for use should direct all processing and user-service activities.

Building and organizing holdings so that they can be easily and effectively used in administration, research, and education should be the primary focus of acquisition activities. Consideration for how documentation may be used should guide all program functions—collections development, collections management, and user services.

A use-oriented approach requires that guidelines for collections management be designed to facilitate the use of holdings by streamlining the processes of arrangement, organization, and description. This model advocates basic intellectual and physical controls over holdings at even the most preliminary stages of processing. It also encourages use of the holdings through promotion of more informative finding aids.

The user services segment of the model stresses that holdings be made available for use in a fair and equitable manner whenever legal, ethical, financial, and physical conditions permit. Means of access and procedures for use of the holdings should be standardized, systematized, and procedurally fair. Archival and records management policies regarding access and use should follow the established practices for reference and research in the fields that are represented in their holdings (e.g., the health, life, and biological sciences).

Introducing Appraisal Standards for Making More Selective Acquisitions

To deal both responsibly and effectively with contemporary documentation in the health fields, archivists are going to have to operate from the premise that "less is more." Because the abundance of documentation available for archival selection is offset by limitations in the financial, physical, and technical resources available to manage that documentation, archivists will have to begin acquiring fewer yet sounder materials. This move to increase quality and decrease quantity—to choose acquisitions more selectively, on a smaller scale—is not only necessary but also beneficial, because it enables archivists to build more durable holdings that are stronger in content.

1. Field research, studies of the literature, and the practical application of trial program models have contributed to the concepts presented in this chapter. The joint archival and records management program at the Johns Hopkins Medical Institutions served as a testing ground for this chapter.

A grant from the National Historical Publications and Records Commission (NHPRC) enabled the staff of the Alan Mason Chesney Medical Archives at the Johns Hopkins Medical Institutions to study contemporary record-keeping practices at academic medical centers throughout the country. The staff conducted two major surveys: (1) an on-site records survey of the Johns Hopkins Medical Institutions (the Hospital, the School of Hygiene and Public Health, the School of Medicine, and the School of Nursing); and (2) a mail survey, the National Records Survey of Academic Medical Centers, sent to 116 teaching hospitals. The hospitals selected for the survey were those designated by the Council of Teaching Hospitals as academic medical center hospitals. The data from these surveys are unpublished; summaries are available upon request.

Because of costs associated with both short-term and long-term preservation activities, decisions regarding the retention of contemporary documentation will have to be made on a more pragmatic basis than ever before. The size of holdings should be readjusted to fit the scale of the available resources, and materials should be acquired only if they can be appropriately managed and made available for long-term use.

Archivists and records managers at academic health centers are forced to meet a two-fold challenge: to preserve a representative selection of vital records that document the corporate activities and mandated functions of their parent institutions; and to select materials of sufficiently high intellectual and physical quality so that they can be effectively utilized for purposes of reference, teaching, and research. To answer this challenge, they need to develop plans that will enable them to acquire representative documentation that is viable both intellectually and physically. In turn, they will have to adapt well-defined acquisition plans and stringent standards of appraisal that are based upon the intellectual usefulness and physical stability of the records. Because the final decisions that are made regarding retention have to be intellectually sound and affordable, these judgments usually entail a significant degree of compromise.

In many cases, acquisition planning may be assisted by statistical strategies for sampling representative and intellectually coherent segments of documentation. It will also benefit from the input of various professionals, ranging from scientists and clinicians to administrators, historians, lawyers, and conservators.

Linking the Administration and Management of Related Curatorial Programs

The creation of administrative linkages between related curatorial programs within an institution is a critical step toward improving the management of these programs as resources for research. Most importantly, the acquisition activities of these programs should be encouraged to complement each other. The establishment of a common intellectual and ethical basis for the operation of related curatorial programs will strengthen their ability to support the research and educational activities of the institution in which they are based. Whether the four major types of curatorial components—contemporary records; historical records; personal papers and manuscripts; and the museum, or objects, component—are dispersed throughout the institution under the aegis of different curatorial programs or are contained within one or two major programs (for example, archives and records management), their administrative cooperation will facilitate the use of their collective holdings for reference and research activities.

Because related information concerning a particular subject is often presented in different types of documentation in various formats and media, communication and cooperation among curatorial programs is essential if researchers' needs are to be met. A shared body of policies, procedures, and terminology can form the basis for effective cooperation among the individual repositories within the institution. Integrating the administration of the various curatorial programs not only increases the accessibility and use of holdings but also improves the efficiency and quality of collections management procedures by promoting adherence to a common set of intellectual and ethical standards.

Rapprochement between archival programs and records management programs is a particularly important example of cooperation and communication between different types of collecting components that share related responsibilities. Never before have these two curatorial disciplines been so constrained to set limits and to make critical choices about the nature and extent of their accessions. Joining forces in the development of policies and procedures will assist both programs in meeting this challenge.

In archival theory and practice, records management has traditionally functioned as the staging process in which the fate of institutional records is decided. Scheduling records has largely served as a deferral process that preserves records until a final decision can be reached about their retention or disposition. Conventional records management programs have usually made provisional schedules for archival retention and then passed the final decisions on to the administrators of archival programs. As a result, records languish for years in a state of institutional purgatory until their statutes of limitation expire, at which time they are reassessed to determine their archival value.

Unfortunately, institutions in the health fields can no longer afford to wait so long before making decisions about contemporary records. Instead, a rigorous and accelerated form of decision making is needed to hasten the appraisal and accession processes both in records centers and in archival repositories. As John Dojka and Sheila Conneen (1984) proposed in their work at Yale, records management may be used by institutions as a preliminary tool for archival appraisal. Such cooperation between archival programs and records management programs enables both to function more coherently and to meet their institutional objectives more effectively.

Taking an Activist Approach to Planning and Preservation

Prospective planning is one key to more efficient means of acquisition, maintenance, and use of holdings. Archivists will have to assume an active role in planning activities at both institutional and repository levels in order to identify and protect valuable documentation.

By becoming more involved in issues regarding the retention and disposition of current institutional documentation, archival programs and records management programs may eventually have greater input in policies that affect the generation and maintenance of institutional records. Thus, as archivists become more actively involved in institutional policy decisions that affect records manage-

ment practices, they achieve more control over the selection of the institutional records that are to be scheduled for archival preservation.

Archivists will also have to assume a proactive approach as they face the new challenge of preserving, storing, and accessing data and information that are stored in a wide variety of formats and fragile media. As archivists deal more frequently with twentieth-century materials, they have begun to recognize that many of the costly preservation problems they face could have been avoided if simple preventive measures in handling the materials had been instituted at the proper time.

In responding to these preservation challenges, archivists are going to have to take a strong stand on prevention and encourage early intervention to protect documentation that is vulnerable to damage and deterioration. For instance, they should encourage their constituents—from chief executive officers to bench scientists—to store paper records in clean and controlled environments to avoid the onset of mold and insect problems. They should be encouraged to follow the example of the publishing industry's intervention in helping libraries deal with the problems of acid paper in twentieth-century books, by recommending that vital documents such as contracts and the minutes of governing bodies be issued on low-acid paper to avoid the inevitable investment of effort and costs associated with deacidification.

Archivists should also extend their preventive maintenance concerns to include other types of media—especially electronic media. They must ensure that documentation that is stored in computer tapes and disks is regularly "refreshed" through transferal of data and information from one computer medium to another as computer systems are upgraded or replaced. This process requires not only that the transfer be carried out but also that the necessary equipment be maintained so that the upgrading can be accomplished. In preserving data and information that is stored in electronic media, the costs of refreshment must always be weighed against those of long-term retention of paper back-up files. As a further step, archivists should join other concerned consumers in efforts to lobby the computer industry to develop more effective and less costly provisions for the long-term preservation of fragile media.

Promoting the Standardization and Integration of Descriptive Information

In unifying the administration of related curatorial holdings, an important step is the integration of an automated information system to manage the listing and description of holdings at the collection level. This process begins with the standardization and integration of the manual inventories and finding guides within the different programs and is followed by the automation of these various listings.

The institution-wide adoption of a common scheme for the organization of documentation and a standardized body of terminology and procedures for describing documentation are prerequisites for the development of computer applications for archival programs in the health fields. Once the policies and procedures of the various curatorial programs are standardized and integrated, conversion to computerization becomes a realistic goal.

Computerized information systems are vital tools for managing the large scale and diversity of late twentieth-century documentation. By making information about a wider selection of materials more accessible to users, computerized systems for reference and access greatly enhance the research and educational use of the different curatorial holdings.

REDESIGNING ARCHIVAL PROGRAMS TO INCORPORATE CHANGES IN THEORY AND PRACTICE

Archival repositories at institutions in the health fields must design programs that will document the mandated functions of their respective institutions in a balanced and effective approach. The development of such approaches demands a fundamental understanding of how documentation is used in the activities of these functions. Being able to recognize which materials are nonessential is as important as knowing which are essential. Strategies for finding and removing redundancies and irrelevant materials are as critical as those for locating and preserving significant documentation.

To develop strategies for selecting and preserving key documentation at institutions such as academic health centers, archivists must first gain an overview of the universe of documentation that exists and of the forces that created it. Knowing how and why the materials were created is an essential step toward understanding the nature of the materials themselves—intellectually, physically, and technically. Learning how to recognize data and information that may be recycled for other studies is, of course, critical. In designing acquisition plans, archivists will have to address the role of their institutions in the larger context of education, science, and health care; study their institutional administrative structures; and analyze the mandated functions of their institutions. The classification model for institutional functions that is presented in chapter 1 may be followed to identify core documentation in specific types of institutions.

Designing a Focused, More Effective Program through Strategic Planning

If archival repositories at institutions in the health fields are to launch viable and dynamic programs, they must first engage in strategic planning to define the scope and mission of the program. The quality and effectiveness of the proposed program are highly dependent upon the implementation of a strategic plan. The goal of strategic planning is to develop a highly focused program that is appropriately scaled to fit the needs and resources of the parent institution.

The strategic plan should be both visionary and pragmatic: it needs to incorporate a clear and far-reaching vision for the program while taking into account the level of resources available to the program. To be effective, the plan needs to address the intellectual and ethical issues that affect the program and its staff, users, contributors, and parent institution, as well as technical and economic issues. It must evaluate basic requirements for facilities, equipment, and staffing, and it must set priorities for the development, management, and use of the holdings.

In the long term, the strategic plan may be used to chart the course of development of the archival program. In most institutions the archives staff does not have the authority to make final decisions about their program's scope and scale. Because such decisions entail the commitment of institutional resources, administrators in charge of space and budget allocations should be included in the strategic planning process. Indeed, a wide variety of groups should be included among the strategic planners. Representatives of the archives staff, the faculty, and the administration should also be encouraged to participate.

Periodic review of the strategic plan (preferably every five years) will help to keep the program focused and in touch with the changing priorities of the parent institution. Faculty members, administrators, and other relevant institutional figures should participate in this review and make recommendations for changing and improving the program.

Defining the Mission and Scope of the Archival Program

As archivists confront the challenges of late twentieth-century documentation and the complexities of their parent institutions, they will need to revise the mission of their programs and make them more proactive in both concept and practice. Mission statements should articulate a more active and focused response to the informational and cultural needs of the parent institutions in particular and the health fields in general.

Thus, the mission of an archival program is to enhance the mandated functions of the parent institution through the preservation, management, and resourceful use of selective institutional documentation. It should advance the activities of education and research in the health care fields by making its holdings available for study outside the immediate institutional community whenever legally and ethically possible.

Recorded and material evidence acquired by the archival program should be maintained and made available for use as (1) aids in the current operation and administration of the parent institution, (2) a means of commemorating that institution's role in the history of the health fields, (3) resources for research, and (4) tools for teaching and other educational activities.

Unifying Curatorial Policies and Procedures

To bring related curatorial activities under better intellectual and physical control, strategic planners must first assess the full range of actual and potential collecting activities that exist in their institutions. They should examine not only formalized programs but also the various types of informal collecting that have evolved. Once they have located programs with related holdings, they must then begin to establish appropriate administrative linkages between the various curatorial jurisdictions.

To respond more directly to institutional needs, this curatorial consortium, which may include archives and records management programs as well as manuscript and museum programs, must interact with the administrative strata that exist within their respective institutions: the executive level, the departmental level, and the office level. Interlocking committees and outreach activities such as publications and exhibits are among the strategies for reaching the various administrative levels. The objective is to build institution-wide consensus for the scope of collecting activities.

Although general policies and procedures should be defined by the consortium, the physical and intellectual management of doc-

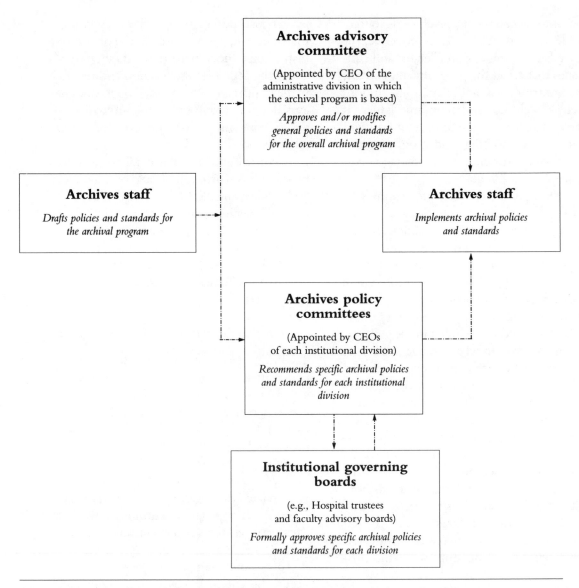

Fig. 6.4 **Flowchart of the role of committees in the administration of archival programs.** Because of the legal, technical, and intellectual complexities that surround archival materials in the health fields, academic health centers and other institutions in the health fields should develop a committee network to inform and monitor the policies that govern the operation of their archival programs.

umentation should occur within the context of its specific curatorial jurisdiction. A unified set of general policies should be adopted by the related curatorial programs. Policies and procedures for the common areas of curatorial practice (collections development, collections management, and user services) should flow out of a common collecting goal for the institution.

Establishing a Network of Institutional Committees

To establish processes of accountability and encourage greater administrative effectiveness, the design of an archival program should incorporate the role of committees. The administration of archival programs in the health fields requires an active committee process to define and monitor its key policies and procedures. Because an archival program acquires documentation on behalf of its parent institution, it needs the input of institutional committees to ensure that the policies and procedures it develops are consistent with the institution's mission, administration, and mandated functions. Institutional committees should play a major role in setting policies for acquisitions and setting standards for the appraisal and use of archival materials.

Because of the large scale and the complexity of most institutions in the health fields—and of academic health centers, in particular—a network of two types of committees should be incorporated into the design of the archival program. An overarching advisory committee should be planned, together with individual policy committees to work with each major institutional division such as the hospital, the medical school, the school of nursing, and the school of public health.

The advisory committee should set overall policies and standards for the archival program. It should be composed of leading members of the faculty and staff of the parent institution as well as distinguished figures from outside the immediate institutional community. A policy committee should be convened for each institutional division. Each policy committee should include key members of the faculty and staff from the institutional division that it represents. The role of these committees is to establish specific policies and standards for the collection and use of documentation from their respective institutional sectors. (See Fig. 6.4.)

Making Provisions for Accountability

The administration and management of an archival program require the resolution of many complex ethical, regulatory, and legal issues. To prepare for handling the broad range of sensitive issues that daily confront archival programs, it is necessary to build a solid infrastructure of ethical guidelines. A set of directives should be drafted at each institution to guide planners in formulating ethically sound policies and procedures for the administration of an archival program. The legal and ethical rights of institutional administrators, faculty members, staff members, students, patients, and human research subjects must be guaranteed in practices of collections development, collections management, and user services. The following ethical directives should guide policy making for archival programs in the health fields.

Ethical Directives for the Development of Holdings

- Select a range of documentation that fairly represents the policies, programs, and activities of the creating institutional body.
- Choose all documentation for the purpose of promoting open and honest inquiry.
- Acquire documentation that has relevance to issues in the larger context of the health fields.
- Focus on the selection of documentation that will stimulate research in new areas.
- Make final accession decisions on the basis of the integrity of the documentation (intellectual, physical, and technical).

Ethical Directives for Collections Management

- Protect the legal and ethical rights of corporate bodies and individuals by identifying materials in the holdings that may be legally or ethically sensitive.
- Prevent unwarranted access to legally and ethically sensitive materials by physically and intellectually segregating these materials from other repository holdings.
- Preserve the integrity of the holdings (intellectual, physical, and technical) by ensuring that collections are properly maintained.

Ethical Directives for User Services

- Promote active and responsible use of the holdings.
- Assure all users fair and equal opportunity to access the holdings.
- Apply standardized policies and procedures for access to the nonsensitive holdings.
- Introduce a procedurally fair process whereby an institutional board reviews requests for access to restricted materials.
- Preserve the integrity of the holdings (intellectual, physical, technical) by maintaining proper procedures for use.
- Protect the well-being of staff and users by maintaining proper safeguards in the use of hazardous materials in the holdings.
- Require that users follow proper procedures in citations of materials from the repository's holdings.

Introducing Common Standards for Acquisition, Management, and Use

The profusion of twentieth-century documentation is forcing the archival profession to address the need to limit the size of repository holdings. Because archival programs must operate on a fixed budget for housing and staffing, they cannot expect to collect on an unrestricted basis. As a result, acquisition goals must be physically quantified as well as intellectually justified. The abundance of twentieth-century documentation necessitates a more stringent approach to the development of holdings. A first step is to specify criteria for collecting. These should evolve from and be limited to the mission of the parent institution.

To avoid redundant collecting within the other curatorial programs at an institution, archival planners should work in conjunction with these other programs to develop a master acquisition plan and common standards for appraisal. In turn, the appraisal process should assess materials for their relevance to the designated criteria for acquisitions and evaluate them according to standards of quality that encompass the informational content and the stability, durability, and technical compatibility of the media.

The objective of joint acquisition planning is to hone the focus for collecting at an institutional level. Other joint efforts should be made to pool resources for storage, preservation, organization, and use of the related curatorial holdings. Institutions may improve the quality of their archival and other related curatorial programs through cooperative arrangements for administration and management and at the same time be able to economize. By having an institutional overview of related curatorial holdings, administrators may be able to distribute funding more closely in proportion to common needs of the various programs. The amount of funding allocated should be guided by the evidential and informational value of the curatorial holdings. See Fig. II.5 for suggestions on how to consolidate standards for common areas of curatorial practice.

Facilitating Wider and More Extensive Use of Holdings

In addition to their significance for historical studies, some observational research data from scientific and clinical projects are still viable for current research in their respective or related disciplines. Because few centers for the preservation of observational data have been established at institutions in the health fields, archival programs at these institutions are having to become more involved in the preservation and management of research records. As a consequence, archival programs will have to revise their policies and procedures to facilitate research in the health, life, and biological sciences as well as in the humanities, history, and other social sciences. The activities of collections development, collections management, and user services must assume a high level of scientific sophistication. In terms of outreach, they must make clinicians and scientists, as well as historians, aware of their holdings.

The processing of holdings should be committed to making materials both physically and intellectually accessible for research. By standardizing descriptive processes for the various formats of material; introducing standardized descriptive terms such as the National Library of Medicine's Medical Subject Headings (MeSH), the Library of Congress Name Authority File, and the *Art and Architecture Thesaurus* (AAT); and developing a thesaurus of proper names for the parent institution, archivists and records managers may make descriptive information about the holdings more accurate and specific, from accessioning onward.

User service procedures should be designed to promote the use of holdings whenever legally and ethically possible. Although these procedures should have appropriate safeguards for protecting holdings from abuse, they should also facilitate reference and research activities.

Because many archival patrons in the health fields are now computer literate, users have higher expectations for access to and retrieval of information from both manual and electronic systems. To communicate with users more effectively and to deliver services more proficiently, archival programs will have to develop computerized systems of access and retrieval for all holdings, both hard-copy and electronic. The introduction of computerized databases and networks will serve to make knowledge of the holdings more accessible to a wider range of users.

CONCLUSION

Reconceptualizing the design of archival programs to meet the challenges that are posed by contemporary documentation is a daunting endeavor. However, in this era of new technologies and a rapidly expanding documentation base, archives must reassess and refocus their traditional programs to serve their parent institutions more effectively. By seeking more direct involvement of the faculty and staff of their institutions in the planning and administration of their programs, archives in the health fields may build programs that are more directly responsive to specific institutional needs for teaching, research, and administration.

Because the model for reconceptualizing archival programs calls for a team approach, it is particularly appropriate for institutions in the health fields. Most scientific, clinical, and educational programs at these institutions already operate in a collaborative mode. Therefore, they are more receptive to a team approach in the design of archival programs. The broad range of expertise that is available at institutions in the health fields constitutes a wonderful resource for the team approach. During this period of revolution in the design of archival programs for the health fields, archivists are fortunate to be able to work closely with the originators of the documentation that they are charged to manage.

BIBLIOGRAPHY

BATTIN, P. 1985. Crossing the border: Librarianship in the information age. *Harvard Librarian* 19:8–10.

BELANGER, T. N.d. *The Future of Rare Book Collections*. Malkin Lecture no. 8. In press.

BELLARDO, L.J., AND L.L. BELLARDO, COMPS. 1992. *A Glossary for Archivists, Manuscript Curators, and Records Managers*. Chicago: Society of American Archivists.

BLAKE, J. 1964. Medical records and history. *American Archivist* 27:229–35.

CRAIG, B.L. 1985. The Canadian hospital in history and archives. *Archivaria* 21:52–67.

DANIELS, M.F., AND T. WALCH, EDS. 1984. *A Modern Archives Reader: Basic Readings on Archival Theory and Practice*. Washington, D.C.: National Archives Trust Fund Board.

DOJKA, J. 1980. *Planning and Organizing a Joint Archives and Records Management Program: The Report of the Yale University Archives Record Survey, October 1978–March 1980*. New Haven: Yale University.

DOJKA, J., AND S. CONNEEN. 1984. Records management as an appraisal tool in college and university archives. In *Archival Choices*, ed. N. E. Peace. Lexington, Mass.: Lexington Books.

ELLIOTT, C.A., ED. 1983. *Understanding Progress as Process: Documentation of the History of Post-War Science and Technology in the United States*. Final report of the Joint Committee on Archives of Science and Technology. Chicago: Society of American Archivists.

HAAS, J.K., H.W. SAMUELS, AND B.T. SIMMONS. 1985. *Appraising the Records of Modern Science and Technology: A Guide*. Cambridge: MIT Press.

HACKMAN, L.J. 1985. From assessment to action: Toward a usable past in the Empire State. *Public Historian* 7:23–34.

HIMMELSTEIN, D.U., AND S. WOOLHANDLER. 1986. Cost without benefit: Administrative waste in U.S. health care. *New England Journal of Medicine* 314:441–45.

KOONTZ, H., AND H. WEIHRICH. 1990. *Essentials of Management*. New York: McGraw-Hill.

MCCALL, N. 1992. The strategic plan for the Alan Mason Chesney Medical Archives of The Johns Hopkins Medical Institutions: Meeting the archival challenges of the information age in the health fields. Baltimore: Johns Hopkins University.

MATHESON, N.W., AND J.A.D. COOPER. 1982. Academic information in the academic health sciences center: Roles for the library in information management. *Journal of Medical Education* 57:1–93.

SCHELLENBERG, T.R. [1956.] 1975. *Modern Archives: Principles and Techniques*. Chicago: University of Chicago Press, Midway Reprints.

WILLIAM H. WELCH MEDICAL LIBRARY. 1986. *The Annual Report of the William H. Welch Medical Library, 1985/1986*. Baltimore: Johns Hopkins University.

———. 1987. *The Annual Report of the William H. Welch Medical Library, 1986/1987*. Baltimore: Johns Hopkins University.

———. 1988. *The Annual Report of the William H. Welch Medical Library, 1987/1988*. Baltimore: Johns Hopkins University.

———. 1990. *The Annual Report of the William H. Welch Medical Library, 1989–1990*. Baltimore: Johns Hopkins University.

7

Building Relevant, Well-focused, and Coherent Holdings

Nancy McCall and Lisa A. Mix, with Arian D. Ravanbakhsh

A RATIONALE FOR THE APPRAISAL AND SELECTION OF DOCUMENTATION IN THE HEALTH FIELDS

FOR CONTEMPORARY INSTITUTIONS in the health fields, there is not one simple, prescriptive formula to follow in the identification, selection, and retention of archival documentation. Many different yet equally viable approaches may be taken. Essentially, individual institutions must choose the approach or approaches that will best fulfill the goals they have set for their own particular archival program. In defining the goals of their archival programs, institutions must seriously consider their objectives for the intended use of archival documentation. Approaches to the development of archival holdings should include criteria and standards for acquisition as well as clearly defined processes for the selection and disposition of documentation.

In her discussion of the role of archivists as selectors, Barbara Craig (1992) noted that the archival community has been reluctant to embrace more selective practices of retention. She attributes this reluctance to the unwillingness of archivists to face the consequences of making controversial decisions. Craig laments the perception of appraisal as a moral dichotomy of right or wrong choices and argues that pursuit of right theories of appraisal is philosophically misleading and also highly impractical. Instead, she points to the process of appraisal as the means of discerning real truth and concentrates on ways by which this process may be improved. She cites the appraisal reforms that have been introduced by Hans Booms and in particular praises his concept of documentation planning to systematize the process of appraisal.

It is critical that archival repositories in the health fields have a documentation plan and a systematized process of appraisal and selection. This plan and process must adhere to the mission of the parent institution and the ethos of the scientific and clinical disciplines that are represented in the functions of the institution. By eliciting the active participation of personnel from each institution in the adoption of a documentation plan and standards for appraisal, archivists may transform the act of selection into a decision that is based upon institutional consensus.

Because of the legal, ethical, technical, and intellectual complexities of documentation in the health fields, appraisal and selection processes must be guided by individuals who understand why the documentation under consideration was created and how it was uti-

lized. These individuals may serve as members of standing committees or specially appointed panels of experts; their role is to inform and advise the archival staff about the nature of the documentation. In turn, the archival staff takes the lead in shaping the process of appraisal and selection. Archivists must be able to exercise the judgment to know when to seek the intervention of their institutional peers. The objective of this joint endeavor is to reach consensus on the development of archival holdings. Archival appraisal and selection should be a responsibility that is shared by the archival staff and the personnel of these institutions.

Criteria and standards for selection of documentation at these institutions should incorporate the ethical principles of archival practice as well as the ethics for teaching, research, and health care delivery. They should also encompass the codes of the particular professional practices that are to be represented in their holdings. The original methodologies that were employed in the generation and use of the documentation should serve as a guide for assessing the quantity and quality of documentation to be selected.

SPECIAL ISSUES IN THE DEVELOPMENT OF ARCHIVAL HOLDINGS AT INSTITUTIONS IN THE HEALTH FIELDS

The profusion of contemporary documentation, coupled with the finite nature of the resources available for the preservation, management, and use of that documentation, makes it necessary for archival programs at institutions in the health fields to establish limitations in the development of their holdings. Although traditionalists in the archival profession may urge the retention of broad and inclusive selections of institutional documentation, the size and complexity of contemporary institutions require that this approach be modified and scaled down. The criteria for acquisitions must be narrowed and more finely focused, and standards of appraisal need to be made more rigorous.

In an era when institutions in the health fields are facing severe economic constraints, the selection of acquisitions should be guided by the level of resources that will be available for their preservation, management, and use. When documentation was largely in paper-based media, the existence of resources was not such a critical factor in retention decisions. Now that documentation is in many types of fragile, short-lived media, the availability of resources has become a paramount issue. Whereas documentation in paper-based media may be stockpiled for years until the resources are eventually found for its preservation, documentation in these more ephemeral media have a much shorter life-span, which requires early intervention to ensure both short- and long-term preservation.

The cost of preserving data and information that are contained in some of the fragile media is often prohibitively high; the cost of preservation or of the transferral of data and information to more stable media may exceed the intrinsic value of the documentation itself. Under these circumstances, archival programs are now more than ever compelled to limit the scope of their selection to the scale of their resources.

Another complicating factor in the health fields is that recorded data and information do not constitute the sole source of empirical evidence. In many instances, related specimens, chemical compounds, and equipment may be needed to enable interpretation of recorded data and information. As a consequence archival programs in these fields must also accommodate relevant selections of material evidence when it is needed to augment or interpret recorded documentation in their holdings.

Although archival programs have always had to balance specific institutional reasons for selection of acquisitions against broader cultural concerns, their task is significantly more challenging today. The mere cost of preserving vital administrative materials—many of which are in fragile media —may be daunting. Thus, it is more difficult than ever for archival programs to focus on larger cultural needs. Most of a program's resources may have to be devoted to the preservation of core administrative records.

In addition, the advent of the information age has also altered many of the criteria for the selection of acquisitions. New methodologies and media that evolved in conjunction with the rise of computerization have brought fundamental changes in the production and use of documentation. Data and information collected for one purpose may now be scavenged and more easily used for other purposes and thus may be transformed into a new type of commodity. The recycling of data and information has become a prevalent practice in the health fields: data and information collected primarily for clinical purposes are frequently also used for research and teaching, as well as for administrative studies such as cost analysis and quality control. Acquisition strategies and appraisal practices must now take into account the multidimensional value of the data and information that are contained in documentation. Records that may be utilized for different purposes have more extended value than those that have limited use.

One viable approach is to limit the scope of acquisitions to the parent institutions' main administrative components and its mandated functions. In following this approach, archival programs should first implement strategies to target the types of critical documentation that Schellenberg terms as evidential—documentation that must be maintained for legal purposes and ongoing administrative purposes (Schellenberg 1956). After targeting critical evidential documentation, they should then consider types of documentation that Schellenberg terms informational, from certain topical areas within the mandated functions. Ideally, these areas should encompass topics that have generated widespread activity throughout the institution and the larger context of the health fields.

NEW APPROACHES TO ARCHIVAL APPRAISAL AND SELECTION

In the 1980s several important new approaches to appraisal and selection emerged within the archival profession. Elements of some of these new appraisal theories that have been advanced are incorporated in the approach that is presented in this chapter.

Interinstitutional Collaboration

The idea of collaboration among archival repositories is not new. Archives do not acquire and appraise records in a social vacuum (Craig 1992). An important part of a sound policy on acquisitions is an awareness of the acquisition policies of other repositories in the same field or the same geographic region. Archival programs must now move beyond mere acknowledgment of the acquisition policies of other repositories and actively work with other repositories in designing complementary strategies for the development of their respective holdings. In an age of shrinking resources, interinstitutional collaboration is intellectually and economically prudent.

In the past decade, the impetus for collaboration in the archival field has come largely from archives of science and technology. In 1983, the Joint Committee on Archives of Science and Technology (JCAST) issued a report, *Understanding Progress as Process* (Elliott 1983), defining the major issues confronting the documentation of twentieth-century science and technology. Many of the issues discussed in this report are similar to those facing documentation in the health fields. The increase in the volume and complexity of recorded documentation, the loss of knowledge because important documentation is not preserved, and the lack of adequate resources limit archivists' ability to deal with the information explosion.

JCAST presented a plan that called for cooperation among the industrial sector, the government, academic institutions, and other institutions involved in science and technology. The plan urged that archivists dealing

with the documentation of science and technology take into account the research processes of the disciplines in these fields. It recommended that the creators, the collectors, the custodians, and the users of documentation be jointly involved in the appraisal process (Elliott 1983). It also recommended that discipline history centers (where they exist) play a central role in coordinating interinstitutional plans for collecting. According to this scenario, the history center for a given scientific discipline would be responsible for stimulating and focusing interest in that discipline's history; involving the creators of scientific documentation in the appraisal process; identifying key individuals and projects to be documented, and developing a systematic program to locate the records documenting the discipline's history; acting as an intermediary between the creators of scientific documentation and archivists, as well as working to place collections in the appropriate repositories; and identifying and defining the universe of documentation in its discipline (Elliott 1983).[1]

Documentation Strategy

Concepts of documentation strategy for the fields of science and technology build and expand upon principles laid out in the JCAST report. One premise is that archivists, in appraising records, should consider the total body of available documentation in a given field or region (Haas et al. 1986). This necessitates collaboration among archivists at different institutions in the same field of endeavor or geographic region.

Documentation strategy is meant to be applied to a specific field of endeavor (such as medicine, science, or higher education), to a specific geographic region, or to both (e.g., medicine in New England), rather than to an institution or to a specific discipline. It re-

---

1. For a description of the program of one of the leading discipline history centers, the Center for the History of Physics at the American Institute of Physics, see Hackman and Warnow-Blewett 1987.

quires that archivists look at their institutions within the larger context of the field represented or their geographic region. Rather than focusing on key individuals or projects, the documentation-strategy approach advises archivists to examine key activities and functions and to identify and collect the records that document those activities and functions. In later refinements of the approach, documentation strategists have suggested that if a certain activity or function (student activities at a university, for example) is not adequately documented by existing material, archivists should then actively seek out or, in some cases, create documentation for this function (Samuels 1986; Samuels 1991; Samuels 1992).[2]

Documentation strategy assumes the close collaboration among repositories recommended in the JCAST report. The aim of such collaboration is to ensure that the historical record is not skewed toward some functions and activities at the expense of others, or toward one particular type of institution.

Critics of documentation strategy note several problems with this approach.[3] First, there are no standard appraisal practices for archives to adopt when devising interinstitutional documentation plans. Second, it is unclear who would coordinate interinstitutional plans. In the JCAST report this role is designated for the discipline history centers; however, many fields (medicine among them) have no centralized discipline history centers. Perhaps the most significant criticism of documentation strategy is that the mission of most archival programs is to serve their parent institutions first. Whereas it is important to look at the institution within a larger context, the prime objective of an archival program is to document the parent institution and to retain those archival materials that will be of greatest use to that institution in carrying out its mandated functions. Finally, true documentation strategy requires a great outlay of resources, in terms of both funding and personnel (Boles 1987; Abraham 1991).

Although the limitations of documentation strategy must be acknowledged, some elements of this approach are useful in appraising archival material at academic health centers. Archivists need to look at their parent institutions in a larger societal context and examine the functions and activities to be documented. Because of the increasing volume of material in twentieth-century medicine, archivists will have to select which major functions and subsidiary activities merit documentation, and then appraise records accordingly. In making such a decision, the total body of available documentation should be a factor.

RECOMMENDED APPROACHES
FOR THE HEALTH FIELDS

Documentation Planning

Documentation planning, introduced in chapter 1, draws on the basic concepts of documentation strategy. However, it is grounded in the premise that archives should concentrate on the mandated functions of their parent institutions. In analyzing the functions of an academic health center according to the principles of documentation planning, archivists should first assess the role of the institution within the broader context of the U.S. health care system and its functions (Krizack 1994). The next step is to identify the key functions of the institution. In the case of an academic health center, the primary functions to be documented are health care delivery, research, and education; ancillary functions may include policy regulation and the provision of goods and services.

When developing criteria for acquisitions, archivists should consider how to document the mandated functions of the specific institution, as well as the place of the institution in the larger societal context of the U.S. health care system. Analyses of how acquisitions document the institution's functions and role

2. For a theory of documentation strategy for institutions of higher education, see Samuels 1992.
3. For a cogent and well-informed analysis of recent documentation strategy concepts, see Cook 1992.

in the U.S. health care system should also guide processing efforts and the preparation of finding aids.

Designation of Topical Areas for Acquisitions

One way to focus an acquisitions plan is to designate topical areas for selection. This approach involves targeting certain subject areas and soliciting institutional materials relevant to those areas. In addition to providing a focus for the program, the designation of such areas may increase the archival program's usefulness to the institution, because documentation of special institutional projects serves as a key information resource for those projects.

The choice of topical areas should be broad enough to include a range of undertakings within the mandated functions and major administrative divisions of the institution and should be multidisciplinary with regard to the departments and fields represented. Examples of intrainstitutional, interdisciplinary undertakings include large collaborative projects in areas such as AIDS, genetics, or the neurosciences. The designation of these topical areas for selection of acquisitions should be based upon pre-existing thematic strengths in the archival holdings and the significance of the topical areas in the larger context of society. To prevent additional strain upon the administrative resources of the archival program, the range of acquisitions may be concentrated toward the prevailing types of formats and media that are already in the repository's holdings.

Archival advisory committees, acting in conjunction with groups of subject specialists, should participate in selecting the topical areas of the acqusitions plan. Once a topical area is designated, the archival program should create a system with criteria and standards for the selection of material. After topical areas have been designated, they should be reviewed on a periodic basis, so that the archival program may modify the scope of the acquisition plan if overall institutional activities change.

The Role of Sampling

Chapter 3 of this volume recommends several approaches for sampling patient records. Some of the strategies presented may be adapted to other types of records at academic health centers. Sampling should be considered for any particularly voluminous body of records. For example, in the case of making representative selections from large groups of administrative records the archives may employ processes of systematic statistical sampling or sampling by year. It is pertinent to note that the designation of collecting areas is essentially a form of sampling, in that archivists target for retention records dealing with a particular subject or records derived from a particular activity. In the selection of some types of scientific data, neither systematic statistical sampling nor sampling by year would be appropriate, because researchers working with this kind of data usually need to see a continuous body of work. However, in some instances when selecting data from a single laboratory, sampling strategies may be employed to target the documentation from key experiments. With this approach only the critical data that are needed to recreate the experiments and to verify their results would be retained.

Considerations for Scientific Data

Since the late 1940s, large-scale funding for scientific research has escalated the amount of research documentation generated and retained by institutions in the health fields. Chapter 4 of this volume sets forth strong arguments for documenting research processes by preserving select samples of data. To preserve the intellectual integrity of the experimental research process, the following categories of documentation should be retained: the primary data; documentation of the experimental design and methodology; information on experimental conditions and external factors that might affect results; and the investigators' inferences from and interpretations of the experimental data.

At an academic health center and other institutions in the health fields, the volume of research data and its accompanying administrative documentation is so large that it is feasible to preserve only select portions of these materials. The designation of topical acquisition areas provides one viable approach for the selection of scientific data. However, even within these parameters, the quantity of data is daunting. For example, suppose an institution may choose to designate the Human Genome Initiative as one of its topical acquisition areas. At the Johns Hopkins Medical Institutions, more than one hundred laboratories are currently engaged in research projects involving this initiative. Therefore, archival planners must also be prepared to make choices within the context of the designated topical area when determining which laboratories and which aspects of a project to document.

A deciding factor should be the quality of the data: Were the data collected in a sound manner? Are they comprehensible to those who were not directly involved in the research? Are the materials and methods documented sufficiently? These elements are critical if the data are to be reinterpreted years after the original research or if scientists wish to replicate the original experiments. For use in secondary studies, the data should have the following characteristics: an acceptable level of validity that does not lead to biased inferences; consistency and reliability that are maintained across time periods and changes in location and transferal to other media; and inclusive and comprehensive coverage of the elements under study (Armenian 1987).

Although it is impractical to consider large-scale preservation of research data, the designation of topical acquisition areas provides criteria for selecting specific kinds of data and thus assures that some representative and useful examples of data will be preserved. By including scientific data in its acquisition plan, an archival program may enable a perspective on the research functions of its parent institution.

THE NEED FOR PROACTIVE PLANNING

Archives at institutions in the health fields will have to initiate a proactive approach to acquisition planning to keep pace with the rapidly changing documentation base of these fields. In their planning they must take into account not only the characteristics of the documentation (intellectual, physical, technical), but also the modes in which it is used for research, teaching, and health care delivery. They must consider how their acquisitions may be utilized in the ongoing functions of their institutions (e.g., teaching, research, health care delivery) in addition to their value for historical studies. The ephemeral media of documentation coupled with limitations in funding for storage and processing require a shift in acquisition priorities. The focus must move from the present concentration on selecting the original physical manifestation of documentation to strategies for selecting and preserving the original elements of content. Data and information may be transposed from one medium to another (e.g., paper-based records to computer disks, or computerized records to microfilm or paper printouts).

In acquisition planning the content of holdings as well as their format and media must be projected. Planners will also have to adjust appraisal processes to assess the content as well as the physical and technical status of documentation. The staff of an archives, with the participation of advisory committees, should work together to establish criteria and standards for the information and media to be preserved. Members of the archives staff should also confer, if possible, with the creators of the documentation to be acquired. Proactive planning requires that specifications be made for the format, media, and content of acquisitions.

DESIGNING AN ACQUISITIONS PLAN

Because the holdings of an archival repository ultimately define the nature of the program, the plan for acquisitions should embody a clear and far-reaching vision for the program.

The designation of criteria and standards for selection is therefore a major means for articulating the vision of the program. The scope of an acquisitions plan should be defined primarily by the mission of the archives, which in turn should be an organic outgrowth of the mission of the parent institution. Although each archival repository will have to specify the scope of its acquisitions and establish its own particular criteria and standards for selection, the plan that evolves should incorporate professional standards from the archival and health fields for evaluating the intellectual, physical, and technical quality of the documentation to be acquired. These standards should address the quality of the data and information in the documentation, the organizational state of the documentation, and the nature of its format and medium. To build holdings that are relevant, well focused, and coherent, the repository must apply these criteria and standards consistently.[4]

For an acquisitions plan to serve as a unifying force for the development of holdings, it must define a critical mass of documentation that is of high intellectual, physical, and technical quality and relevant to the aims of the program. The acquisitions plan provides an archival program with a centralized focus and a dynamic for its overall development. It also serves as a practical guide for accessioning and deaccessioning. Because of the tremendous quantity of documentation at institutions in the health fields, a well-defined plan is needed to set priorities and to chart the course of collecting. In repositories that encompass various curatorial distinctions (e.g., records management, archives, personal papers and manuscripts, and museum and object collections) the implementation of an overarching plan for acquisitions will help to focus and to integrate the collective development of holdings. Whereas the plan should be highly specific, it should not be rigid. To remain viable the plan must be flexible and responsive to basic changes that occur in the generation and use of documentation at the parent institution in particular and in the health fields in general. See Fig-

ure 7.1 for an overview on how to tailor an acquisition plan to accommodate the scope of individual archival programs.

The objective of a joint acquisition plan for repositories with related curatorial activities is not to preserve as many different kinds of documentation as possible but to provide a modus for acquiring a coherent body of documentation with significant relationships of intellectual content. The objective of such a plan is to be measured not by the volume of documentation collected but by the significance of the intellectual relationships and the caliber of the materials selected. Smaller quantities of related documentation with coherent intellectual content will have higher value for research and education than do larger quantities of unrelated documentation with uneven intellectual content. A cost savings is also indicated. Archivists and other curatorial professionals may share in joint strategies for collections management and user services as well as for acquisition planning. Separate management of large quantities of disparate documentation is labor-intensive and costly. Unifying the acquisition policies for related curatorial activities at institutions in the health fields will help to build a collective body of materials that are more relevant, well focused, and coherent. Thus, such joint acquisition activity may eventually lead to more returns in research and reference use of the overall holdings.

The design of an acquisitions plan should include provisions for the formats and media of the documentation to be selected, as well as the intellectual and physical controls necessary to preserve that documentation. The formats, media, and volume of the recorded documentation (i.e., inscriptive, visual, and aural records) and material evidence to be selected should be projected early in the development of the acquisitions plan because of the special provisions that must be made for the organi-

---

4. We concur with Barbara Craig (1992) regarding the significance and ongoing importance of studying the documentation itself.

zation, description, storage, maintenance, and use of these materials. See Figure 7.2 for a profile of the formats that may be found at archival repositories in the health fields.

An acquisitions plan should project both the physical scale and intellectual scope of the holdings. It must define the institutional perimeters for the selection of acquisitions and set the levels and rates of growth of acquisitions. The scale of projected holdings should be determined by the availability of resources for the processing, maintenance, and use of acquisitions. To acquire holdings without viable means for maintaining them and making them accessible for use is an example of poor acquisition planning. Holdings will remain inaccessible for reference and research if the means are not available to preserve and manage them.

IMPLEMENTING STRATEGIES FOR APPRAISAL

The appraisal of contemporary documentation in the health fields is a particularly labor-intensive process. Although appraisal requires a team of skilled and well-informed personnel, few archival programs can afford to establish staff positions for appraisal alone. As a result, appraisal activities need to be coordinated as a shared task that may involve different staff members at each stage of the evaluation process. Because of the large scale of contemporary acquisitions and the small professional staffs of archival programs, some aspects of appraisal may have to be delegated to temporary or part-time staff members with little training or experience.

To ensure that procedures for appraisal are conducted properly, clear guidelines should be communicated to all personnel who may be involved in the process. Whereas specially appointed senior staff should have the only authority to make final decisions on appraisal, much of the preliminary assessment may be made by junior staff. It is critical that they have standardized descriptive procedures to follow. Senior staff, however, should not base final appraisal judgments on descriptive infor-

Steps in the formation of an acquisition plan

Step 1

Articulate a philosophical precept to guide all acquisition activities. Base the conceptualization of this statement upon the following mandates:

- Mission of the institution that sponsors the repository
- Mission of the archival program
- Vision for the development of the archival program

Step 2

Define the intellectual scope of acquisition policies. Base intellectual criteria around the following focal points:

- Institutional sites *(e.g., health care delivery facilities, educational institutions, research institutes, etc.)*
- Corporate structure *(e.g., governing boards, central administration, individual departments, etc.)*
- Mandated functions *(e.g., health care delivery, teaching, research, etc.)*
- Topics of specialization that crosscut institutions, corporate divisions, and mandated functions *(e.g., AIDS, Human Genome Initiative, neurosciences, etc.)*

Step 3

Designate the types of materials to be acquired. Base these designations upon the following criteria:

- Compatibility with existing holdings
- Curatorial category *(e.g., contemporary records, historical records, personal papers, object collections)*
- Format *(e.g., recorded documentation, material evidence)*
- Medium *(e.g., paper-based, machine-dependent, etc.)*

Step 4

Specify standards for selecting acquisitions. Include standards for the following values:

- Intellectual significance
- Physical stability
- Technical functionality

Step 5

Project the ultimate scale and rates of acquisition. Base these projections upon the following capacities:

- Housing
- Availability of staff
- Technical resources

Fig. 7.1 **Tailoring an acquisition plan to accommodate the scope of individual archival programs.**

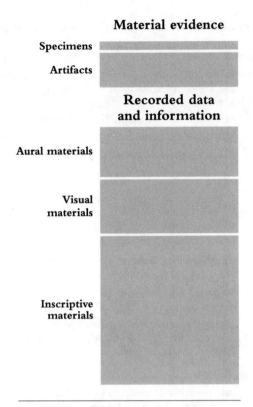

Fig. 7.2 **Representation of formats at archives in the health fields.** Inscriptive and visual materials usually exceed aural materials and material evidence in these repositories.

mation alone. After assessing that information, they should always physically examine the materials under consideration before making a final decision. In addition, they should always document their appraisal decisions before they proceed with accessioning.

DEFINING THE CRITERIA AND STANDARDS
FOR APPRAISAL

Whereas appraisal is both comprehensive and complex, it is essentially an iterative activity. A standardized assessment must repeatedly be made of all incoming materials. The assessment entails numerous parallel processes of evaluation. The materials must be assessed according to the criteria set forth in the acquisitions plan as well as according to standards of

intellectual, physical, and technical quality and terms of ownership and legal status.

Because appraisal is so labor-intensive, efforts should be made to streamline the process as much as possible. Standardizing the descriptive terminology to be used in the preparation of appraisal reports and the format and style for recording the appraisal information, as well as regulating the steps in various evaluative procedures, may make the process more reliable and at the same time accelerate decision-making activities. Parallel assessments should be made according to checklists for topical criteria and standards for value (intellectual, physical, technical). Cost/benefit analyses should also be made to determine whether the intrinsic value of the materials under consideration would offset the costs that would be incurred in their preservation and management. By specifying acquisition criteria and standards of quality and by regulating terminology and formats for recording descriptive information, the appraisal process may be facilitated and made more reliable. By breaking these procedures into a series of well-defined steps, the appraisal process may be computer assisted. As in the case of other archival computer applications, the effort to standardize and regulate appraisal procedures for the purpose of computerization will ultimately make the process more efficient and also more reliable. Through a uniform approach, the appraisal process may be focused and streamlined. Indeed, if standardized controls are imposed on the preparation of the assessment information, appraisal decisions may be better informed and more easily made.

Because of the complexities of documentation in the health fields, the appraisal process cannot be overly simplified. However, a standardized checklist of criteria and standards will help to focus the initial observation and assessment of materials. The responsibility for making final appraisal decisions still rests with the archivist. Because this is a decision that demands professional judgment, it may not be abdicated to a formula or to a machine. Archivists must ultimately assume respon-

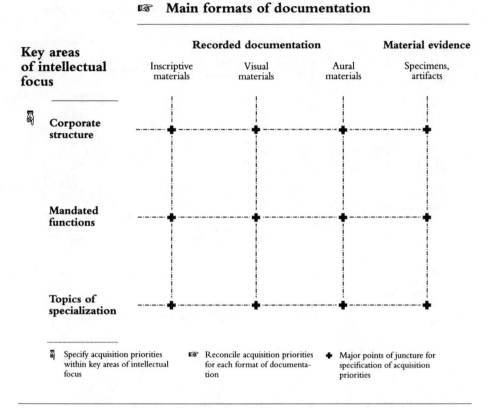

☞ **Main formats of documentation**

Fig. 7.3 **Project the intellectual range of documentation to be acquired within the various formats.** This matrix may also be used to assess the range of formats in extant holdings.

sibility for the development of a repository's holdings through the activities of appraisal. Systematizing appraisal into a procedurally fair process will help to ease the responsibilities of decision making.

The main advantage of systematizing the process of appraisal is that it yields a body of basic information about the intellectual, legal, physical, and technical status of the documentation. Such a body of information is useful in guiding decisions regarding both the selection and the processing of documentation because it yields insights into the intrinsic value of the documentation. Appraisal entails an obligation to identify the salient characteristics of documentation.

A reliable and effective appraisal process also paves the way to better procedures for accessioning, processing, and use. In particular, the assessment narrative may serve as the

Composite of the media in an archival repository

Material evidence

Artifacts
(Multimedia materials, e.g., painting, sculpture, equipment, textiles, etc.)

Specimens
(Chemical and biological materials)

Recorded documentation

Machine-dependent
(Computer disks and tapes, motion pictures, microfilm, audio disks and tapes, etc.)

Paper-based
(Inscriptive records, prints, drawings, still photographs, etc.)

Fig. 7.4 **Profile existing or projected media in holdings.** This type of outline will help to determine the scope of preservation and access needs.

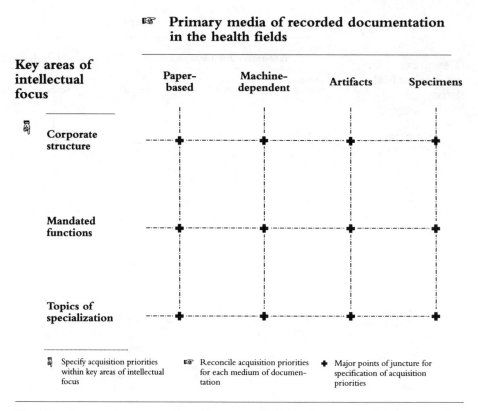

Fig. 7.5   **Project the range of media to be acquired.** This matrix may also be used to assess the range of media in extant holdings.

descriptive entry for accessioning or deaccessioning records. Developing and maintaining a complete and reliable body of information about the intellectual, legal, physical, and technical status of individual acquisitions provides a means for achieving better basic knowledge of the overall holdings. This process also affords a useful source of preliminary information about recently acquired holdings.

CONCLUSION

The development of a well-focused plan for acquisitions and the implementation of a systematized process for appraisal are vital to the formation of a body of useful and long-lasting holdings. Whereas the foundation for appraisal begins on a broad base at the institutional level with documentation planning, the implementation of the appraisal process occurs primarily at the repository level. Standardized

and systematized appraisal procedures should be designed to yield detailed and accurate information about the nature of accessions. When consistently applied, this appraisal process will facilitate the repository's processing activities and provide a preliminary resource for reference and research queries. A fundamental goal of the appraisal process is to provide reliable information about new acquisitions to the repository staff, the institution, and the appropriate scholarly communities. Appraisal in the health fields entails that documentation be classified and described according to principles of the discipline that it may represent.

The development of archival holdings at institutions in the health fields entails balancing the professional, ethical, and legal responsibilities of the parent institution with the overarching need to select a body of documentation that is intellectually relevant, well focused, and coherent. In addition, the media of this body of holdings must be physically stable and durable. The goal is to select holdings that will be useful to the administrative activities and mandated functions of the parent institution in particular and the health fields in general.

BIBLIOGRAPHY

ABRAHAM, T. 1991. Collection policy or documentation strategy: Theory and practice. *American Archivist* 54:44–52.

ARMENIAN, H.K. 1987. Consultant's report to the Johns Hopkins Medical Institutions Records Project.

BOLES, F. 1987. Mix two parts interest to one part information and appraise until done: Understanding contemporary record selection processes. *American Archivist* 50:356–68.

BOLES, F., AND J.M. YOUNG. 1985. Exploring the black box: The appraisal of university administrative records. *American Archivist* 48:121–40.

BOLES, F., WITH J.M. YOUNG. 1991. *Archival Appraisal*. New York: Neal-Schuman.

BRICHFORD, M. 1977. *Archives and Manuscripts: Appraisal and Accessioning*. Chicago: Society of American Archivists.

COOK, T. 1992. Documentation strategy. *Archivaria* 34:181–91.

CRAIG, B.L. 1992. The acts of the appraisers: The context, the plan, and the record. *Archivaria* 34:175–80.

DANIELS, M.F. 1988. Records appraisal and disposition. In *Managing Archives and Archival Institutions,* ed. J. G. Bradsher, pp. 53–66. Chicago: University of Chicago Press.

DOLLAR, C.M. 1984. Appraising machine-readable records. In *A Modern Archives Reader: Basic Readings on Archival Theory and Practice,* ed. M. F. Daniels and T. Walch, pp. 71–79. Washington, D.C.: National Archives Trust Fund Board.

ELLIOTT, C.A., ED. 1983. *Understanding Progress as Process: Documentation of the History of Post-War Science and Technology in the United States.* Final report of the Joint Committee on Archives of Science and Technology. Chicago: Society of American Archivists.

ENDELMAN, J.E. 1987. Looking backward to plan for the future: Collection analysis in manuscript repositories. *American Archivist* 50:340–55.

FISHBEIN, M.H. 1987. Reflections on appraising statistical records. *American Archivist* 50:227–34.

HAAS, J.K., H.W. SAMUELS, AND B.T. SIMMONS. 1985. *Appraising the Records of Modern Science and Technology: A Guide.* Cambridge: MIT.

HAAS, J.K., H.W. SAMUELS, AND B.T. SIMMONS. 1986. The MIT appraisal project and its broader implications. *American Archivist* 49:310–14.

HACKMAN, L.J., AND J. WARNOW-BLEWETT. 1987. The documentation strategy process: A model and a case study. *American Archivist* 50:12–47.

HAM, F.G. 1984. The archival edge. In *A Modern Archives Reader: Basic Readings on Archival Theory and Practice,* ed. M. F. Daniels and T. Walch, pp. 326–35. Washington, D.C.: National Archives Trust Fund Board.

———. 1993. *Selecting and Appraising Archives and Manuscripts.* Chicago: Society of American Archivists.

KEPLEY, D.R. 1984. Sampling in archives: A review. *American Archivist* 47:237–42.

KRIZACK, J.D., ED. 1994. *Documentation Planning for the U.S. Health Care System.* Baltimore: Johns Hopkins University Press.

PEACE, N.E., ED. 1984. *Archival Choices: Managing the Historical Record in an Age of Abundance.* Lexington, Mass.: D. C. Heath and Co.

PHILLIPS, F. 1984. Developing collecting policies for manuscript collections. *American Archivist* 47:30–42.

RAPPORT, L. 1984. No grandfather clause: Reappraising accessioned records. In *A Modern Archives Reader: Basic Readings on Archival Theory and Practice,* ed. M. F. Daniels and T. Walch, pp. 80–100. Washington, D.C.: National Archives Trust Fund Board.

REED-SCOTT, J. 1984. Collection management strategies for archivists. *American Archivist* 47:23–29.

SAMUELS, H.W. 1986. Who controls the past? *American Archivist* 49:109–24.

———. 1991. Improving our disposition: Documentation strategy. *Archivaria* 33:125–40.

———. 1992. *Varsity Letters: Documenting Modern Colleges and Universities.* Metuchen, N.J.: Scarecrow Press.

SCHELLENBERG, T.R. 1984. The appraisal of modern public records. In *A Modern Archives Reader: Basic Readings on Archival Theory and Practice,* ed. M. F. Daniels and T. Walch, pp. 57–70. Washington, D.C.: National Archives Trust Fund Board.

SINK, R. 1990. Appraisal: The process of choice. *American Archivist* 53:452–58.

YOUNG, J.M., COMP. 1985. Annotated bibliography on appraisal. *American Archivist* 48:190–216.

8

Promoting and Facilitating Wider Use of Holdings

Deborah McClellan and Nancy McCall, with Anne Slakey

A MAJOR GOAL of this book is to promote greater awareness and use of archival resources in the health fields. Whereas earlier chapters have focused on the intellectual significance of archival materials for research and education, the present chapter concentrates on ways repositories may facilitate access to and use of their holdings. If repositories in the health fields are to build holdings that include patient information and other kinds of sensitive information, they will have to protect privacy, proprietary, and other legal rights of individuals and corporate bodies; at the same time they will be required to facilitate access to the intellectual content of the materials. Repositories with holdings from the health fields must, therefore, be prepared to develop responsible and effective policies for access and use. In turn, a number of procedures for reference, research, and outreach will have to be adjusted to reflect the objectives for access and use.[1]

The user service activities of archival repositories—reference, research assistance, and outreach—constitute the primary pathways to use of the holdings. Therefore, the policies and procedures that relate to these activities must be conceptualized to enhance means of access. At archival repositories, the scope of user service activities is determined mainly by the nature of the holdings, by the corresponding legal and ethical requirements that govern their access and use, and by the kinds of users and the ways in which they employ the holdings for reference and research.

Because archival holdings are mostly unbound, unpublished, and irreplaceable, a closed-stack system of access is a managerial necessity. As a result of this controlled, closed-stack access, user service activities in archival programs are particularly labor-intensive. In effect, the user services staff of an archives functions as a human bridge between the repository's patrons and its holdings. The bridging provided by the staff is both intellectual and physical: patrons interact with the user services staff to identify and select pertinent documents from indexes and inventories; and the staff members then locate and retrieve the documents, oversee their use, and subsequently ensure their safe return to the stacks.

BRINGING USERS CLOSER TO THE CONTENT OF DOCUMENTATION

Although archives and libraries may employ different types of procedures for reference, research assistance, and outreach, these procedures usually emanate from a shared philosophy of service. Archives and libraries devoted to the same special disciplines face a common set of objectives for user services. Research practices in these disciplines often place similar demands upon the user service activities of archives and libraries. Because of the related demands for reference, research assistance, and outreach that must be met by libraries and archives in the health fields, these repositories should work closely together in the development of their respective policies for user services.

The higher expectations for services are providing an impetus for change in the user service activities of archives in the health fields. As libraries in the health fields endeavor to bring their patrons closer to the content of publications, the demand grows for archival programs to bring their users closer to the content of archival holdings. Archives in the health fields, therefore, will have to reconceptualize their overall approach to user services. To facilitate modes of research, libraries in the health fields provide access to a wide array of current medical knowledge that has been abstracted from recently published literature. The user-friendly systems for reference, research assistance, and outreach that are employed by libraries in the health fields should serve as models for archives in the same fields.

However, as the holdings of libraries shift from books and journals to include videos, databases, etc., library models for user ser-

---

1. One of the major impediments to the preservation and use of research resources in the health fields has been the reluctance of archival and manuscript repositories to deal with the issues of confidentiality that affect access to these materials. Many repositories have refused to collect documentation that includes patient and human-subject materials. As a result, a key segment of documentation in the health fields is being lost and overlooked.

vices must address new issues pertaining to copyright and ownership of intellectual information. Libraries as well as archives now face many different regulations for access and use. Because libraries in the health fields must focus greater attention on the element of content, they are now facing new kinds of regulations that pertain to the right to reproduce intellectual information. Thus, in conjunction with their patrons' demands for more proficient means of access and retrieval, the user services staffs of archives and libraries in the health fields are having to face greater and more complex responsibilities regarding rights of access and use. As methodologies of research and clinical practice in the health fields demand that archives as well as libraries bring users closer to the data and informational elements of content, both types of repository have to face a daunting array of legal and regulatory requirements regarding access and use.

In designing a model for user services, archival repositories in the health fields must devote special attention to policies for access and use. Policy makers will have to weigh the necessity of restrictive controls for access against archival programs' obligations to facilitate the activities of reference, research, and outreach.

This chapter presents a model for use of archival holdings from the health fields. The objective of the model is to remove unnecessary impediments to the use of documentation and at the same time to implement better controls for the protection of proprietary and private information. The intention is to introduce procedures that will facilitate access to and use of scientific, clinical, and social information in documentation and at the same time prevent unwarranted disclosure of personal identities and proprietary information. This approach fosters open intellectual inquiry within the bounds of legal and ethical requirements.

DEVELOPING A MODEL OF REFERENCE FOR ARCHIVES IN THE HEALTH FIELDS

Archival reference practices have traditionally placed the burden of obtaining data and information upon the requester. Thus, the function of the reference staff has been to provide documents from which a selection of pertinent data and information may be obtained. In this process, the requester is expected to identify and abstract the data and information that are needed. The conventional role of the reference staff is to serve as guides to documentation and not as abstractors and disseminators of content. This limitation of the staff's role places the responsibility for interpretation upon the user, not upon the reference staff. This practice has evolved from the archival tenet that documents should be allowed to speak directly to users without the interpretation of an intermediary.

With the rapid expansion of computer and reprographic technologies and means of telecommunications, various new forms of business and professional correspondence have emerged. As a result, the user services staffs of archival repositories have had to assume more of an interpretive role in the selection, reproduction, and transmission of documentation. Because of the increased availability and use of these new technologies and means of communication, archival reference policy, which was previously directed almost exclusively toward on-site users, has now been forced to adapt its procedures to accommodate the remote user. In response to requests from off-site users that are transmitted by a variety of means—including conventional mail, telephone, electronic mail, and telefacsimile—reference staffs now must assume the responsibility not only for selecting relevant documentation but also for choosing the most appropriate means of reproduction and transmission of this documentation.

Additional factors, including the presence of a broader range of formats and media in archival holdings, and changing expectations of the user population, are prompting archives in the health fields to provide an expanded set of user services. Throughout the course of their daily work, personnel in the health fields have become accustomed to obtaining rapid and easy access not only to documentation but also to relevant abstracts of its content. Many of the activities of research, teaching, and health care delivery are now supported by sophisticated data and information systems. Because of the prevalence of highly effective automated data and information systems in hospitals, libraries, and laboratories, the personnel from these institutions who patronize archival repositories expect equivalent access and retrieval services.

As archival programs in the health fields begin to adapt archival reference practices to meet the current needs of users, they may draw upon models for user services that are now employed at libraries in the health sciences and related fields. Of particular relevance to archival programs is the mode in which these models for user services operate. They essentially function as brokerages for data and information. Their activities are geared to provide selections of data and information directly to users rather than merely to locate the documentation in which the data and information may be found. However, the user services of these libraries are supported by elaborate infrastructures of computer-based systems that permit data and information to be rapidly retrieved and transmitted to users.

Although archival programs cannot expect to develop in a few simple steps the level of computerized services that currently exists in health science libraries, they may at least begin by borrowing from the philosophic and the organizational concepts for these computerized services. Archives and libraries in the health fields share a common mission to bring users closer to the elements of content. To use published and unpublished documentation more effectively in research and teaching, the data and information elements of the content must be made more easily accessible.

As is discussed in chapters 5 and 9, archival

programs have an enormous task ahead as they develop computerized systems. However, the challenge of computerizing archival reference systems is particularly daunting. As a first step, archival programs may begin with a number of manual procedures to facilitate access to the content of documentation. By first revising manual systems of access and retrieval, they may provide more proficient services and at the same time begin groundwork for the eventual computerization of these systems.

Some preliminary steps may be undertaken to prepare finding aids for conversion to computerized systems of access and retrieval. The format for each type of finding guide should be standardized, and common descriptive practices should be employed. The features of the library model for reference that are, perhaps, most applicable and most useful to archival reference in the health fields are the descriptive rules, procedures, and vocabulary that are employed. Use of the Medical Subject Headings (MeSH) in practices of archival description in both manual and computerized systems leads to greater precision and standardization of terminology. (See part III for a more extensive discussion of the role of description.)

In the effort to make clinical and scientific documentation more accessible for research, archival programs must follow the precedents of the library-based system and discipline-specific procedures for managing data and information. By having to focus on the data and information elements of documentation, both archives and libraries in the health fields are now compelled to manage their holdings at the molecular level of content.

CONSIDERING THE ROLE OF REFERENCE IN PROGRAM DESIGN

The user services division of an archival program should interact on a regular basis with the other functional divisions of the program —collections development and collections management. The quality and effectiveness of the overall archival program may be greatly enhanced by linking user services more closely to these other program divisions. The bridging that this division extends to users also serves as a means of obtaining feedback about the program. The direct interaction that occurs between patrons and the user services staff provides an opportunity for the staff to assess patrons' needs and to observe how the holdings are being employed for reference and research. By compiling and analyzing user statistics and assessing comments from users, the archives staff may learn firsthand about the strengths and flaws of their program.

As the main link between the patrons and the holdings, the members of the user services staff perform an important quality assurance function for the archival program. Since they are the first to observe the use of newly processed collections, they are often in a position to recognize problems involving the organization and description of these materials and to suggest improvements. In their direct interaction with users, members of the user services division staff serve as major emissaries of the archival program. In this capacity they convey to the users not only data and information from the holdings but also the ethos of the program.

One of the key objectives of the model for reference is to make archival holdings in the health fields more accessible for research. A particular goal is to open clinical and scientific holdings for aggregate study while making responsible provisions for protecting the rights of individuals and corporate bodies and preventing disclosure of private and proprietary information.[2] Considerations for the protection of rights and the promotion of research should be reconciled in both the policies and procedures for an archival program. The process will entail an overhaul of each functional division—collections development,

collections management, and user services. Whereas the overall effort to develop more proficient and responsible means of access is extremely labor-intensive to implement, the system is efficient and manageable when once in place.

PLANNING FOR USER SERVICES

Whether the user services policies of an existing archival program are being revised or a new program is being implemented, the first planning step should be a rigorous assessment of both the repository's holdings and its users. The status of the holdings should be considered, as well as projections for acquisition. The composition of the user population—both current and potential—should be evaluated. Areas of research and types of methodologies to be employed should also be reviewed. Once this assessment has been made, more relevant policies and more effective procedures for access and use may be developed. The practices and expectations of the users should help determine the types and levels of services to be provided. See Figure 8.1 for an approach to follow in planning for user services.

Assess the intellectual scope of the repository's holdings.

Ascertain the various types of research that may be conducted with these holdings (historical, sociological, epidemiological, biostatistical, etc.).

Develop policies that are appropriate for the particular type of research to be conducted.

Introduce procedures that will enable smooth and effective access to holdings.

Target a relevant audience of potential users and promote the specific research opportunities that exist.

Fig. 8.1 **An approach for promoting and facilitating wider use of archival holdings.** For archival programs to assume a more dynamic role in the advancement of knowledge, efforts must be made to explore the types of research opportunities that exist within repositories and to improve means of access to critical research materials.

2. The practice of opening patient information and human-subject information for forms of aggregate research is common in the health fields. Well-developed models of access exist for these forms of studies. The models for archival access that are presented in this chapter are based upon established procedures for access in the health fields.

An effort should be made to evaluate the intellectual scope of the holdings as well as the range of their formats and media. To ensure appropriate controls over access and use, policies and procedures regarding user services must make provision for the range of content and also the representation of formats and media. A preliminary gauge of the intellectual scope of holdings may be made through an assessment of the types of documentation that are included. Archival repositories at institutions in the health fields usually include in their holdings documentation that reflects the mandated functions of their institutions. Since the most common functions are research, teaching, and health care delivery, the documentation from these institutions is largely scientific, educational, and clinical in content. The documentation varies greatly in terms of format and medium. Included are examples of recorded documentation (inscriptive, visual, and aural) as well as samples of material evidence. The media range from conventional paper-based documentation to microfilm, floppy disks, and other forms of machine-readable materials.

Together, the content, format, and medium of documentation determine the users' primary mode of access to that documentation. Because access to and use of clinical, scientific, and educational documentation are subject to many specialized requirements, considerable planning must go into the development of appropriate policies and procedures for user services. Whereas the format of documentation largely determines the means of intellectual access, the medium primarily controls the means of physical access. For instance, if an archives has extensive holdings in microfilm and in computer media, special technical accommodations will have to be made to facilitate access to these media: microfilm readers and computer terminals will be necessary equipment for the repository's reading room.

Determining how and by whom documentation will be used is the next phase of assessment. Because a major objective of user services activities is to encourage research use of repositories' holdings, efforts must be made not only to identify and publicize resources for research but also to facilitate research through appropriate policies and procedures. Whether existing policies and procedures are being revised or new ones are being developed, the intention should be to focus and streamline processes of access. Regulations for access should reflect the basic principles and purposes that must be served. They should meet program objectives as well as legal, ethical, and regulatory requirements. Because user services activities entail documentation of procedures, planners should try to avoid redundant record-keeping practices. Policies and procedures should be reasonable, articulate, and easy to follow.

UNDERSTANDING THE CONDITIONS THAT REGULATE ACCESS

Most of the mandated functions of institutions in the health fields generate documentation that may require protection in the form of restricted access. Such controls are necessary to ensure the preservation of confidentiality and privacy, as well as compliance with specific restrictions that have been imposed by terms of ownership, professional codes of ethics, and federal, state, local, and institutional regulations concerning access and privacy. Many types of clinical, scientific, and educational documentation include information that deserves these guarantees: for example, medical records and photographs of patients, promotion and tenure records of faculty members, academic records of students and trainees, legal records, research records with human-subject information, and various forms of proprietary information such as protocols for patent applications and technical licensing. See Figure 8.2 for an overview of the conditions that regulate access to archival holdings.

Privacy

The preservation of an individual's privacy is perhaps the most common reason for restricting access to archival materials. The term *privacy* means, in essence, the right of an individual to be left alone. It encompasses the right to solitude or seclusion; freedom from intrusion into, or public disclosure of, one's personal affairs; freedom from publicity that places one in a false light; and protection from the appropriation of one's name or likeness for another's advantage (Peterson and Peterson 1985).

Most of the restrictions proposed by donors of personal papers fall within the scope of privacy considerations. These stipulations generally are intended to prevent the embarrassing disclosure of private facts concerning the donor or other individuals whose names or likenesses appear in the donated materials. Members of archival staffs need to be sensitive to these concerns and to accommodate donors' wishes whenever these appear to be reasonable and consonant with good archival practice. An archives that accepts donations may also find that its commitment to respecting privacy will sometimes require it to impose additional restrictions that its donors did not stipulate. In appraising personal paper collections, staff members need to be keenly observant and on the alert for sensitive materials, and prepared to discuss the implications of these sensitivities with the prospective donors.

In instances when donors do not apply restrictions to collections of personal papers that contain patient records, for example, the repository that accepts the collection must assume responsibility for protecting the privacy of the patients and assign the appropriate restrictions where necessary. If the archives staff is aware of the presence of patient records or other similarly sensitive documents, such as human-subject files from research projects, in collections that are being donated, they must alert the donors of the need to restrict access to these materials. Because the privacy of patient and human-subject information is widely

Rights to privacy—Personal information in documentation that society commonly deems to be private (e.g., in patient records, research records involving human subjects, student records, personnel records, etc.) is to be guaranteed regular and ongoing protection. This information should be routinely restricted and access granted only when ethical conditions permit.

Proprietary rights—The confidentiality of proprietary information such as trade and business secrets, research protocols, and applications for patents and technical licenses is usually time dependent. Access is to be limited for the time specified in contractual agreements.

Rights of donors—Agreements regarding access and use that repositories negotiate with donors are to be honored in accordance with the stipulations that both parties have reached.

Corporate mandates—The mission and governance policies of the institution in which an archival program is based are to be honored in the administration of regulations on access.

Regulatory and legal codes—Regulations and laws that govern access and use of archival materials are to be obeyed. Relevant codes include those that apply to medical records, student records, copyright, etc.

Professional codes of conduct—The codes of the professions represented in the holdings of the repository are to be respected. Their positions on protection of privacy and freedom of inquiry should be honored whenever they are applicable.

Respect for open intellectual inquiry—In regard for with the ethos of research, open intellectual inquiry is to be promoted whenever ethical, legal, and regulatory conditions permit.

Respect for safety and health—Archival staff and users are to be guaranteed protection, both from substances in the holdings and from conditions in the repository environment that may be hazardous.

Respect for preservation and maintenance of archival materials—Archival holdings are to be guaranteed protection from physical damage, loss, and disruption of order.

Fig. 8.2 **The ethical foundation of archival policies and procedures for access.** Policies and procedures must embody ethical consideration for the rights of corporate bodies and individuals, including the subjects of research, archival users, and staff.

guaranteed by laws, institutional regulations, and the ethics of the health professions, access to these types of documentation must be controlled by the repositories that house them and administer their use. Repositories at institutions in the health fields are usually bound to uphold their institutional policies regarding access to patient and human-subject information and must therefore regulate access in compliance with these policies.[3]

If a donor does not agree to the terms of the restrictions to be imposed by the repository, the archives staff should, of course, first try to arbitrate the dispute and reach a decision that will be satisfactory to both parties. In some cases the donor may choose to remove the sensitive materials from the collection under consideration. However, most donors of collections that contain patient and human-subject information are aware of the privacy rights that are involved and want to act in good faith to protect this information.[4]

Sometimes neither the donor nor the archives staff may be aware of the presence of sensitive materials until the collection is actually being processed. When these materials come to light during processing, the archives staff should contact the donor or the donor's heirs and negotiate terms of access. Such a situation only underscores the need for thorough appraisal of collections before they are accepted by repositories.

Issues of privacy often involve more than a single individual, because certain revelatory information may also be a source of embarrassment or pain to an individual's immediate family and their descendants. Even though the right to privacy ceases at death, an archives needs to be cautious about lifting access restrictions on personal paper collections upon the death of a donor. It is often necessary to prevent disclosure of private information long after the donor has died, in order to protect the privacy of other living individuals who may be adversely affected.

The need to protect the privacy of patient and human-subject information, of course, applies not only to donated materials but also to all archival holdings, however they are acquired. The principles of restricted access for patient and human-subject records that relate to donated papers are equally relevant to all materials acquired by the archives of an academic health center that may contain this type of information—photographs, administrative records, faculty and staff correspondence files, and, of course, case files and laboratory records. The content of the materials must be carefully evaluated to preserve the privacy of the individuals mentioned therein. Although

3. Donations of personal papers to repositories at institutions in the health fields and donations of personal papers to large autonomous repositories such as the National Archives or the Library of Congress involve different sets of issues. These larger autonomous repositories generally have the administrative latitude to be able to accommodate a donor's personal wishes on access. The donor conditions surrounding the Thurgood Marshall papers and the Sigmund Freud papers at the Library of Congress are a case in point. However, the smaller repositories that are part of large, complex institutions such as hospitals or medical schools are obligated first to comply with institutional policy on access. When the donor's wishes conflict with institutional policy and the differences cannot be resolved, the repository is not administratively in a position to accept the collection.

4. Another factor in the need for repository-imposed restrictions involves the nature of the information being protected. Whereas the Librarian of Congress recently argued against curator-imposed restrictions in the instance of the Thurgood Marshall papers, this case differs in significant respects from situations involving the personal papers of physicians and clinical investigators. The content of the Thurgood Marshall papers falls into a category of public interest information. In our democratic society a long precedent exists for the disclosure of public interest information. It may be argued that it would serve the public's interest to know how Supreme Court decisions were debated in the inner offices of the justices as well as in the public arena of the courtroom.

However, patient and human-subject records fall into a category of private information. In our society a precedent also exists for the protection of private information. It may be argued that allowing open access to records that deal with human subjects in research and with patients of health practitioners would infringe upon the right to privacy of those individuals and their families. In legal and ethical codes, a long tradition exists for the protection of patient and human-subject information. To allow open access to patient and human-subject records would violate laws as well as the ethics of the health professions.

Archivists who are in charge of holdings that contain patient and human-subject records face a daunting situation. On the one hand, legal and ethical codes require that they protect the privacy of the individuals who are represented in these records. On the other hand, strong precedents exist in the health fields for research involving the collection of clinical data and information. Archivists in the health fields are, therefore, in a position to protect the disclosure of private information while at the same time promoting open inquiry for intellectual studies.

specific regulations exist only for certain types of documents and information (for example, students' academic records), all materials nevertheless deserve equal protection from unwarranted invasion of privacy. Simple adherence to a donor's well-intended stipulations or to regulatory requirements does not always guarantee adequate protection of privacy. Instead, the fulfillment of legal requirements must often be accompanied by consideration of ethical codes that protect the privacy of individuals. Private institutions have more flexibility to negotiate donor-based restrictions than do public institutions.

Legal and Institutional Restrictions

Although federal, state, and local regulations regarding privacy and access to information impinge most directly on access policies at public institutions, private institutions are also bound by governmental regulations concerning access to institutional records. In addition, both public and private institutions must impose restrictions on access to various forms of institutional documentation in order to protect the privacy rights of individuals and the intellectual property of the institution. Measures must be taken to protect the privacy of faculty, staff, students, patients, and human subjects; as well as proprietary business information, trade secrets, and protocols for patents and technical licensing. Most institutions in the health fields impose special regulations for the protection of privacy in the following types of documentation: student records, patient records, research records, personnel records, and house staff records. Many of these institutions also regulate access to the following other types of documentation for the purpose of protecting intellectual property and proprietary business information: grant and contractual proposals, protocols for patent and technical licencing applications, and sensitive current fiscal records.

Essentially, most of these restrictions are lessened over the passage of time. According to case law in the United States, an individual's right to privacy ceases at death. However, in terms of both philosophy and practice, many institutions have taken steps to protect the privacy of individuals for periods of time after their deaths. They have imposed these measures largely out of consideration for the privacy of the individuals' families and the privacy of other parties that are named in the records. For instance, some educational institutions have policies for protecting the privacy of student records for a certain number of years after the death of the student. Likewise, health care delivery facilities usually also regulate access to patient records after the death of patients. At most institutions in the health fields many regulations regarding access to intellectual property and proprietary business information may be lifted after a certain passage of time because much of this information becomes less sensitive over time. In fact, after patents, technical licenses, and copyrights have been issued there is a greater need to open their files for purposes of accountability, verification, and ongoing research.

The laws and regulations regarding access to institutional records at institutions in the health fields centers primarily around the following three areas of legal activity:

- The Family Education Rights and Privacy Act
- Medical records laws
- Institutional ownership of intellectual property

The discussion that follows provides a summary of the major issues in these three areas.

The Family Education Rights and Privacy Act   The Family Education Rights and Privacy Act of 1974 (commonly known as FERPA, or the Buckley Amendment) applies to any educational institution that receives funds under any federal program administered by the U.S. Department of Education; therefore, it affects all public schools and universities and nearly all privately supported universities and professional schools.

The purpose of this act is to define who may or may not gain access to students' academic records. While it guarantees students aged eighteen or over the right to review their own educational records, the statute also prevents the disclosure of personally identifiable information to outside parties (except a limited number of defined groups) without the students' express consent. Only directory information—for example, a student's address, telephone number, date and place of birth, field of study, participation in extracurricular activities, and the awards and degrees he or she has received—is considered unrestricted information that can be released to any individual without prior approval by the student.

The Buckley Amendment does, however, include several provisions that make it feasible for an archives staff to release additional academic information under certain circumstances. In particular, the statute permits the release of records to "organizations conducting studies for, or on behalf of, educational agencies or institutions for the purpose of developing, validating, or administering predictive tests, administering student aid programs, and improving instruction, if such studies are conducted in such a manner as will not permit the personal identification of students and their parents by persons other than representatives of such organizations" (FERPA sec. 1232).

This exception may be construed broadly to include all types of education-related research conducted using student records, provided that the identities of the students are not disclosed. Furthermore, under these provisions it is possible to allow access to academic records for purposees of research without the students' consent, provided that the researcher enters a legally binding agreement not to release any personally identifiable information. Also of interest to institutional archives is the fact that the statute sets no time limit on the duration of the restrictions concerning disclosure; in addition, it is not clear whether the amendment is retroactive. Fortunately, the early court cases that have tested the application of this statute have generally taken a relatively liberal, common-sense ap-

proach to the interpretation of the law (Peterson and Peterson 1985). Among the important implications of these test cases is the strong suggestion that the records of deceased individuals need not be restricted under this statute.

A violation of the Buckley Amendment may result in penalties that include the withdrawal of federal funding. Because institutions in the health fields (public and private) are heavily dependent on federal aid and need to protect their funding base, they have tightly regulated access to student records. Sometimes their regulations are even more stringent than those stated or implied by the statute itself. Given the probable existence of additional institutional constraints, and the ambiguities of the amendment, it is wise for an archives staff to obtain the advice of the parent institution's legal counsel before granting access to any academic records, except in the most straightforward cases.

Medical Records Laws In defining the legal terms of access to medical records, there is at the federal level no broad-sweeping statute equivalent to FERPA. However, at the state level there are many corollaries to FERPA that regulate access to medical records. Whereas these state laws are not uniform in terms of language and the specific issues that are addressed, they do emanate from a common concern to protect the privacy of patient information. S4-305 of the Health–General Article of the Annotated Code of Maryland, which addresses disclosure of medical records, is a direct corollary to FERPA. The areas covered by this particular law are similar to the areas that are usually covered in the various medical records laws in the individual states. While we urge archivists who are responsible for the management of patient records in their holdings to obtain copies of their own state laws governing medical records, we also recommend that they follow the regular discussion in the medical literature on the topics of confidentiality and the disclosure of patient information. These articles are usually good sources of information about court rulings in individual cases dealing with disclosure of patient information. When confronted with a particularly complex issue regarding access to patient records in their holdings, archivists may wish to do a search of the medical literature for articles that deal with disclosure issues that are similar to those that they are facing. Bibliographic data bases such as MEDLINE and HISTLINE are excellent resources for quick and comprehensive searches of current literature for pertinent articles about confidentiality and disclosure of patient information.[5]

Other Laws and Regulations Some other federal and state regulations that have direct implications for archives are those controlling the creation and disposition of official records related to federal or state-funded grants and contracts (e.g., the progress reports of clinical trials or basic research grants funded by U.S. agencies such as the National Institutes of Health). Because these records are subject to the federal Freedom of Information Act or to related state laws, they may generally be considered to be in the public domain. However, proprietary information (e.g., business-related information or technical information that is covered by patent laws) and personnel information (e.g., the salaries of hospital employees) within these records must be protected from unwarranted disclosure.

Institutional Ownership of Intellectual Property In recent years the role of institutions in the ownership of intellectual property has become a paramount legal concern in the health and scientific fields (Nelkin 1983). Because rights of access to and use of intellectual property are usually defined in terms of ownership, archivists must have a basic understanding of some of the current issues that affect the ownership of intellectual property at institutions in the health fields.

As more academic and research institutions in the health fields enter the medical marketplace, many new issues regarding the ownership of intellectual property have arisen

(Lucier and Matheson 1992). Interinstitutional collaboration in research also raises a host of new legal concerns about the ownership of intellectual property. Another major aspect of the intellectual property rights discussion involves the ownership of research data when principal investigators move from one institution to another (Horowitz with Moore 1990; Waldeman 1990).

Although there is ongoing debate in the scientific community over rights of intellectual property, consensus has been reached in several areas regarding the role of institutions and sponsored research. The institution that sponsors a research project is entitled to ownership of the data and information that were created or collected in the course of the project. Despite the source of funding, the institution that sponsors the research project controls the ownership of the data and information from the project. Thus, when a principal investigator moves to another institution the sponsoring institution may claim possession of the original research data but permit the investigator to take copies of it.

A principal investigator is entitled to the rights to traditional works of authorship, such as articles and books, that may result from the sponsored research. However, the patents to inventions and the technical licenses for products, such as computer software, that may result in the course of sponsored research are considered the property of the institution that sponsored the investigation.

In some instances, institutions in the health fields also engage in contractual work with industrial corporations. When negotiating contracts for these joint ventures, the ownership of trade secrets and business property is usually clearly specified. The parties involved may tag the components of intellectual infor-

---

5. Robert J. Levine of Yale University and Rene C. Fox of the University of Pennsylvania have written extensively on the ethics of research with patients and human subjects. Collectively their articles constitute a corpus of ethical thought for research in the health fields that involves patients and human subjects.

mation that are to be held confidential and specify conditions for these in the contract that is negotiated.

Donor Stipulations

Individuals who donate materials to archives rarely give them unconditionally; likewise, departments and offices transferring institutional records to a repository seldom do so without imposing conditions. Some donor-generated and institutionally generated restrictions are time-dependent: for example, the donor or an authorized institutional administrator may propose to restrict access to certain information for a specified period of time (e.g., until fifty years after the death of the donor or institutional personnel). In most instances, the conditions imposed usually stem from legitimate concerns about privacy. Some conditions may, however, emanate from personal biases of the donor. Therefore, the conditions proposed by donors must be carefully evaluated and negotiated to comply with legal and ethical codes.

Archives must also be prepared to reject restrictions that are clearly frivolous or are so complex to administer that they would make the donated materials virtually useless for scholarly research. Any restrictions that prohibit certain individuals or groups of individuals from gaining access to the donated materials would be in violation of the principle of equitable access. It is ultimately the responsibility of the archives to ensure that the restrictions that are imposed will be ethically and legally sound. The archives also bears an obligation to inform the donor about the conditions it intends to impose on access.

Because an archives is ethically bound to honor the donor-generated restrictions to which it has agreed, any and all proposed stipulations must be carefully considered before a private gift or institutional deposit is accepted. Furthermore, the negotiations concerning access restrictions should be carried out before legal ownership has passed to the archives. An archives is free to refuse to accept a prospec-

tive donor's gift if the proposed restrictions on access cannot be met, just as a donor is free to withdraw an offer of archival materials if he or she cannot accept the conditions for access that the archives has proposed.

The receipt of gifts and the negotiation of conditions must be well documented. To record the receipt of gifts and the accompanying conditions, some repositories rely upon formal deeds of gift, while others prefer to retain a body of correspondence that documents the details of the transactions. Standardized deed-of-gift forms tend to be limiting because they do not easily accommodate exceptions. Whereas the agreements to accept gifts usually involve special conditions, it is more effective to document transactions by compiling a file of pertinent correspondence. The deposit of institutional documents from official institutional divisions is usually recorded by formal, standardized transfer agreements.

Hazards to Users or to Archival Materials

In some instances, access to archival materials has to be restricted for physical rather than intellectual reasons. Because archival holdings are essentially irreplaceable, the risks posed by physical handling should also be addressed when specifying conditions for access. Restrictions may need to be imposed when certain materials are too fragile to withstand regular use. Out of concern for preservation, a repository may have to limit the handling of documents and artifacts that are in a poor state of conservation. Access may also have to be limited when items are too heavy or too bulky to be safely transported to areas where they can be examined by users.

Because archives bear a responsibility to protect users and staff, conditions on access should afford protection from exposure to hazards that may be in the holdings. For instance, mold- or insect-infested documents or materials with other forms of contamination will require special treatment in order to make them safe for reference and research use. When hazards cannot be eliminated from archival materials, the repository should provide appropriate means of protection to those who need to handle the materials. If hazards are suspected, the archives should obtain expert advice and take the recommended precautions to protect both staff and patrons.

Whenever selections of archival materials have to be withheld from direct examination because of their fragility or the hazards they pose, the archives should make every effort to provide researchers with pertinent descriptions of the materials. This information may include transcriptions, photographic reproductions, and cataloging data.

RECOGNIZING AND MANAGING INFORMATION THAT REQUIRES PROTECTION

In imposing restrictions on access, archival practice has focused on specific types of records that usually contain information that is commonly regarded as private (for example, student records or hospital charts) or proprietary (trade and business secrets). This approach is effective in that it identifies and isolates aggregate groups of records which by nature of definition contain certain types of information that are regarded as being private and proprietary. As discussed earlier, documents containing trade and business secrets become less sensitive over time. However, documentation with private information remains sensitive for a much longer period of time. Whereas mass restrictions for specific record types may guarantee protection for the privacy of individuals, they at the same time pose a monolithic impediment to research. Because records involving patients and human subjects contain information that may be needed for ongoing studies, it is important to consider ways that these records might be released for some purposes of research. The issue then becomes how to permit legitimate research while protecting the privacy of individuals. If personal identifiers are protected, then researchers may be given access to the intellectual content of records. The thrust of the decision then focuses on the merit of the proposed research. In establishing criteria and

standards for reviewing applications for access, the following issues should be addressed:

- Protection of personal identifiers
- Purpose of the research
- Quality of the research plan
- Credentials of those who are to conduct the research

Physical and Intellectual Controls for Sensitive Information

To ensure the identification and appropriate handling of sensitive documentation, measures must be taken as early as the appraisal stage to flag these materials. At the accessioning and processing stages additional steps should be taken to assess the content of this documentation. By the time this documentation reaches the jurisdiction of user services, it should be clearly identified and procedures for access should be specified.

The Role of Collections Development

The appropriate handling of sensitive documentation begins at the stage of appraisal. It is important for archival staff to consider how the sensitive materials will fit into the overall acquisition plan for their repository. They should then consider what special arrangements may be needed to ensure that access to the documents, their personal identifiers, and other sensitive information will be guaranteed protection.

Staff members need to examine any donations being offered to the archives for the presence of sensitive documentation. At the same time, the donor's proposed stipulations regarding restrictions on access should be considered. It is imperative that the final terms of all donor-imposed restrictions be established and clearly documented before any materials are formally accepted and accessioned. After the sensitive information is assessed, the staff should stipulate the specific precautions that need to be taken to protect that information.

Once all of these factors have been considered, the archives staff should weigh the burden of managing the relevant legal and ethical concerns against the intrinsic intellectual and cultural value of the materials (McCall 1992). Archives should not acquire materials that place an undue strain upon the staff and the resources of the repository, nor should they accept donations encumbered with restrictions that cannot reasonably be met. Rather, an archival program should accept materials only when its staff has the resources to administer and manage them appropriately.

The Role of Collections Management

Accessioning should follow after the appraisal decision has been reached. At this stage requirements should be specified for the physical and intellectual management of the materials. If materials contain sensitive information and thus need special controls, this fact should be noted here and at further stages of processing.

Appropriate processing of materials containing sensitive information is critical to the protection and preservation of confidentiality. Each archives needs to ensure that sensitive information is segregated physically and intellectually so that it may be properly managed by the user services staff. Provision must also be made for authorized users to study restricted materials under conditions that would prevent unauthorized access by other visitors to the archives.

At all stages of proccessing, sensitive materials should be clearly labeled as such, so they may easily be identified by any member of the staff. Chapter 4 of *Archives and Manuscripts: Law* (Peterson and Peterson 1985) provides an excellent set of guidelines for the physical and intellectual protection of sensitive materials.

Unprocessed materials may contain sensitive information that has not yet been identified and protected. It is, therefore, necessary to restrict access to unprocessed materials. In some instances, segments of unprocessed materials may be screened for sensitive information and processed on a provisional basis so that new accessions may be made more readily available for research.

A particularly important consideration with regard to access is the preparation of catalog records and finding aids. Disclosure of the presence of sensitive information must be made in generic, not specific, terms. For example, the entry in the finding aid may specify that a series is restricted because it contains patient records. However, the names of the patients or other personal identifiers should not be published in a finding guide.

Archives staff members must be scrupulous in ensuring that confidential information is not disclosed in catalog records, finding guides, and inventories. In the finding aids that are accessible to users, they should describe only the types of materials that are restricted (e.g., patient records, student records). They should, however, maintain inventories with individual file listings for internal staff use. An example of a finding guide entry may be as follows: "records of psychiatric patients, 1889–1941, 2 linear feet, arranged alphabetically and chronologically." Only staff members should have access to a separate list that includes the names of all the patients whose records are part of that restricted series. If a researcher who is interested in a particular individual asks the staff if that individual's records are included in the series, the staff bears an obligation to inform the researcher whether or not the records are there but must refrain from discussion of content. Archivists must protect sensitive information and at the same time not suppress knowledge of its existence.

It is, therefore, the responsibility of an archives staff to ensure that any finding aids for users clearly indicate (without divulging sensitive details) the existence of restricted categories of materials. For example, an entry in a published finding guide may read, "Series XVII. Confidential correspondence and medical records, 1922–1976. (Restricted.) Apply to user services staff for access."

Although the reference staff is most directly involved in overseeing users' dealings with restricted materials, the collections management staff has a major role to play in the processing of sensitive documentation. The administration of restricted holdings may be greatly facilitated if the policies for processing restricted materials are coordinated with policies for access. The collections management staff and the user services staff should, therefore, work together to develop joint policies for the processing and management of restricted holdings. Strategies for collections management must ensure that the appropriate physical and intellectual controls are applied in the organization and description of sensitive documentation.

The performance of the staff is of paramount importance in the administration of sensitive documentation. The staff must be knowledgeable about the intellectual, legal, regulatory, and ethical issues that are involved and be able to determine the types of restrictions that are needed. Only through their observation and judgment will sensitive materials be flagged and identified: their assessments and their judgments are critical factors in the execution of policies and procedures. Therefore, a major part of the planning for the administration of access entails the selection, training, and supervision of staff.

DEFINING ETHICAL OBLIGATIONS
REGARDING ACCESS

If archives at institutions in the health fields are committed to supporting the mandated functions of these institutions—health care delivery, teaching, and research—they have an obligation to promote the use of documentation from these functions in ongoing reference and research. Because this documentation invariably includes sensitive materials that require protection, the archives must develop policies and procedures that will protect privacy and at the same time promote research. Since each request for access to sensitive materials must be considered on an individual basis, a formal review process should be instituted for the purpose of evaluating individual requests. In establishing such a process, the archives needs to address the general legal, ethical, and intellectual dimensions of

access, as well as the specific rights of the individuals and corporate bodies that are involved.

According to the code of ethics of the Society of American Archivists (1992), archivists are obligated to "respect the privacy of individuals who created, or are the subjects of, documentary materials of long-term value, especially those who had no voice in the disposition of the materials. They neither reveal nor profit from information gained through work with restricted holdings." In addition, the obligation of archivists to promote access to holdings is also addressed in the SAA code of ethics: "Archivists answer courteously and with a spirit of helpfulness all reasonable inquiries about their holdings, and encourage use of them to the greatest extent compatible with institutional policies, preservation of holdings, legal considerations, individual rights, donor agreements, and judicious use of archival resources. They explain pertinent restrictions to potential users, and apply them equitably."

Three basic principles regarding access are contained within this statement: (1) The archives staff has a clear duty to respect the legal, ethical, contractual, and institutional constraints that limit or prohibit access to certain holdings. (2) For an archives to be of service to its parent institution, it must make its holdings as open and accessible as possible so that they will be used. (3) Any policies developed to encourage the use of archival holdings and provide for their protection must be applied uniformly and fairly.

Archivists in the health fields bear an obligation to promote the research use of scientific, clinical, and educational documentation whenever legal and ethical conditions permit. They must explore the intellectual resources of their holdings and define the research potentials that exist. Because the scientific and clinical data from many disciplines in the health fields may be recycled and utilized in ongoing research, archivists should facilitate the active use of scientific and clinical data in their holdings (Sieber 1991; Cordray, Pion, and Boruch 1990).

Archives at institutions in the health fields should always have policies of equal access: any individual has the right, and should be given the opportunity, to request access to unrestricted records and to apply for access to materials that are restricted. Information about available holdings should be freely obtainable by all users, and policies and procedures regarding access should be clearly set forth.

At the same time, an archives must respect the restrictions that limit access to specific holdings. To institute a procedurally fair process for reviewing applications for access to restricted materials, archives should adopt a peer review model to weigh the legitimacy of each request.

Fairness is at the heart of decisions about access. The peer review process must be discriminating but not discriminatory in reaching decisions regarding access to specific materials. Its decision-making process should not be influenced by irrelevant factors such as the race, gender, religion, or ideology of the person making an access request, and regulations concerning the use of protected materials must be applied equitably.

To prepare guidelines for access to the holdings of individual repositories, archivists must first articulate and then ascribe to a set of ethical principles that pertain to the access issues associated with their own specific holdings. They must base these principles upon the ethical code of the Society of American Archivists and also the ethical codes of other relevant professions. For instance, archivists who are responsible for the administration of documentation from institutions in the health fields should take into account the ethical codes of various health professions that are represented in their holdings. They bear an obligation to identify the specific ethical principles that should be incorporated in the administration of access to the particular documentation in their custody (MacNeil 1993,

197). In her recently published book *Without Consent: The Ethics of Disclosing Personal Information in Public Archives* (1993) Heather MacNeil also recommends following a set of ethical guidelines that Alice Robbin proposed for protecting personal privacy in data archives (Robbin 1978, 15–17). MacNeil notes that the standards proposed by Robbin may also be applied to other types of archives because they enshrine the commitment of archivists to fundamental principles regarding access to confidential information. Some of these principles are as follows:

- Address the social and professional codes and the moral standards of the communities that they serve.
- Assume responsibility for protecting the trust of individuals who have provided personal information with the understanding that their rights to privacy would be guaranteed.
- Provide competent administration and appropriate security of confidential information to prevent unwarranted disclosures.
- Define conditions for protecting confidential information.
- Make public announcements of the conditions for protecting confidential information (MacNeil 1993, 197).

In the health fields there exists a precedent for use of documentation with human-subject and patient data in research. The policies that have evolved in the health fields to protect disclosure of personal identifiers in scientific and clinical research may also serve as models for archival practice. Although the introduction of enciphering devices for computerized records promises to protect disclosure of personal identifiers in patient and human subject records, archivists will continue to deal with the protection of personal information in hard copy records.

ESTABLISHING GUIDELINES FOR ACCESS

To develop policies for access, archives at institutions in the health fields may benefit from the body of access-related policies that have evolved in areas of research, teaching, and health care delivery. These policies are designed to foster legitimate research and prevent the disclosure of personal information (Boruch et al. 1991). By borrowing from established policies in the field, archival programs may develop policies for access that combine the ethical standards of the archival and health professions.

Policies and Procedures

It is not feasible for an archives to depend upon a series of detailed anticipatory rules to meet any and all questions about access: the legal and institutional environment is in a constant state of change, and the scope of the access requests varies greatly. Because it is so difficult to anticipate future requests and needs for protection, it is important for archives in the health fields to avoid narrowly defined rules and regulations. The most useful approach is to develop policies and procedures that will provide a basis for decision making. The mission statement for the archival program should define the repository's philosophy regarding access. It should set forth the program's stand on reference and research by articulating the balance to be struck between open intellectual inquiry and the protection of personal and proprietary information. Also important is a set of ethical directives to guide policy formulation and the execution of procedures. See Figure 8.2 for a compendium of the ethical directives to be incorporated in policies and procedures for access.

The procedures for administration of access should be standardized and systematized to enable even and efficient handling of all requests. The procedures may be divided into a sequence of basic steps to be followed. See Figure 8.3 for an example of the procedures

Step 1

Registration of researcher—Archives are to be open and accessible to all individuals on an equal basis. A standardized policy and procedure for the registration of all researchers should be introduced. Registration information includes name, address, institutional affiliation, and purpose of research.

Step 2

Reference interview—The reference staff is to inquire about the registrant's research objectives and help to identify which materials in the repository's holdings will best serve those objectives.

Step 3

Application for access—Provisions are to be made for two different forms of application: a standardized policy and procedure for access to *unrestricted* materials, and a standardized policy and procedure for access to *restricted* materials. In both forms of application the intended use of information from the requested archival holdings is to be cited.

Step 4

Review of application—Two means of review are to be followed: one for review of applications for access to *unrestricted* materials and the other for review of applications for access to *restricted* materials. Staff members may be authorized to process requests for access to unrestricted materials, but an institutional committee of peers should be convened to review and make decisions about requests for access to restricted materials.

Step 5

Managing terms of access—Reference staff are to direct users to follow the repository's regular policies on the handling and use of archival materials, as well as any special stipulations that may have been made by the review committee, and should monitor the activities of the users.

Fig. 8.3 **Steps for administering access.** Archives staff are to follow an equitable and procedurally fair process in reviewing applications for access. They should maintain records of this process to demonstrate administrative accountability.

that an archival repository should adopt for the administration of access.

In specifying the terms of policies and procedures for their repository, archivists should address the following issues:

- Who is authorized to negotiate with prospective donors about imposing specific restrictions on the donated materials?
- At what stage will sensitive materials be identified and protected information be marked and physically segregated?
- How will sensitive materials be marked and segregated?
- What resources (e.g., a committee on access, legal experts) are available for consultation and decision making regarding access requests, and what procedures should be followed in acting on their recommendations?
- How will individual requests be documented?
- What information should be obtained about each requester's educational and professional background, research plan, and proposed use(s) for the requested materials? (See Table 8.1.)
- What review process(es) should be followed once a request has passed an initial screening? (Presentation to a review board or a committee on access? Consultation with a legal representative of the donor or other affected individuals?)
- What assurances will be required of those who are approved to use protected materials? (A nondisclosure agreement? A prereview of the material to be published?)

The Committee on Access

A particularly valuable resource for the administration of restricted access requests is a peer review committee. The structure and function of this committee may be modeled on the concept of the internal review board (IRB), a multidisciplinary group of experts at a medical institution that reviews proposed research projects involving human subjects. The overall function of an archival committee on access is analogous to that of the IRB: to review the proposed research and the credentials of individuals who wish to conduct research that has ethical and legal implications. In the case of archival research, those implications are the result of access to personal and proprietary information.

In appointing a committee on access, an archival program should strive for a multidisciplinary composition. Ideally the members of such a committee should be drawn from among the parent institution's clinicians, basic scientists, historians, and legal experts, as well as other archivists and curatorial experts; the group should always include one member of the archives staff, who presents to the committee the specific access request being considered. The variety of viewpoints represented by such a diverse group helps to balance discussion and decision making. Because each access request is different, an archives may wish to vary the exact composition of the committee to match the expertise of the members to the specific request being considered. See Figure 8.4 for an overview of the responsibilities of a committee on access. In the administration of access, the role of the archives staff is to serve as facilitators who set in motion a procedurally fair review process.

Legal Counsel and Other Experts

Archivists must be well informed about federal, state, and local statutes as well as institutional regulations that pertain to access. This endeavor is made more complex by the fact that statutes affecting access cover a wide spectrum, from freedom-of-information acts and sunshine laws to contractual and grant laws, property laws, and tax laws. Moreover, these laws and regulations are in a constant state of flux.

To keep abreast of changes in statutes and regulations, staff members should regularly consult their institution's legal counsel for guidance and support. Legal counsel should be consulted on policy formulation for the archives and issues pertaining to individual applications for access as they arise.

Topical experts should be consulted on issues pertaining to the intellectual content and physical condition of documentation under review for access. A network of topical experts is an invaluable resource for the review process.

IMPLEMENTING AND UPHOLDING GUIDELINES FOR ACCESS

The user services staff provides the critical link between a repository's holdings and the individuals who seek to use those holdings. If an archives is to encourage the use of its holdings and maintain high ethical standards, the user services staff must see that all users are given an equal opportunity to apply for access to both restricted and unrestricted information, and that all applications for access are handled on an equitable basis and according to established procedures.

When the user services staff receives applications for access to restricted archival holdings, they must begin a preliminary review process. Staff should start by discussing the request with the applicant. Some of the questions that may be appropriate to ask of a researcher are presented in table 8.1.

Formal applications for access to restricted materials may be divided into two categories on the basis of the type of study being proposed. One category is for aggregate studies that do not involve the disclosure of personal identities. The other involves the disclosure of personal information. Most requests in this category are for biographical studies.

The review of applications for studies that do not involve disclosure of personal identities may be expedited when chances for disclosure are minimized. Some studies employ coding mechanisms to identify the individuals in order to prevent disclosure of their names and at the same time permit wider use of the research data and information. Also, a number of computer applications now enable the stripping of personal identifiers in copies

Table 8.1. Questions for researchers requesting access to patient records

1. What sort of data and information will be gathered from the medical records?
2. How many records do you anticipate using?
3. How do you plan to identify those records?
4. How do you plan to record data and information from those records?
5. Will associated persons, such as research assistants, be assigned to review records for this project?
6. Has this project been reviewed and approved by a national peer-review organization? (If so, the archives may be reasonably well assured that the historical project is carefully thought out.)
7. Do you plan any publications from this research? Where? (These questions will help identify a well thought-out research plan.)
8. List other archival and printed sources that you have consulted. (This question will both establish that the archives need to be used and document the fact that the scholar has done the appropriate preliminary research.)
9. Attach a brief (no more than two pages) description of the proposed research, including a timetable, and a curriculum vitae. Include any other information or publications that may assist us in evaluating your application.

Note: This table was prepared by Joel Howell.

of files that are to be made available for aggregate research. In such instances the personal identifiers are preserved in the original file in case follow-up contacts have to be made, and a copy with identifiers stripped is thus made available for research. However, the handling of records in hard copy with personal identifiers is more complex because there are usually no feasible ways of removing the identifiers without defacing the original materials or engaging in a labor-intensive process of photocopying the documents and deleting identifiers on the photocopied document. One approach is to make these materials available to researchers who have been approved for aggregate studies with the condition that they are not to disclose any personal identifiers.

The responsibility of the review committee is to evaluate and act on the following:

- Credentials of the applicant

- Design of the applicant's research plan

- Relevance of the materials requested to the objectives of the proposed research

- Ethical, regulatory, and legal implications of the proposed research

- Argument for restrictions

- Argument for open intellectual inquiry

- Terms of the review decision

Fig. 8.4　**The peer review model for evaluating requests for use of restricted archival materials.** This model is borrowed from the health fields where the peer review process has been widely employed to adjudicate issues that involve complex legal, ethical, intellectual and technical problems. Because most requests for access to restricted archival materials in the health fields involve issues of a similar nature, this same type of peer review process may be utilized as a prototype for archival adjudication.

All requests involving aggregate studies of patient and human-subject records should be peer reviewed whether or not the personal identifiers have been stripped or coded, or remain intact. Even when names are removed, it may be possible to establish personal identifiers through other types of relevant information. As a result, all researchers who have been approved for aggregate studies should be required to sign a nondisclosure statement agreeing not to release personally identifiable information from the materials to be studied. The researcher is thus enabled to utilize the intellectual content of the materials while the archives protects the privacy of the individuals who are identified in the documentation. By facilitating access to clinical and other sensitive holdings for aggregate study, archival programs open new avenues of research at their repositories.

Nondisclosure statements should be negotiated through legal counsel. However, when a repository has negotiated a nondisclosure statement through legal counsel, some re-

searchers might still violate the terms of the agreement. In the instance of a violation, having a signed legal agreement demonstrates that the repository acted in good faith and places the onus of responsibility on the researchers. To prevent the disclosure of private information in a publication, a repository would have to seek a court ruling. Since it is difficult to quantify the extent of the damages suffered in the publication of private information, the courts are reluctant to rule on enforcement. Hence the best advice is not to rely primarily on the promise of protection from a nondisclosure statement, but to invest more effort in reviewing the intended products of the applicant's research.

The archives staff must always confer with appropriate experts to determine whether the research protocol is viable for the materials to be consulted. Requests that involve the disclosure of personal information require not only the review of subject experts but also the review of legal counsel. Usually the disclosure of personally revealing information involves permission from those who would be affected by the disclosure of the requested materials (e.g., the subject of a biography, if living, or the subject's immediate relatives).

Studies involving personally identifiable information that is intended to be published (such as individual case studies or biographical accounts) require a different source of advice and consent. Because of the privacy-related issues involved in such research, appropriate permission(s) must be obtained before applications are even reviewed. Permissions must be obtained from the subjects of research or their heirs or legal representatives before the request is submitted to a committee on access.

CONCLUSION

This chapter discusses the changing scope of user services at archival repositories in the health fields. It also defines an approach to user services that will help to accommodate the information needs in those fields. The policies and procedures set forth reflect a strong pro-use theme, one that advocates access whenever legal and ethical conditions permit.

Because of the unusual quantity of materials with legal, regulatory, and ethical restrictions at archival repositories in the health fields, the administration of policies and procedures for access is particularly complex. These holdings are also intellectually challenging because of the scientific, technical, and clinical range of the subject matter. Members of user services staffs at archives in the health fields must, therefore, combine a broad-based knowledge of the fields that are represented in the holdings with excellent research and interpersonal skills and a strong commitment to archival ethics.

The user service activities of an archival program in the health fields entail careful planning and vigilant management if the repository is to operate responsibly and effectively as an information resource. The ultimate purpose of this chapter is to assist archivists in the health fields to plan, establish, and manage user service activities within the context of their particular institutional settings. Readers should select the administrative and managerial elements that will work best in the framework of their own archival programs.

ACKNOWLEDGMENTS

The authors wish to thank Susan Abrams for editing an earlier version of this chapter, and Karen Butter, James Wirth, Ruth Simmons, and Heather MacNeil for reading various drafts.

Concepts for this chapter have evolved largely out of the policies of the Alan Mason Chesney Medical Archives and the activities of its user services division. Special thanks go to Paul McHugh, who has chaired the program's committee on access for more than a decade, and the attorneys of the General Counsel's Office of the Johns Hopkins University, who have advised on access decisions over the years. We are particularly grateful to Patricia Friend and Frederick DeKuyper, of the General Counsel's Office.

BIBLIOGRAPHY

BARRITT, M.R. 1986. The appraisal of personally identifiable student records. *American Archivist* 49:263–75.

BLUMBERG, B.S. AND R.C. FOX. 1985. The Daedalus effect: Changes in ethical questions relating to hepatitis B virus. *Annals of Internal Medicine* 102:390–94.

BORUCH, R.F., A. REISS, JR., J. GARNER, K. LARNTZ, AND S. FREELS. 1991. Sharing confidential and sensitive data. In *Sharing Social Science Data,* ed. J. Sieber, pp. 61–86. Newbury Park, Calif.: Sage.

CORDRAY, D.S., G.M. PION, AND R.F. BORUCH. 1990. Sharing research data: With whom, when, and how much. In *Proceedings of the Workshop on Data Management in Biomedical Research.* Washington, D.C.: U.S. Department of Health and Human Services.

FAMILY EDUCATIONAL RIGHTS AND PRIVACY ACT (FERPA). 1974. In *United States Code,* title 20, sec. 1232.

FOX, R.C. 1974. Ethical and existential developments in contemporaneous American medicine: Their implications for culture and society. *Milbank Memorial Fund Quarterly—Health & Society* 52:445–83.

FOX, R.C. AND D.P. WILLIS. 1983. Personhood, medicine, and American society. *Milbank Memorial Fund Quarterly—Health & Society* 61:127–47.

GESELBRACHT, R. 1986. The origins of restrictions on access to personal papers at the Library of Congress and the National Archives. *American Archivist* 49:142–62.

GREENE, M.A. 1987. Developing a research access policy for student records: A case study at Carleton College. *American Archivist* 50:570–79.

HOLBERT, S.E. 1977. *Archives and Manuscripts: Reference and Access.* Basic Manual Series. Chicago: Society of American Archivists.

HORN, D. 1989. The development of ethics in archival practice. *American Archivist* 52:64–71.

HOROWITZ, F.D., WITH C.W. MOORE. 1990. Ownership, access, and retention of data: Some general issues and differences among disciplines. In *Proceedings of the Workshop on Data Management in Biomedical Research.* Washington, D.C.: U.S. Department of Health and Human Services.

LEVINE, R.J. 1986. *Ethics and Regulation of Clinical Research.* Baltimore: Urban and Schwarzenberg.

————. 1988. Protection of human subjects of biomedical research in the United States: A contrast with recent experience in the United Kingdom. *Annals of the New York Academy of Sciences* 530:133–43.

————. 1989. Institutional review boards. *British Medical Journal* 298:1268–69.

————. 1991. Informed consent: Some challenges to the universal validity of the Western model. *Law, Medicine, and Health Care* 19(3–4):207–13.

————. 1992. Clinical trials and physicians as double agents. *Yale Journal of Biological Medicine* 65(2):65–74.

————. 1993. New international ethical guidelines for research involving human subjects [Editorial]. *Annals of Internal Medicine* 119:339–41.

LUCIER, R.E., AND N. MATHESON. 1992. *Synopsis of an Invitational Symposium on Knowledge Management.* Sponsored by Council on Library Resources; Johns Hopkins University; University of California, San Francisco.

MCCALL, N. 1992. Models for access to medical records. Paper presented at the annual meeting of the Society of American Archivists, Montreal, September 1992.

MACNEIL, H. 1992. *Without Consent: The Ethics of Disclosing Personal Information in Public Archives.* Metuchen, N.J.: Society of American Archivists and Scarecrow Press.

NELKIN, D. 1983. *Science as Intellectual Property: Who Controls Research.* New York: Macmillan.

PETERSON, G.M., AND T.H. PETERSON. 1985. *Archives and Manuscripts: Law.* Basic Manual Series. Chicago: Society of American Archivists.

ROBBIN, A. 1978. Ethical standards and data archives. In *Secondary Data: New Directions for Program Evaluation,* ed. R.F. Boruch. San Francisco: Jossey-Bass.

SIEBER, J., ED. 1991. *Sharing Social Science Data.* Newbury Park, Calif.: Sage.

SOCIETY OF AMERICAN ARCHIVISTS. 1992. *SAA Code of Ethics for Archivists.* Chicago: Society of American Archivists.

TOMES, J. 1990. *Healthcare Records: A Practical Legal Guide.* Healthcare Financial Management Association. Dubuque: Kendall/Hunt.

VAN CAMP, A. 1982. Access policies for corporate archives. *American Archivist* 45:296–98.

WALDEMAN, H. 1990. Ownership, access, retention, and sharing of research data produced by PHS grants or contracts and CRADAS. In *Proceedings of the Workshop on Data Management in Biomedical Research.* Washington, D.C.: U.S. Department of Health and Human Services.

PART III

STANDARDIZING AND UNIFYING THE MANAGEMENT OF HOLDINGS

A MAJOR DIFFICULTY confronting archival programs in the health fields is the lack of common procedures for collections management. To launch a more focused approach to the administration of their holdings, archival programs will have to redefine and streamline some of their basic collections management practices. They must adjust the principles for collections management to accommodate not only the scale of twentieth-century documentation but also the broader intellectual scope of this documentation, its changing formats and media, and its projected patterns of use. Moreover, policies for managing documentation in other types of curatorial programs in the health fields should also be reconceptualized to improve both the classification and the description of documentation. Collections management procedures for each of the curatorial jurisdictions should be revised to deal with changes in the documentation of the health fields. See Figure III.1 for an overview of the information infrastructure for collections management.

The impetus for a joint approach to collections management is to enhance the ability of institutions and repositories to manage holdings more effectively across the different curatorial jurisdictions and throughout their common areas of curatorial practice. If related standards of intellectual and physical control are introduced in the management of the various curatorial jurisdictions, their overall holdings will be made more accessible for use, both by the staff of repositories and by their patrons. The goal of more effective controls for curatorial holdings requires a transformation in collections management practices: the intellectual and physical control for common areas of curatorial practice should be standardized and unified. A common vocabulary of description should be introduced, as well as standardization in

Donor file—accounts of gifts and loans made by individuals or institutions. Each file includes information needed to contact the donors (e.g., names, titles, affiliations, addresses), a brief list of the materials given or loaned, and dates of receipt.

Accessions log—a system of registration for receipt of accessions. Arranged chronologically by the date received, the log documents acquisition activity and may be used to compile accession statistics. Accession numbers are assigned to each entry. These numbers may in turn be used as identifier tags as accessions are processed and catalogued.

Accession file—collection of essential information about each accession. It should include specifics on provenance, access status, information content, and condition. It may be used to inform processes of accessioning, preliminary arrangement, and cataloging. These files may be maintained separately or combined with collection files.

Collection file—a system that is designed to collect vital information for the management of a repository's holdings. Arranged by titles of record groups and collections, this system incorporates a wide range of documents that are to be maintained for legal, regulatory, and ethical purposes; it also includes information pertaining to the content, arrangement, and condition of these holdings. A separate file is maintained for each record group and collection.

Restricted access file—a system for administering restriction requirements. Arranged by titles of record groups and collections with access restrictions, these files contain information about the conditions of restriction; they also document requests and special waivers for access. These files may be incorporated into the collection files or be maintained as a separate file series.

Shelf list—a list of record group and collection titles, with storage locations. It is to be maintained in both electronic and hard copy. A portable, hard copy list is useful in storage and retrieval activities. Care should be taken to maintain only one active master list to which all additions and changes are made.

Repository catalog—a listing of all holdings by collection and record group title. Entries are to include a brief description of individual collections and record groups and also note the types of finding guides that exist.

User service files—a system for managing user service activities. These files are to include the patron registry and reference correspondence. They may be used to monitor the scope of reference and research activities, and may also help the staff determine priorities for processing and acquisition.

Fig. III.1   **The information infrastructure for collections management.**

the format and style for recording descriptive information. Procedures for common elements of collections management, from appraisal and accessioning to processing and cataloging, should be unified and standardized. See Figure III.2 for a list of the tools that may be applied to standardize description.

To achieve greater unity through the various curatorial practices in the health fields, many issues associated with the compatibility of descriptive terminology, formats for description, and stylistic conventions will have to be resolved. The lack of standardized descriptive procedures for the wide spectrum of documentation in the health fields poses a daunting challenge. If related documentation in the various curatorial jurisdictions is to be linked intellectually, current curatorial practices will have to embrace a common language for description as well as a common format and style for recording descriptions. By borrowing from conventions of bibliographic description for the health fields and from formats for recording description in different areas of curatorial practice, curatorial professionals have the opportunity to forge common descriptive standards for documentation in the health fields.

Although reforms in curatorial practice must ultimately be addressed through the professional curatorial associations, they nevertheless begin with new applications in the work place. To foster collections management reform at repositories in the health fields, archivists may start by exploring the current intellectual resources for standardizing descriptive practices.

The use of the MARC (machine-readable cataloging) format is one means of providing a common format for intellectual and physical description. MARC, a standardized format for recording descriptions, was originally developed in the library field. It has since been adapted for use in cataloging archival and manuscript collections. (The adaptation is known as MARC-AMC [machine-readable cataloging, archives and manuscripts control].) Although no specific version of MARC has been developed for cataloging museum collections, existing formats have been adapted for cataloging some types of material evidence (Gerstner 1992).[1] The MARC format has provisions for the basic types of documentation in the health fields, from recorded evidence to material evidence.[2] It accommodates the description of inscriptive, visual, and aural documentation as well as the description of objects and specimens. Plans are under way to integrate the various versions of MARC (e.g., AMC, audiovisual media, etc.) into one format to be used for all library, archival, and museum materials.

Although an authority file for specific institutional nomenclature must be tailored for individual institutions, the National Library of Medicine's Medical Subject Headings (MeSH headings) can be immediately utilized at all repositories in the health fields for the purpose of standardizing the terminology of topical information. For nonmedical terminology and proper names, the Library of Congress subject headings and Name Authority File should be consulted. Many archives, including the National Archives and Records Administration (NARA), also use the *Art and Architecture Thesaurus* (AAT). The AAT is used particularly in conjunction with entries on the Research Libraries Information Network (RLIN).

In developing both universal and institutional subject headings, the processing staff of an archives should collaborate with the cataloging staff of the parent institution's medical library. Because the library usually has a sys-

MARC (Machine Readable Cataloging) format—a standardized format developed in the library field, originally for recording descriptions of published materials. The MARC format contains categories for the description of inscriptive, visual, and aural documentation. MARC-AMC (Archives and Manuscripts Control) is a refinement of the MARC format that is used in cataloging archives and manuscript collections. Consensus has not yet been reached in the adaptation of MARC format for cataloging museum objects; archives and libraries with material evidence in their holdings may, however, adapt the MARC format to accommodate this category of materials. (Many institutions already catalog objects using the MARC Audiovisual Media format.) A standardized entry format based on MARC should be employed by all of the curatorial components within an archival program.

Authority file—a thesaurus of standardized terminology to be used in descriptions of repository holdings. An authority file indicates the standard subject headings for universal terms, proper names, and institutional names. The following sources should be consulted in preparing authority files for individual repositories:

- **Medical Subject Headings (MeSH)** may be immediately employed at every repository in the health fields for the purpose of standardizing the terminology of topical information;

- **Library of Congress subject headings** should be used for nonmedical subjects, and the *Library of Congress Name Authority File* for proper names;

- **Institutional subject headings** should correspond with those used by the institution's medical library. The library usually has a system in place for universal subject headings and an authority file for institutional subject headings. Adoption of the library's system not only provides the archives with ready-made terminology but also ensures a compatible vocabulary for the institution's library and archival descriptive practices.

Archives, Personal Papers, and Manuscripts **(APPM)**—a cataloging manual, adapted from the Anglo-American Cataloging Rules (AACR2), for use in archives and manuscript repositories. The manual provides a standard for archival bibliographic description.

Fig. III.2 **Tools for standardizing description of curatorial holdings in the health fields.**

---

1. A project whose goal is to catalog medical object collections using MARC format is currently under way in Ohio. Based at the Cleveland Health Sciences Library, the project involves seven repositories with object collections in the health sciences, and was funded by grants from the National Library of Medicine and the National Endowment for the Humanities.

2. Philip D. Spiess II, in a personal communication to the editors, has stated that he does not wholeheartedly endorse the use of MARC format applications for cataloging museum objects because of its bibliographic origins. He cites the inadequacies of bibliographic description for artifacts and specimens as being the major drawback to the MARC museum applications. He advocates the use of MARC format only in conjunction with the prescriptions in the *Common Databases Task Force* report.

tem in place for universal subject headings and an authority file for institutional subject headings, its cataloging staff may be able to help catalogers in other curatorial areas to adapt MeSH and Library of Congress headings to their specific needs. The adoption of the library's system not only provides other curatorial areas with ready-made terminology but also ensures compatibility between the library and the various collecting components. The combination of a standardized format and a standardized vocabulary of description creates a powerful tool for the integrated management of curatorial holdings. The application of this tool will also provide a means of profiling the intellectual and physical status of curatorial holdings.

Whereas the MARC format and MeSH headings should be employed in all descriptive procedures for the various curatorial jurisdictions, the main point of linkage should occur at the cataloging stage. A standardized entry based on the MARC format should be employed by all curatorial jurisdictions. The cataloging standard applicable for MARC-AMC data elements is AACR2/APPM (*Anglo-American Cataloging Rules,* 2d ed., Archives, Personal Papers, and Manuscripts). At the institutional level, a common thesaurus should be compiled for the vocabulary to be used in catalog entries. This thesaurus should include an authority list of institutional names and of terms to be used to describe formats and media of documentation, as well as a dictionary of MeSH headings. Catalog descriptions should be created only for collections and/or record groups, not series or individual items.

The entry format should be designed in anticipation of preparing a joint catalog of an institution's curatorial holdings and the computerization of the catalog in the form of a relational database. However, the database should be conceptualized and designed before the entry format is standardized so the entry may be adjusted to fit the requirements of the relational model. See Figure III.3 for an overview of the curatorial practices to be coordinated.

Although MeSH headings are widely accepted as the standard subject headings for bibliographic description in the health fields, they are also commonly used in many other descriptive procedures in these fields, from the development of knowledge management bases to the regular recording of research data and clinical information. The MARC format is also gaining acceptance in other curatorial areas: as the archival, manuscript, and museum fields begin to computerize many of their descriptive procedures, they are accepting the MARC format as their standard format for description. The use of these standardized means of description throughout the curatorial programs in the health fields will improve the ability to access and use their holdings. To stay abreast of new developments in computerization, archivists must keep pace with the professional literature. One of the best sources for keeping apprised of advances in computer applications in the archives and museum field is *Archives and Museum Informatics.*[3]

As the health fields become more densely computerized, curatorial programs in these fields are having to adapt accordingly. Not only must they computerize procedures to manage their holdings more effectively, but they also have to accommodate both the collection and the management of computerized documentation. To increase knowledge of their holdings and to deliver services more proficiently, these programs will have to convert to computerized systems of access and retrieval for both hard-copy and electronic

3. *Archives and Museum Informatics* is a quarterly newsletter that reports on developments in information technologies, theories, and techniques relevant to archives and museums. This newsletter includes the following features: articles; conference reports; international notices of professional meetings; publication reviews; news on institutional information systems, databases, and other applications of technology; software reviews and news; and standards—reports on initiatives toward standards for technologies and professional practice. Edited by David Bearman, *Archives and Museum Informatics* is a major forum for communication that links the archival and museum professions. Bearman also edits a series of technical reports— *Archives and Museum Informatics Technical Report*—that are in-depth studies for archives and museum professionals involved in automation.

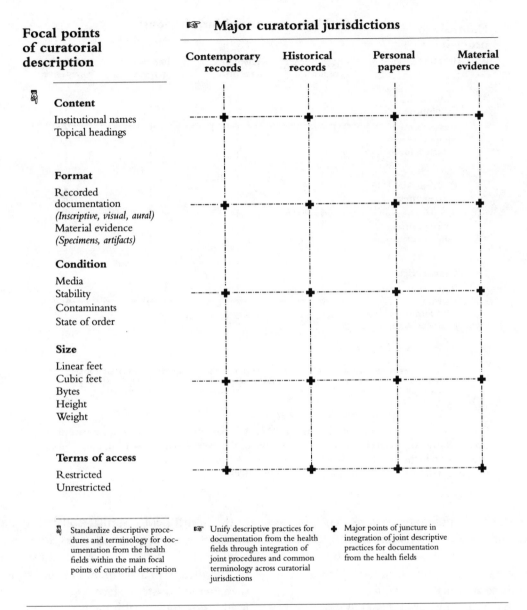

Focal points of curatorial description

☞ **Major curatorial jurisdictions**

	Contemporary records	Historical records	Personal papers	Material evidence

🖐 **Content**

Institutional names
Topical headings

Format

Recorded documentation
(Inscriptive, visual, aural)
Material evidence
(Specimens, artifacts)

Condition

Media
Stability
Contaminants
State of order

Size

Linear feet
Cubic feet
Bytes
Height
Weight

Terms of access

Restricted
Unrestricted

🖐 Standardize descriptive procedures and terminology for documentation from the health fields within the main focal points of curatorial description

☞ Unify descriptive practices for documentation from the health fields through integration of joint procedures and common terminology across curatorial jurisdictions

✚ Major points of juncture in integration of joint descriptive practices for documentation from the health fields

Fig. III.3   Coordinating practices of curatorial description for the health fields. To promote a common vocabulary and greater precision in curatorial descriptive practices for the health fields, terminology must be standardized and uniformly applied within the main focal points of curatorial description.

documentation. Moreover, they must focus on making information about their holdings more accessible to a wider range of users through participation in computerized databases and networks. Both computerization and telecommunications technologies should be employed to enhance the transmission and dissemination of information from the holdings.

The various areas of curatorial discipline—records management, archives, manuscripts, and museums—may begin to prepare their programs for the era of computerization by standardizing and unifying their basic descriptive procedures. A first step is to rationalize the process by which descriptive information is collected and recorded so that it may be more easily adaptable to the logical con-

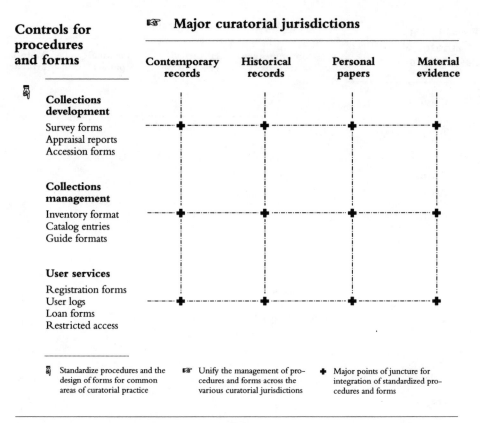

Fig. III.4 **Coordinating procedures and forms for the curatorial management of documentation in the health fields.** To enhance the overall management and use of documentation in the health fields, controls should be employed to standardize procedures and the design of forms for common curatorial practices.

straints of computer applications. The precedents set by the MARC format and AACR2 rules in curatorial practices and by MeSH headings in bibliographic description indicate that these are reliable and effective tools. The time has come for the staffs of curatorial programs to become acquainted with these tools and to learn how to use them to make their programs viable for the information age. See Figure III.4 for an overview of the forms and procedures that may be coordinated for computerization.

Curatorial programs in the health fields possess the intellectual and technical potential for standardizing and integrating their collections management procedures. The actual implementation of these procedures depends on a joint endeavor with curatorial professionals, technological experts, and practitioners

in the health fields. Similar collaborative enterprises, ranging from the development of bibliographic databases to the construction of knowledge management and information management systems, have already succeeded in libraries in the health fields.

Because the curatorial professions in the health fields face related challenges in the computerization of descriptive practices, they are in a position to work toward common solutions. It is already apparent that some library-based models may be adapted by other curatorial jurisdictions.

As the knowledge base of the health fields expands and the means of scientific communication change, the curatorial boundaries of descriptive practices begin to blur. Archivists, records managers, and manuscript and museum curators are beginning to borrow bibliographic controls to standardize and integrate the management of their holdings. At the same time, librarians are shifting their collections management focus from printed text on paper to encompass different formats and media. As they deal with new forms of documentation, librarians face issues that are similar to those that other curatorial professionals are confronting. To manage these new materials of nonverbal communication, librarians and other curatorial colleagues must lay the groundwork for describing the new knowledge base of the health fields.

BIBLIOGRAPHY

DARLING, L., ED., AND D. BISHOP AND L.A. COLAIANNI, ASSOC. EDS. 1983. *Handbook of Medical Library Practice.* Vol. 2, *Technical Services in Health Science Libraries.* Chicago: Medical Library Association.

EVANS, M.J., AND L.B. WEBER. 1985. *MARC for Archives and Manuscripts: A Compendium of Practice.* Madison: Historical Society of Wisconsin.

GERSTNER, P. 1992. A stethoscope among the books, a scalpel in the archives: Cataloging artifacts in the historical collection. *Watermark* 16 (1): 1–3.

HENSEN, S.L. 1989. *Archives, Personal Papers, and Manuscripts: A Cataloging Manual for Archival Repositories, Historical Societies, and Manuscript Libraries.* Chicago: Society of American Archivists.

NATIONAL LIBRARY OF MEDICINE. 1986a. *Locating and Gaining Access to Medical and Scientific Literature.* Report of Panel 2. Bethesda, Md.: U.S. Department of Health and Human Services.

———. 1986b. *Medical Informatics.* Report of Panel 4. Bethesda, Md.: U.S. Department of Health and Human Services.

———. 1986c. *Obtaining Factual Information from Data Bases.* Report of Panel 3. Bethesda, Md.: U.S. Department of Health and Human Services.

SPIESS, P.D., II. 1993. Letter to volume editors, 4 August.

9

Computerizing Basic Archival Functions

Lisa A. Mix

THE EVER-INCREASING LEVEL of computerization in the health fields presents both a challenge and an opportunity to archival programs at academic health centers. Because the majority of archival patrons at academic health centers are now computer-literate, users have high expectations for access to and retrieval of information from both manual and electronic systems. To communicate with users more effectively and deliver services more proficiently, archival programs can take advantage of computerized systems of access and retrieval for their holdings, both hard-copy and electronic. Efforts can also be profitably directed toward making knowledge of the holdings more accessible to a wider range of users through local and national databases and networks.

PLANNING FOR THE COMPUTERIZATION OF ARCHIVAL FUNCTIONS

Assessing Program Needs

Planning for computerization is most effectively undertaken within the context of strategic planning for an archival program. Plans for computerization will grow out of the mission statement of the archives, and the mission of the parent institution. To determine the computerization needs of an archival program, planners should first ask some basic questions concerning the functions of that program: What are the administrative responsibilities of the archives? What types of material (e.g., historical records, personal papers, photographs) are under the archives' jurisdiction? Does the archives administer a records management program? Is the archives responsible for a fine arts or object collection? How extensively is the archives used for research? Only after answering these basic questions can planners begin to tackle the bigger questions: which archival functions can be improved through automation, and how can automation improve these functions?

Richard Kesner's *Automation for Archivists and Records Managers* (1984) includes a thorough discussion on planning for automation through assessing program needs. Kesner presents a planning matrix for automation, listing all the possible archival functions classified into categories such as "collection development," "physical control," "intellectual control," "reference services," "general administration," "grants administration," and "publications" (Kesner 1984, 30–31). His follow-up volume, *Information Systems: A Strategic Approach to Planning and Implementation* (1988), advocates planning and implementing comprehensive information systems

within the context of strategic planning for an institution. Taken together, Kesner's two books constitute a good resource for those who seek to develop plans and implementation strategies for automation in an archival setting.

Establishing and Adapting Effective Manual Procedures

It is important to plan for computer resources at the outset of an archival program, even if archival functions are not to be computerized from the start. In fact, it is likely—and maybe even preferable—for an archival program to use manual systems and procedures in the beginning. However, it is wise for archival procedures to be designed with the idea of eventual conversion to computer format; effective manual systems can serve as the basis for effective automated systems. Even if the archival program has no immediate plans to computerize (and the program will most likely computerize in phases), archival systems and procedures for user services, processing, and administration should still be developed with computerization in mind. This foresight will help archivists standardize procedures and will encourage the design of appropriate and functional forms.

Developing and using effective manual forms and procedures will enable the staff to work out some of the potential problems in the system before computerization. This approach will also enable the staff to determine the requirements of an automated system. Kesner (1988) recommends that in computerizing a previously manual function the staff consider the last three years of activity.

It is important to bear in mind, however, that computer systems have the potential to be far more flexible and capable than their manual forebears. Instead of merely reproducing a manual system in automated form, an archival program should utilize new automated systems to perform functions that were impractical with manual systems (Weir 1988).

Using Institutional Resources

Well-established institutional computer systems can work to the archivist's advantage. Some of the most innovative and state-of-the-art applications of computerization are being carried out at academic health centers. Therefore, archivists who want to explore and design new forms of computerization will often find that excellent resources are available within their own institutions.

The archives staff should be sure to establish contact with individuals in their institution who can provide helpful advice concerning the process of computerization. They can usually gain valuable advice at the outset from the information systems department or the computing center. The library is also a good source of technical assistance at this stage, especially if automated systems have already been established there. If one of the divisions of the health center has established a particularly effective computing system, the administrators of that system should be contacted for help.

Obtaining Computer Consultants

If no one on the archives staff has a thorough knowledge of computers, a consultant should be hired to supervise the planning and implementation of computer systems. It is far better for an individual who is well acquainted with computers to oversee initial computer purchases than for the uninitiated to attempt to sift through the complex market of hardware and software.

It is possible that the archival program's consulting needs regarding computers can be met within the parent institution; this alternative will be less expensive than hiring an outside consultant. However, it may be necessary to hire someone outside the organization who also has some background in archives or library science, to ensure that the consultant is attuned to archival concerns: an understanding of basic archival principles is as important as a thorough knowledge of computer technology. Although computer consultants can

charge dearly for their services, the advice of a carefully chosen consultant is well worth its cost.

Involving Archives Staff Members

The needs and job functions of the archives staff are key elements in planning for computerization. The size of the staff will, of course, help determine the number of computers needed. Planners also need to look at staff members' job responsibilities and determine how each staff member will be using a computer. They should look closely at day-to-day staff activities and archival operations and then solicit suggestions from staff members regarding computer needs. For example, if (as is often the case in a small operation) some staff members "wear several hats" and perform a variety of archival duties, those individuals will need computers capable of performing a variety of tasks, and with the capability of accommodating several different software programs. Staff members whose main computer need is good word-processing capabilities, for example, will need less powerful computers.

ARCHIVAL USES OF AUTOMATION

Administration

Probably the most straightforward use of computers for archival administration is for word processing. Most word-processing programs are fairly easy to learn and require little knowledge of computers. A good word-processing program can significantly speed up the production of routine correspondence, form letters and reports. It is especially useful for the preparation of grant proposals and grant reports, because certain basic information (about the institution or about the grant project) is often presented repeatedly in a number of proposals and reports.

Processing and Cataloging

Both word-processing programs and database programs have direct applicability to processing and cataloging activities. A word-processing program can be used for correspondence, for preparing finding guides and procedures manuals, and, to a limited extent, for cataloging the collections in an archives, although a database program is better suited to this task. However, if resources are limited and a good word-processing package is all that is available, then such a package will suffice. In such a case, planners should work out a cataloging format with carefully defined terms and use the word-processing program to prepare lists and inventories of archival materials. The word-search feature will provide keyword- and name-searching capacity. Obviously, the program's level of effectiveness for cataloging will vary according to which particular word-processing program is used.

Database programs are suited to many of the tasks of processing and cataloging. With a database program, one needs to enter a set of data only once, and then it can be manipulated in a variety of ways. Unlike a word-processing program, a database program does not require that the data be entered in any particular order; furthermore, the data can be retrieved in an order chosen by the user. For example, if thorough and accurate information about a collection is captured at the accession point and entered into a database, the information can then be printed out by accession number, donor name, location, collection name, or any other designated field. As the cataloging progresses, subject, keyword, and name fields can be added to a database. Thus, a researcher could search for all the material related to a given subject or produced by a particular individual.

Once an archives has worked out a computerized cataloging format, it should consider sharing information about its collections through a larger database. For example, if its parent institution's library has an on-line catalog, the archives should consider integrating its cataloging information into that catalog. Also, the archives should consider using the MARC-AMC (machine-readable cataloging, archives and manuscripts control) format to enter information about its collections into a local or national bibliographic network so that users offsite will know of its holdings.

Despite some shortcomings, MARC-AMC has become the professional standard for computerized cataloging of archival material. The advantages of the MARC-AMC format are that it offers a standardized format for a cataloging database and that it is flexible enough to provide for the needs of different sizes and types of archival institution. A MARC record may contain information on any level of archival description, from a single item to an entire record group. Furthermore, the MARC format is the format accepted by national bibliographic networks such as RLIN (the Research Libraries Information Network). An archival cataloging database that is recorded in MARC-AMC format and incorporates the use of Medical Subject Headings (MeSH) should readily accommodate the research needs of most users of archives at institutions in the health fields (Evans and Weber 1985; Weir 1988; Bearman 1989; Gertz and Stout 1989; Honhart 1989).

An important point about MARC format is that it is not a program, but a form for structuring data. A cataloger arranges information about archival material, using MARC's order, fields, tags, and designated vocabulary. That data can then be put into many different computer environments: a database program, a word-processing program, or ASCII format (indeed, a computer environment is not strictly necessary—the data could be entered on paper forms or cards). However, MARC cataloging works best in a computer system specifically designed for this use. There are a few commercial MARC-based software packages available; in addition, most libraries' on-line catalogs are designed around the MARC format (though not necessarily MARC-AMC). While one can, theoretically, use the MARC format with any database program, it is very cumbersome to do so with an off-the-shelf database package that was not specifically designed for cataloging.

User Services

Obviously, many uses of the computer for user services will depend on how effectively the computer has been used in processing and cataloging the collections. The user services staff will have to retrieve (or assist the users in retrieving) the information input by the processing staff. It is therefore advisable that the reference staff work closely with the processing staff in developing computerized finding guides, to make the finding guides as easy to use as possible.

Automated text-retrieval programs can be used to retrieve information entered by the processing and cataloging staff. Text-retrieval programs access files in a variety of formats (e.g., word processing, database, ASCII text). Such programs are particularly helpful if the catalog and the finding guides are in a word-processing format (i.e., without the benefits of database search and report capabilities). Text-retrieval programs can perform searches much faster than can word-processing programs (which depend on word-search functions). Furthermore, text-retrieval programs allow for Boolean searching and synonym searching. Some reference archivists prefer text-retrieval programs to databases because the former allow for more free-form searches that correspond to the types of question that researchers ask in the reference room.

A key aspect of user services is outreach, or making the holdings of the archives known to researchers both within and outside of the parent institution. Computer technology affords some excellent opportunities for outreach. On-line bibliographic networks such as OCLC and RLIN are established avenues for reaching users through research libraries. However, the Internet and the proposed National Research and Education Network (NREN) provide the means to reach users more directly, without using libraries as an intermediary. The finding aids and catalogs of an archives (or, if resources permit, the holdings themselves) can be loaded onto a Gopher site that can be accessed by anyone with an Internet account. The archives can also communicate with potential users by posting information about the holdings on relevant bulletin boards and newsgroups (Michelson and Rothenberg 1992).

Records Management

Many aspects of the records management process lend themselves to database applications. Records survey forms, transmittal forms, and disposition schedules can easily be converted to computerized form. Linking these forms in a relational database effectively streamlines the records management operation. Such a database allows the records management staff to sort information by location, originating department, span dates, receipt date, disposition date, or record type. The information can be used to generate inventories, shelf labels, or notices and reports to originating departments. Furthermore, laws and regulations governing the retention of records can be entered into a table in the database, enabling the staff to generate automated schedules for retention and disposition. Such an automated records management system can confer an important advantage: standardization (Kesner 1988).

CHOOSING HARDWARE AND SOFTWARE

The computer market is potentially confusing and is constantly changing. However, the task of choosing appropriate computer systems and software becomes less daunting if an archives considers certain basic issues during the selection process. The following checklist presents some of the issues and questions to be addressed:

Hardware-specific Issues

- Is the system expandable? It is important to look beyond immediate needs. No doubt the archives will need to add more functions and programs to its computers in the future, and the memory and disk space available should be able to accommodate more than just the current needs. Planners should avoid getting locked into a dead-end system.

- Is this model of computer still a strong contender in the market, or is it being phased out to make way for something newer and more powerful? This is sometimes a hard judgment to make, and may require some careful research. One indicator of a computer's future is the extent to which new software is being written for use on that machine.

- If several computers are to be purchased, are they all compatible with each other? Whenever possible, the computers purchased by an archives should also be compatible with computers elsewhere in the institution, or at least with those in departments with which the archives will need to share data. Sometimes, in the case of large institutions, so many different systems are being used that it is impossible to have compatibility with everyone. However, the archives can check to see if one particular system is more widely used than others. It may also be useful to invest in some conversion utilities.

- Can the computer accommodate the necessary number of peripheral devices? Monitors, keyboards, and printers are all peripheral components, and each requires a free port on the back of the computer. Sufficient capacity should be included to permit the addition of a modem, a mouse, a connection to a LAN (local area network) or data switch, or some other device.

Software-specific Issues

- Is the software going to meet the needs of the user(s)? Will it readily do what is needed, or will it require extensive modification?

- Can the software be used on a network? If networking arrangements are being planned, either within the archives or within the parent institution, this question must be considered.

- Is the software widely used throughout the institution? More important, is it used by departments with which the archives may need to share data?

Issues concerning Both Hardware and Software

- What relevant experiences have others had? Planners should talk to others in the parent institution and elsewhere who are using the system that the archives is considering. (Any reliable dealer will give references.) They should find out what users like about it and what problems they have encountered.

- Is good technical support offered? Is there a number to call when users are having problems? Sooner or later staff members will need to call for technical support, because no computer system is completely problem-free. Many companies now have twenty-four-hour toll-free numbers for technical support. Talk to other users and find out just how helpful, reliable, and accessible a program's technical support is.

CONVERTING DATA SETS TO COMPUTER FORMATS

In addition to continuing to maintain their extensive collections of historical records and personal papers, twentieth-century archives in the health fields are likely to be the designated repositories for large collections of scientific and clinical data. Fortunately, computerization can offer some solutions to the challenges posed by these collections. It is unlikely that archives will have the resources to preserve huge data sets in paper-based media. Indeed, it may be undesirable to do so, as such data sets (unless extremely well indexed) are almost impossible to use in paper form. Clinicians and scientists wishing to use data collected previously by someone else generally prefer to have the data in a machine-readable, easily manipulated form.

Large sets of hard-copy data can be rendered more usable by a process of retroconversion—that is, conversion of the data to a machine-readable form. This conversion can be done in a number of ways. One way is to enter the data into a computerized database, a process that is not as simple as it might sound. It requires first developing a database that will preserve the integrity of the original data while making it accessible to modern researchers. Then someone must be hired to key in the data. Archivists should not fall into the trap of regarding such data entry as a mindless task, one that can be contracted with a local temporary employment agency. The conversion of scientific and clinical data requires thought and, in many cases, a good deal of interpretation. Those entering the data should be able to understand the process by which the data were originally generated.

Retroconversion is not a task to be undertaken lightly. It requires a substantial outlay of money and staff time, which should be weighed against the research value of the data. Rather than use permanent members of the archives staff for such a project, it is often more viable to subcontract the work to a reputable contractor. Several firms specialize in the retroconversion of data, and will work with the archives staff in developing a database and converting the data.

Another way of converting hard-copy data to a machine-readable format is to scan the data into an optical disk system. Used wisely, optical disk systems make retrieval of and access to archival information much more productive.

CD-ROM (compact disk–read only memory) disks resemble audio compact disks. A CD-ROM disk holds 550 megabytes of data, which can be stored as images or as text. An advantage of the CD-ROM system is that there are standards for CD-ROM disks, in terms of both the physical medium and the file structure. In fact, many systems can read the same disks. Also, once a master disk containing information is created, negative "stamper" disks can be made, which in turn can be used to make distribution copies without generational loss in quality. A CD-ROM disk can store up to 270,000 pages of single-spaced text and thus provides more than enough space for most archival collections. However, because images take up so much more digital storage space than text does, a CD-ROM disk's capacity is not adequate for storing large collections of images. (For detailed discussion of optical disk systems, see Cong Bui 1984; Allen 1987; Dayhoff 1988; Gasaway 1988; Morariu and Whitney 1988; Weir 1988; Stielow 1992.)

A few words of caution should be added about optical disks. First, the scanners used to input the data vary in reliability; thus archivists should be extremely careful about quality control. Second, the question of long-term preservation is a very big unknown. Because optical disks are a relatively new storage medium, no one knows for certain how long the data on a disk will last. Manufacturers and vendors of optical disk systems consider the term *archival* to mean having a life-span of fifty years, whereas archivists generally understand the term to imply permanent preservation of data. When this discrepancy is brought to the attention of vendors, they often point out that the optical disk will in time be superseded by a superior method of storing data; that is, the medium itself will last longer than the system that supports it. This possibility, however, opens up a whole new world of unknowns. Archivists will need to keep abreast with new technologies as they emerge. However, it is unlikely that resources will be available to convert everything to new media; a significant amount of data could end up relegated to obsolete media, readable only by extinct technology (Michelson and Rothenberg 1992; Stielow 1992).

ACCESSIONING AND MANAGING COMPUTERIZED RECORDS

Computerized records pose complex challenges for archives. The records exist in a diversity of formats, each with special requirements for documentation, preservation, and handling. When an archives accepts a collection of records in computer format, those records should be well documented. That is, they should be accompanied by sufficient information to tell someone how to access and use them (Kesner 1988; Michelson and Rothenberg 1992; Stielow 1992). Otherwise, the archives is taking up precious space with unusable records.

Machine-readable records have special preservation requirements. Magnetic media, such as computer tapes and magnetic disks, have a limited life-span. An archives accepting such media should be equipped to store these items properly, with proper climate controls. Because machine-readable media are unstable, even with proper storage controls, the archives should "refresh" the data periodically. A schedule should be devised whereby data on magnetic media are copied onto fresh media. If the data are not regularly refreshed, the records will eventually become unusable.

By definition, machine-readable records require some type of machine interface to allow users to access and manipulate the data and information contained in those records. This absolute dependence on compatible hardware and software is problematic because computer technology changes rapidly. Computer files acquired by an archives are likely to have been created using obsolescent hardware and/or extinct software packages. There are two ways to deal with this situation. One is to recreate the environment in which the data files were originally produced. This entails maintaining the old hardware needed to read the files. Extinct software poses an even thornier problem: the archives must either retain old software packages or try to recreate the behavior of the software (Michelson and Rothenberg 1992).

The option described above is not feasible for most archival programs. Maintaining old hardware is cost-prohibitive, and the struggle against software dependence is ultimately futile. A more proactive approach is to work with the creators of the data to ensure that critical data are updated to current formats. This requires some appraisal effort when the files are created, since the archives staff and the data creators must decide which data files warrant such conversion. However, this approach accords well with a proactive program for appraising and managing current records in any format. Moreover, this approach can give the archival program a key position in the institution's information flow (Stielow 1992).

With the proliferation of personal computers, floppy disk files have become as ubiquitous as paper. Little attention has been given in the archival literature to the management of personal computer files. One very useful study is Jean K. Brown and Linda L. Ruggerio's 1989 article "Establishing Policy and Standards for Decentralized Electronic Information Management at the University of Delaware," which presents a plan for gaining administrative control over personal computer files in an academic setting.

INTERACTING WITH INSTITUTIONAL COMPUTER SYSTEMS

Kesner (1984 and 1988) recommended that archivists impose themselves on the planning process of their parent institutions. It is vital for archivists to become familiar with the computer systems in place at their institutions and to take an active role in the planning process. At an academic health center, an archivist will find at least one—and very probably more than one—very sophisticated system already in place. The extent to which these systems are centralized will vary according to the specific institution, as will the effectiveness of the systems. The archivist should try to determine, to the fullest extent possible with the resources at hand, the variety of computer systems that exist within the institution and the degree to which these systems are linked. For example: Is there one centralized network to which all computer systems are connected in some way? Are there several different computer systems arranged along functional lines? Is the institution so decentralized that every department or division has its own system? Chances are, the archivist's institution will fall somewhere within these three alternatives. It is also quite likely that, as in other areas of academic medicine, the computer systems will be in a state of constant transition and evolution. Archivists can use this information about institutional computer systems to fit the archival program into the existing networks and systems. Firsthand knowledge of their parent institutions' situation and the needs of their own programs will enable archivists to take an active role in influencing future institutional decisions about computerization.

BIBLIOGRAPHY

ALLEN, M. 1987. Optical character recognition: Technology with new relevance for archival automation projects. *American Archivist* 50:88–99.

AMBACHER, B. 1988. Managing machine readable archives. In *Managing Archives and Archival Institutions,* ed. J. G. Bradsher, pp. 121–33. Chicago: University of Chicago Press.

BEARMAN, D. 1989. Archives and manuscripts control with bibliographic utilities: Challenges and opportunities. *American Archivist* 52:26–39.

BLAKE, J.B. 1971. Automation and the control of historical sources. In *Modern Methods in the History of Medicine,* ed. E. Clarke, pp. 260–76.

BLUM, B.I. 1987. How to implement systems. *MD Computing* 4:50–55.

BROWN, J.K., AND L.L. RUGGERIO. 1989. Establishing policy and standards for decentralized electronic information management at the University of Delaware. *ARMA Quarterly,* April, pp. 34–47.

CONG BUI, D.N. 1984. The videodisc: Technology, applications, and some implications for archives. *American Archivist* 47:418–27.

COOK, M. 1986a. *Archives and the Computer.* 2d ed. London: Butterworths.

———. 1986b. *The Management of Information from Archives.* Hants, England: Gower.

DOLLAR, C.M. 1984. Appraising machine-readable records. In *A Modern Archives Reader: Basic Readings on Archival Theory and Practice,* ed. M. F. Daniels and T. Walch, pp. 71–79. Washington, D.C.: National Archives Trust Fund Board.

DURR, W.T. 1988. At the creation: Chaos, control, and automation—Commercial software development for archives. *Library Trends,* Winter, pp. 593–607.

EVANS, M.J., AND L.B. WEBER. 1985. *MARC for Archives and Manuscripts: A Compendium of Practice.* Madison: Historical Society of Wisconsin.

GASAWAY, M. 1988. Image processing: Advances in insurance document management. *Insurance Software Review,* Spring, pp. 24–34.

GERTZ, J., AND L. STOUT. 1989. The MARC Archives and Manuscripts Control (AMC) format: A new direction in cataloging. *Cataloging and Classification Quarterly* 9:5–25.

HONHART, F.L. 1989. MicroMARC:amc: A case study in the development of an automated system. *American Archivist* 52:80–86.

KESNER, R.M. 1984. *Automation for Archivists and Records Managers: Planning and Implementation Strategies.* Chicago: American Library Association.

———. 1988. *Information Systems: A Strategic Approach to Planning and Implementation.* Chicago: American Library Association.

LEWIS, R.C. 1987. A decision maker's guide to information transfer in the health care industry. *Topics in Health Care Financing* 14:69–76.

MCKEEHAN, N. 1989. Research databases: A new direction in collection development. *Bulletin of the Medical Library Association* 77:252–55.

MICHELSON, A. 1987. Description and reference in the age of automation. *American Archivist* 50:192–208.

MICHELSON, A., AND J. ROTHENBERG. 1992. Scholarly communication and information technology: Exploring the impact of changes in the research process on archives. *American Archivist* 55:236–315.

MORARIU, J.A., AND M.A. WHITNEY. 1988. Videodisc technology and biomedical communications. *Journal of Biocommunication* 15:6–9.

NOLTE, W. 1987. High-speed text search systems and their archival implications. *American Archivist* 50:580–84.

SALTON, G. 1988. *Automatic Text Processing: The Transformation, Analysis, and Retrieval of Information by Computer.* Reading, Mass.: Addison-Wesley.

SIMBORG, D.M. 1984. Local area networks: Why? what? what if? *MD Computing* 1:10–20.

SMITH, J.W., AND J.R. SVIRBELY. 1988. Laboratory information systems. *MD Computing* 5:38–47.

SPROULL, L., AND S. KIESLER. 1991. *Connections: New Ways of Working in the Networked Organization.* Cambridge: MIT Press.

STIELOW, F.J. 1992. Archival theory and the preservation of electronic media: Opportunities and standards below the cutting edge. *American Archivist* 55:332–43.

WEIR, T.E. 1988. New automation techniques for archivists. In *Managing Archives and Archival Institutions,* ed. J. G. Bradsher, pp. 134–47. Chicago: University of Chicago Press.

ZUBOFF, S. 1988. *In the Age of the Smart Machine.* New York: Basic Books.

10

Making Provisions for the Management of Contemporary Records

Nancy McCall and Lisa A. Mix, with John Dojka and Gerard Shorb

RECORDS MANAGEMENT FUNCTIONS as a Janus-like discipline that focuses in two directions—toward the present in one facet, and toward the future in another (Angel 1968). In scheduling contemporary documentation for retention and disposition, records management practices must consider future evidential and informational uses of this material. As a consequence, records management programs occupy a pivotal position in the appraisal and preservation of institutional documentation. Today they face a plethora of new issues that are associated with basic changes in the composition and use of documentation in the health fields.

The transformation of traditional means of intellectual communication holds special implications for the practices of records management. With the rise of nonverbal communication in the health fields, many new forms of nontextual documentation have evolved. Various forms of visual as well as aural documentation now coexist with textual documentation in institutional records centers. Because of the increase in nonverbal documentation at institutions in the health fields, records managers at these institutions are having to develop retention and disposition schedules for textual as well as nontextual documentation.

Another issue facing records management practice is the fragile and ephemeral physical composition of contemporary documentation. Retention and disposition decisions must now focus on the life-span of the media of documentation. The limited life-span of some contemporary documentation presents a major challenge to records scheduling practices. Records managers may no longer rely on the incubation of time in making their retention and disposition schedules. To guarantee the preservation of documentation in fragile media, some scheduling decisions will have to be adjusted to meet the needs of their life-span. As a result, records managers will have to accelerate their processes of scheduling. Because they can no longer afford the passage of time to inform their decision making, they will have to act more promptly in the present. In turn, archival programs are having to accession more current documentation in multivariate formats and in fragile media.

Another factor involving time is also af-

fecting both archival and records management practice. In the health fields in particular, the use cycle of documentation has greatly accelerated. Some records may now pass rapidly from creation to highly active use to less active use in a relatively brief span of time—sometimes in just a matter of days. On the other hand, the records in some areas of research such as longitudinal and latitudinal studies have a greatly extended use span that often encompasses decades. The phenomenon of the brief use cycle is a particularly difficult issue for both records management and archival practice to address because their appraisal concepts are focused around much more extended cycles of use. With the prevalence of accelerated use cycles, an accumulation of recently retired records is being channeled from records centers to archives at a steady rate. This means that both archivists and records managers are faced with the dilemma of dealing with masses of newly created documentation. Whereas both archivists and records managers have relied upon longer periods of maturation for documentation in their appraisal practices, they are now having to force faster and more concentrated assessment processes.

The increasing pressure to make appraisal decisions more swiftly and decisively has profound implications for both archival and records management practices. Without the passage of time to modify and inform their decision making, both archivists and records managers are now compelled to make irrevocable disposition decisions in haste. Compounding the situation in the health fields is the high value that administrators and investigators place on the use of current data and information in the quest for new knowledge. They ascribe value largely on the basis of active use. Therefore, as the use of documentation decreases, the perception of its value also changes. These presentist standards—that current, active information has the highest value—threaten the very survival of knowledge in the health fields.

Archivists and records managers must join together in a mutual effort to protect information resources from premature loss. The value of documentation depends more on its intellectual quality than its age. For instance, epidemiologists have demonstrated that retrospective as well as prospective studies are needed to study patterns of morbidity and mortality. In order for the health professions to address current problems and set future goals, they must have a better grasp of the origins of current issues in the health fields. Records managers and archivists who are engaged in the fast-paced and quick-response mode of appraisal practices for contemporary documentation from the health fields bear an enormous responsibility. Their decisions regarding disposition and retention of documentation will affect future studies in various disciplines. Their misjudgments may result in large losses or great redundancies of information. On the other hand, their astute judgments may contribute to the preservation of documentation that researchers will be able to use for the advancement of knowledge.

Never before have acts of appraisal been so consequential. In previous eras, when documentation was in more durable paper-based media, records managers and archivists could defer many problematic choices and set collections aside for future generation to make the final disposition or retention decision. Such deferrals of judgment may no longer be made. The physical fragility of much contemporary documentation demands a mode of quick response. Archivists and records managers must accelerate their appraisal activities in order to select and preserve key documentation.

Archivists, as Nina Matheson advised in chapter 5, must assume a more active role in the computerization activities of their institutions so as to assure that critical documentation in electronic media is selected and scheduled for preservation. We urge that they also take an activist role in the records management activities of their institutions. Archivists and records managers must begin to work

more closely together as a group. They also should start to interact on a more regular basis with the clinicians, scientists, and educators who are generating contemporary documentation at their respective institutions. The collaboration of curatorial professionals (archivists, records managers, etc.) and clinicians, scientists, and educators is needed to identify, select, and preserve key segments of documentation.[1] To encourage greater collaboration between archivists and records managers, this chapter addresses the joint responsibilities that they must now assume in the management of contemporary documentation.

OVERVIEW OF RECORDS MANAGEMENT PRACTICES AT ACADEMIC HEALTH CENTERS

Studies by the archives staff at the Johns Hopkins Medical Institutions have indicated that many different types of management practices exist for contemporary records at academic health centers.[2] The term *records management* applies largely to the management of administrative records. However, systems also exist to manage other types of records, such as patient records, pathology records, laboratory records, radiological records, etc. Records management programs range from types that are formalized and highly structured to those that are informal and unsystematic. Some records management programs are centralized to serve the overall institution, whereas others are decentralized and serve compart-

1. This approach is based largely upon the recent precedent of knowledge management in the health fields. Knowledge management recommends the emergence of partnerships in scientific communication in which investigators in the health, life, and biological sciences; computer scientists; software engineers; and research librarians share responsibility for the collection, structuring, representation, dissemination, and use of knowledge.
2. The National Records Survey of Academic Medical Centers was conducted in 1987 as part of the Johns Hopkins Medical Institutions Records Project, funded by the National Historical Publications and Records Commission. A survey was sent to 116 U.S. academic medical centers to gather information about administrative record keeping, patient records, and computerization. Seventy-eight academic medical centers responded.

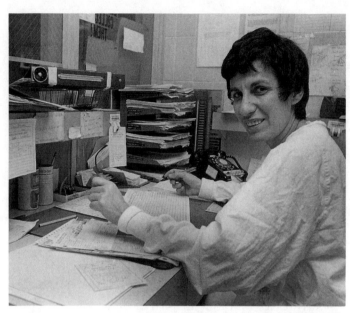

Fig. 10.1 Patient records at the Johns Hopkins Hospital.
Handwritten, paper-based records still comprise a significant portion of the records at academic health centers. *Source: Alan Mason Chesney Medical Archives, the Johns Hopkins Medical Institutions.*

mentalized areas. Institutions that are federally or state controlled have the highest rate of formalized and centralized programs. In most government-run institutions, records management is mandated by law. Private institutions, on the other hand, have long held a laissez-faire attitude toward records management.

When formal programs are in place at private institutions, they tend to be loosely structured and decentralized. In instances where no formal programs exist, contemporary records are managed in an ad hoc manner by individual departments or divisions. Because many accreditation requirements and regulatory requirements carry stipulations about the retention and disposition of specific records, a reactive form of records management is practiced at most private institutions, usually at the departmental level.

As regulatory, accreditation, and legal requirements for record keeping have intensified in recent years, private academic health centers in turn have issued more formal institution-

wide guidelines concerning the retention of contemporary records. Now that insurers link the reimbursement for the delivery of health care services to management of the patient record, and granting agencies make the management of research data a condition for funding, private academic health centers are having to assume more administrative responsibility for the retention of patient records and research documentation.

The profusion and the complexity of late twentieth-century documentation in the health fields place a tremendous burden on records management programs at academic health centers. Whereas traditional models for records management are designed for central administrative settings and encompass the full spectrum of institutional documentation, they are not easily adapted to the decentralized administrative environment of academic health centers. The volume of records generated each year in an academic health center is so great that most of these institutions are able to select only a small fraction of the overall output for permanent retention. Because traditional records management models do not provide adequate organizational concepts for academic health centers, new approaches must be developed for these institutions.

REDEFINING CONCEPTS OF RECORDS MANAGEMENT FOR THE HEALTH FIELDS

The term *records management* refers to a system that controls the recorded information an organization needs to do business (Robek, Brown, and Maedke 1987). The practice of records management is grounded in the concept that the records of an institution have a "life cycle" composed of distinct phases: creation, highly active use, less active use, and disposition (preservation or destruction). Records are created, used for some purpose, stored for future use, and finally either destroyed or deposited in an archives. The life-cycle concept provides an analytical framework for breaking the records production, records handling, and records storage activities of an institution into component parts so that problems can be isolated and effective solutions implemented (Dojka and Conneen 1984).

In the information age, the life-cycle concept is applicable to some of the records created at an academic health center, but not to all. Whereas administrative records tend to follow the life-cycle pattern and can be managed in keeping with it, quantitative research data and clinical records demand a different approach. In appraising and managing clinical and research documentation, archivists must consider the multidimensional uses of the data and information in the documentation. Data sets may be used for a variety of purposes in addition to those for which they were originally created. Some sets of high-caliber data may be reused five, twenty, or one hundred years after they are created, and thus they do not have a typical life cycle.

Most traditionalists in the field of records management continue to focus on the physical management of documentation. However, in the past decade the health fields have shown greater interest in applications of information management because they offer more accessibility to the content of documentation. Because records management is limited mainly to the control of documents containing information rather than the information itself, it is becoming a less viable practice for the health fields. The major functions of these fields are increasingly dependent on information management practices. The Association of American Medical Colleges, the Association of Academic Health Centers, the Medical Library Association, and the Association of Academic Health Science Library Directors have advocated ambitious information management programs for health institutions. Their recommendations include comprehensive planning coupled with the automation, standardization, and integration of information resources (Association of American Medical Colleges 1982; Association of American Medical Colleges 1986; Association of Academic Health Centers 1984; Palmer et al. 1986). In practice, however, most institutions

have found it financially and administratively difficult to support centralized and broadly inclusive programs in either records or information management.

It is clear that elements of information and records management practices will have to be combined to achieve more effective intellectual and physical control of contemporary documentation. However, the main challenge is to design a conjoint model that will be both workable and affordable. A new paradigm is therefore required for the administration of records and information management practices. By pooling resources and redistributing responsibilities for management of contemporary documentation, institutions may be able to introduce more effective and cost-efficient practices.

The following approach recommends the redistribution of administrative responsibility along functional lines. In this model, the functional units of an institution would assume greater responsibility for the administration of their own records. For instance, research units would bear primary responsibility for the administration of research documentation, clinical units would bear primary responsibility for the administration of clinical documentation, etc. However, policy for the overall administration of institutional documentation should be formulated at the central administrative level of the institution. Thus, policy making is unified at the corporate heart of the institution, and the actual administration of documentation (intellectual and physical) is decentralized to the departmental level.

A monolithic approach to records and information management is not feasible because of the quantity and complexity of documentation at institutions in the health fields. Rather than promulgate one overarching system for the management of all institutional documentation, administrators must be able to accommodate the inclusion of many different types of systems for records and information management. To address the diverse records and information needs that exist within these institutions, the model presented calls for a multifaceted approach that involves a coalition of major institutional systems for records and information management.

Because of their responsibility for preserving key strains of institutional documentation, archival programs have a major role to play in this coalition. They must function as the conscience of the institution and help to set objectives and standards for the preservation of institutional documentation. Archivists should actively participate in policy formulation for the management of contemporary documentation at the central administrative level. At the departmental level, archivists must work with records and information managers to appraise contemporary documentation and to assure that pertinent materials are preserved. To be more effective in meeting their responsibilities for the preservation of critical institutional documentation, archives must add a component to their programs for the acquisition of contemporary documentation. The following sections of this chapter are devoted to the design and management of contemporary records components for archival programs.

Dealing with Administrative Decentralization

In view of the quantity, diversity, and complexity of contemporary records at academic health centers, a highly centralized and inclusive approach to records management is not feasible. A monolithic approach intended to control record-keeping procedures throughout an institution and to normalize the scheduling and physical management of contemporary records would collapse under the weight of the infrastructure needed to implement and maintain it. Instead, a decentralized approach in which individual institutional divisions manage their own records in accordance with basic institutional guidelines is the most workable option for today's academic health center.

Allocating the responsibility for control of contemporary records to the institutional components that generate them appears to lead to more effective management of the records. At academic health centers, the success of record-keeping systems that evolve in the workplace may be attributed to the involvement of personnel who best understand the record-keeping objectives. These in-house systems tend to be especially responsive in areas regarding access, retrieval, and use. On the other hand, records management systems that are imported to the workplace are not as responsive to department-specific needs. Usually these imported systems have to be reconfigured to become workable.

An attempt to normalize all institutional record-keeping practices would not only be costly and labor-intensive, but it would be an essentially futile endeavor because so many of the record-keeping needs in the health fields are highly specialized and usually discipline specific. Institutions should not waste resources in an attempt to alter and normalize records systems that are smoothly functioning and serving them well. Instead, they should seek to adopt the effective systems that have evolved in individual workplaces as examples for other institutional divisions with similar types of records to follow.

One important consideration in the design of record-keeping systems at academic health centers is the usability of the system. The best models for record keeping in the health fields are largely user-driven, and records systems that have a high rate of use must, of necessity, be user friendly. Specific considerations for access and retrieval, and controls for quality of information content, are usually incorporated in their basic design. These systems also make provisions for the physical and intellectual management of the records. Thus a hybrid form of records and information management is being practiced in the largely decentralized settings of academic health centers.

As technology has introduced processes that enable large collections of data in electronic media, new appraisal issues have arisen for both archival and records management programs. Because of the technology and expertise required to maintain electronic records,

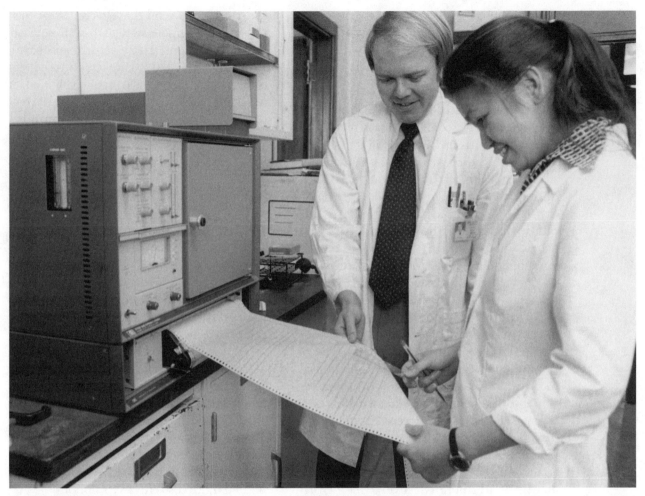

Fig. 10.2 **A gas liquid chromograph, 1977.** Some machines, such as this one, produce paper-based documentation, as well as documentation in electronic form. *Source: Alan Mason Chesney Medical Archives, the Johns Hopkins Medical Institutions; photograph by Joseph Sullivan.*

these programs will not be able to assume a major custodial role for electronic records in general and databases in particular. Although archival and records management programs must make provisions for the selection and preservation of electronic media and research data, they will have to balance their choices within the larger context of their other acquisition priorities. They must not allow these materials to dominate their programs. Records managers and archivists should therefore collaborate with computer and subject experts to devise appraisal strategies for data in electronic records. Archival and records management programs should ultimately function as resources for information about their institution's electronic record systems. Rather

than take on the responsibility for the large scale maintenance of electronic record systems, they should serve as a clearinghouse for information about these systems (Cook 1992).

The same approach holds for large sets of research data (whether or not these databases are in electronic form). While there are circumstances in which archival and records management programs may have to accession sets of research data, these programs should not attempt to take on the research functions of a data center. Again, these programs should attempt to serve as resources for information about databases rather than take on the custodianship of the databases themselves. Records management and archival programs must balance their acquisition priorities with overall institutional needs and not skew their programs to any one medium or topical subject.

Responding to the Regulatory Environment

The regulatory environment has contributed to the rise of records management in the health fields. The recent increase in regulatory requirements has had an especially significant impact on records management activities at academic health centers. Because the records of research, education, and health care delivery are among the most heavily regulated records in the country, their generation, maintenance, and use is tightly controlled.

Although the regulatory environment has encouraged standardization in some record-keeping practices, the lack of a consolidated set of requirements for the health fields has fostered a great deal of redundancy in the production of records. Many different yet overlapping regulations require the collection of the same kinds of data and information. Despite efforts to reduce the redundancy in regulatory requirements for record keeping, the extent of duplication is still daunting. Like measures to deal with other record-keeping issues, measures to deal with regulatory redundancy are more effective at the departmental level than at the institutional level.

Because the creators of the records are most knowledgeable about applicable regulations, most institutions have decentralized the administration of regulatory compliance and distributed it to the departmental level. As a result, the burden of regulatory compliance is placed directly within the sphere of activities being regulated. In conjunction with this shift of administrative responsibility, some of the best record-keeping systems have evolved in the most heavily regulated departments. The need to meet stringent compliance standards involving the maintenance of records has served as an impetus for the development of better record-keeping systems.

The departments that are most heavily regulated usually have systems in place that maintain the records needed for active and ongoing use on site and send those records that may be retired to remote storage to wait out statutes of limitations. Those departments have a strong incentive to separate seldom-used records that are being held until expiration of regulatory and legal limitations from current records that are actively used on a regular basis. The costs of storing records with minimal requirements for access and retrieval at remote locations are considerably lower than those associated with the maintenance of systems for on-site access and retrieval of intensely used records.

Linking the Management of Contemporary Records to Archival Programs

The proliferation of contemporary records in the health fields has challenged both public and private institutions to find new and better ways of managing their records. The quantity of records produced today requires greater storage space and more sophisticated systems of access and retrieval than ever before. Because of the additional financial burden associated with the management of contemporary records at academic health centers, both private and public institutions have incentives for finding more cost-effective solutions.

Policies for managing contemporary records at these institutions should incorporate two goals: they should make provisions for retaining records of enduring value, and they should establish appropriate disposition procedures for records of limited value. These provisions call for a means of prospectively identifying and tracking records with potential long-term value. The use of such an approach will assist records management and archival programs in identifying and appraising records that may have long-term value for research, teaching, and clinical care.

To implement this approach archivists and records managers need to collaborate in the design of prospective selection processes. The role of the archival program is to make provisions for the acquisitions of more contemporary records. To deal more effectively with their acquisition plans, archival programs must begin to intervene earlier in the appraisal and selection of contemporary records. They should start to accession some records directly from their departments of origin and thus bypass an interim stay in a records storage center. Contemporary records from categories that are specified in the archival acquisition plan should be considered for this mode of early selection. By intervening earlier in the selection of contemporary records, archival programs may be able to take prompter action in their preservation and organization. Archival programs should designate a special collecting component for the selection and management of contemporary records. The contemporary records component should be administratively linked to the institution's records management program. However the contemporary records program may be administered, the objective is to gain intellectual control over contemporary records of enduring value.

The collaboration between archivists and records managers should be mutually beneficial in numerous respects. For example, a well-defined archival acquisition plan will help records managers to set their own retention priorities. The imposition of records management files and forms practices will help to ensure that the files to be scheduled for archival retention are coherent, complete, and well organized. Eventually the body of knowledge that archives staff members build in the course of working with the creators, users, and managers of current institutional records will help them to define appraisal standards for contemporary documentation.

Setting Priorities

Because they are immersed in ongoing efforts to meet current regulatory and accreditation requirements, few academic health centers have been able to take stock of their contemporary documentation base and assess these records as resources for ongoing and future activities. Although much contemporary documentation generated at academic health cen-

ters has only limited value over time, a significant portion does have ongoing value for the purposes of administration, teaching, research, and patient care. The challenge is to identify the records that have ongoing value to the institution and to make appropriate provisions for saving and utilizing this documentation while arranging for the disposition of nonessential records. To manage the profusion of contemporary records more effectively, the custodians and administrators of institutional records may consider saving only a very small portion of the institution's contemporary documentation. They are constrained to retain only what the parent institutions will be able to afford to preserve after they have fulfilled their ethical, legal, and regulatory obligations.

In designing a contemporary records component for an archival program, it is important to gain an overview of the parent institution's contemporary documentation base. A survey of the institution's major records and information systems should, therefore, be undertaken. This survey should be directed at the larger *system* level rather than the *record group* and *series* levels in order to provide a look at the broad spectrum of the institution's key record-keeping and information management systems. Thus, an archival program will have a better vantage of the institution's contemporary documentation base. This survey should help the archival program prioritize its selection of contemporary documentation. All selections of contemporary documentation should, however, be based on the archives' acquisition plan. The survey results may also serve as a reference guide to the institution's key record-keeping and information systems.

Taking a Selective Approach in the Acquisition of Contemporary Records

The need to retain fewer records should not be cause for despair. Having to save less may actually provide the motivation for developing more creative and purposeful approaches to selection of contemporary records.[3] To preserve a small yet coherent segment of the contemporary documentation base, a highly selective acquisition approach must be applied. Institutional functions may still be well documented on a small scale, provided that relevant criteria for selection are applied. Some institutions may want to concentrate on documenting their corporate history, whereas others may focus on preserving scientific and clinical documentation. Institutions must recognize the potential uses of their contemporary documentation in order to develop more selective approaches for the acquisition of contemporary records. (Selection approaches are discussed more fully in chapter 7 of this volume.)

Final decisions about the retention and disposition of contemporary institutional records should be made in conjunction with the archival acquisition plan that is to be devised by the committee process outlined in chapter 6. The archival staff should also attempt to place bodies of records that have significant research value yet do not fit the scope of the archival program's acquisition policies in other appropriate repositories within the institution or at other institutions.

PLANNING AND DESIGNING A CONTEMPORARY RECORDS COMPONENT

In designing procedures for the management of contemporary documentation, both archivists and records managers must invest more effort in the development of intellectual controls. To deal more effectively with their custodial responsibilities, records managers must shift their focus from the end stage of the record life cycle toward greater concentration on the anterior phase of the cycle. Because of their complexity and quantity, it is no longer possible to manage institutional records after they accrue. Prospective controls must be introduced to manage contemporary documentation more effectively.

Management procedures must now be imposed at the inception of records creation. In order to make this shift of focus from posterior to anterior control, appraisal practices will have to move from a reactive, retrospective mode to a more proactive, prospective mode. To bring the role of appraisal to the beginning stages of record creation, archivists and records managers will have to work more closely with each other and with the creators and users of the records.

Because of the complexity of issues to be addressed—from the nature of content and potential for interactive use to the technology of records creation, maintenance, and communication—a collaboration of experts from many fields must be involved. Archivists and records managers are going to have to conduct formal studies on these issues to develop professional standards for the appraisal of contemporary documentation.

In appraising contemporary records, archival and records management practices will have to place more concentration on the content of documentation. A major objective in selecting documentation from the health fields is to assure that the integrity of its content is maintained. Appraisal standards should revolve around the kinds of data and information that are needed to verify the outcome of health care delivery and research activities. Appraisers must, therefore, be able to evaluate documentation in terms of the data and information of its content. Establishing a component for contemporary records entails practical as well as theoretical planning.

To begin designing a collecting component for contemporary records within the context of an archival program, an archives must first project that component's scope and levels of growth. An advisory committee alone does not have the authority to make final decisions

3. Timothy Ericson contends that Daniel Boorstin's discussion of fertile verges has special implications for archivists as they face new problems. Boorstin writes that the "new mixtures and new confusions" that each generation in history faces may compel them to find creative and new solutions. The sheer quantity of contemporary documentation is forcing archivists to consider more selective approaches in the appraisal and selection of contemporary documentation. (Ericson 1992).

about such matters; because these decisions require the commitment of institutional resources, administrators in charge of space and budget allocations must also be brought into the planning process for the contemporary records component.

Even though an archival program may be in a position to obtain outside funding for renovating storage space and hiring additional staff, the availability of internal resources should also be guaranteed. The archives staff needs to have an administrative forum in which to discuss the goals for the contemporary records component and the commitment of institutional resources that will be needed. The program's goals must ultimately be defined in conjunction with an assessment of internal and external resources. Once it is established, the contemporary records component should be reviewed by the appropriate institutional committees at least every five years to ensure that it remains consistent with institutional goals and objectives.

In large, decentralized institutions, a primary objective of contemporary records components should be to provide a general assessment of the current status of institutional documentation. Because these institutions are composed of many disparate parts, it is important to maintain an overall intellectual picture of the institutional documentation base. The overview should focus on the documentation from key functional activities such as teaching, research, and health care delivery. It should also assess the range of formats (recorded documentation and material evidence) and media that are included.

Clarifying the Objectives of the Program

The objectives for a contemporary records component should be defined at both the institutional level and the archival program level. They need to address the intellectual as well as the physical issues associated with the management of contemporary records. To be effective, the implementation of planning should be scheduled around both long- and short-term goals. The overall scale of the component and the eventual scope of its holdings should be determined by the availability of resources (both external and internal) for the component's operation.

The mission statement for the contemporary records component should provide the ethical and intellectual basis for the component's operation. This statement should be designed to reflect both the mission of the parent institution and the mission of the archival program with which it is affiliated. It should summarize the basic institutional responsibilities for contemporary records and incorporate a visionary ideal toward which the component aims.

Adopting a Decentralized Focus

Most academic health centers practice administrative decentralization. The contemporary records component should be planned to work within this context. In the same way that individual departments operate under the general authority of the central administration as autonomous units with functional linkages to related departments, contemporary records components need to be designed to operate within a decentralized administrative setting. Such a setting can work to the advantage of the archival program.

The responsibility of the contemporary records component for maintaining core administrative documentation demands that the component have a close working relationship with the central administration. However, the component must also be responsive to the documentation needs of individual departments. Because most individual departments are organized around the functional activities of teaching, research, and health care delivery, selection strategies for individual departments should be designed to follow these basic functions.

This decentralized approach occurs on two levels. The general areas to be targeted for records scheduling are best defined at the institutional level and are usually negotiated with the central administration. The specific kinds and extent of documentation to be selected are to be determined at the departmental level. Terms must be negotiated on an individual basis with different departments.

In coping with a decentralized administration, the contemporary records component needs to maintain a balance between the priorities of the institution and those of the departments. This component must be flexible enough to incorporate significant change at the central administrative and departmental levels and yet be strong enough to resist being subsumed by the demands of one or the other. The advisory and policy committees discussed in chapter 6 may help run the gauntlet between the central and departmental areas. These committees will provide a forum for discussion and design of policy for disposition and retention of contemporary records.

The constant need to address the overarching objectives of the institution with those of the archival program helps to focus the acquisition priorities of the contemporary records component. Indeed, the need to alter the component's policy in response to new institutional objectives may provide intellectual stimulus and encourage reexamination of theory and the risking of new solutions.

Because this administrative strategy offers the potential for innovation as well as for stabilization, it is a viable approach for large, decentralized settings. However, the implementation of this strategy depends upon effective interaction among the program staff, the advisory and policy committees, the offices of the central administration, and the individual departments. An effort should be made to harness the cooperation and collaboration of many people from different levels of the institution.

ESTABLISHING INTELLECTUAL CONTROLS

Documenting Major Record-keeping Systems

One of the first steps in establishing intellectual control of the contemporary institutional record base is to document all major insti-

tutional record-keeping systems. A survey should be undertaken to develop an accurate log of all the key record-keeping systems within the institution (e.g., surgical pathology; laboratory medicine; unit-patient records; satellite patient records; house staff records; student records; and administrative records). A listing of the extant record systems is a valuable information resource for documenting current institutional activities as well as for planning for future acquisition strategies. Ascertaining the kinds of record systems that exist and their departmental locations should be key aims of this listing. This type of finding aid will provide a broad overview of the institutional record base as well as an opportunity to locate specific record-keeping systems. Entries should focus on the major research resources that exist. Because collecting and maintaining data—particularly observational data—is costly and time consuming, institutions should encourage and facilitate the use of existing research data whenever possible. One way for an institution to encourage the sharing of existing data in research is to have the contemporary records component of the archives compile and regularly update a listing of the research data that are available. Policies for access and use of these data should be developed and administered by the departments in which they are based.

The enormous size and rapid growth of the documentation base at academic health centers makes it unfeasible to conduct an inclusive survey of all institutional documentation. A viable alternative is to conduct a survey that focuses on representative selections from the broad spectrum of the institutional documentation base. In designating the documentation to be surveyed, planners should target both the central administrative level and the departmental level, and should include the main functional areas of teaching, research, and health care delivery.

The survey should identify documentation according to type, format, and medium. It should focus on the quality of evidential and informational content and should specify how documentation is created, used, and maintained. Details about how the documentation is organized and how it is used, how long it is in active use, and how long it is kept should also be collected in the survey. The regulatory status of documentation should be assessed, in addition to its physical and technical status. The institution's objectives in health care delivery, research, and teaching should guide the selection of criteria for the survey.

The contemporary records component of an archival program should function as an information clearinghouse for institutional records systems and also serve as a unit for the preservation of key contemporary documentation. Selections of documentation should be guided by the acquisitions plan for the archival program. Whereas global surveys of the institutional documentation base may provide a useful source of reference for the archival program in general and its contemporary records component in particular, more detailed inventories of individual groups of documentation will be needed in order to develop specific records schedules.

Appraising Records

Appraisal affords an excellent opportunity for an archival program's historical records component and its contemporary records component to collaborate on a joint approach that will enhance each other's acquisition objectives. Appraisal is the common ground on which the two components may meet and form an effective alliance. For both components, appraisal should serve a major gatekeeping function. The archival program should standardize and unify appraisal policies for the two components.

As discussed earlier, the acquisition plan for the contemporary records component should evolve from the overarching acquisitions plan for the repository. By employing common criteria and standards for the selection of historical and contemporary records, an archival program may develop two strains of holdings that will complement each other.

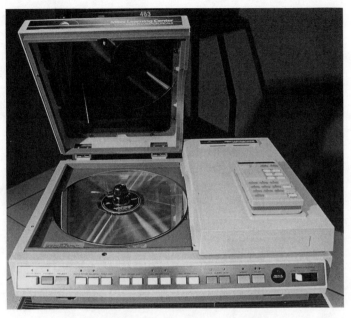

Fig. 10.3 **A videodisc machine.** Many of the new media are machine-dependent. *Source: Alan Mason Chesney Medical Archives, the Johns Hopkins Medical Institutions.*

The appraisal process consists of a dual evaluative review. Records are first assessed in terms of their relevance to the criteria of the overall acquisition plan; they are then evaluated according to common standards of intellectual, physical, and technical quality.

Because of the great quantity of documentation produced at academic health centers, the contemporary records component of an archival program must strictly limit its focus to only those materials that fall within the scope of the archival acquisition plan. Such an approach introduces records-scheduling strategies that are compatible with the repository's objectives and requires that the contemporary records component become involved in the intellectual issues of the archives acquisition plan at an early stage in program planning. By linking records scheduling to the context of archival appraisal, a clear focus may be established for the selection and preservation of contemporary records.

When contemporary records are scheduled, they must be assessed and monitored according to the repository's appraisal standards. They must be evaluated for their intellectual, physical, and technical quality.

Within the diverse documentation base of academic health centers, the quality of documentation varies significantly. Many of the materials are not viable for long-term retention because of deficiencies in their physical or intellectual composition. Even documentation from the areas designated in the acquisitions plan may contain flaws. For instance, some of this documentation may have a limited life-span because it is physically fragile or is recorded in a rapidly deteriorating medium. Another segment of this documentation may be imperiled because its media are dependent on equipment that is rapidly becoming obsolete.

When records are scheduled for informational purposes, the freedom exists to base retention decisions solely on the quality of the documentation. However, when records are scheduled for evidential reasons, retention decisions must be based on legal and regulatory requirements. They must be retained regardless of their quality. Thus, a dichotomy exists in the scheduling of records: records that must be retained for evidentiary purposes may be intellectually flawed, physically fragile, and inaccessible because of obsolete and incompatible technologies. When different generations of computer technology and inconsistent controls are employed in the production and maintenance of evidentiary records, their long-term survival may be in jeopardy. While it is possible to employ highly selective, quality-driven processes in the acquisition of informational materials, the selection of evidentiary materials must still be guided by the scope of legal and regulatory requirements. In some instances these requirements may permit the transferal of data and documentation from an unstable medium to another that is more durable. Archivists and records managers, however, must engage in more prospective planning with the creators of key evidential materials to assure that proper controls are employed in their generation and maintenance.

Scheduling decisions in general require a rigorous assessment of the overall quality of the documentation. When documentation of high intellectual quality from key acquisition areas is in a medium that is rapidly degrading or one that may be read only by special equipment that is becoming obsolete, scheduling decisions must include provisions for the transfer of the data and information to a more stable and usable medium. On the other hand, when documentation with content of low intellectual quality (i.e., data that are fragmented, inaccurate, or incomplete) from key acquisition areas is found, it should always be assessed for its evidential importance as well as its intellectual significance. If this flawed documentation does not have to be maintained for legal and regulatory reasons and is not viable for use in reference and research, it should be eliminated whenever conditions permit. Records scheduling is the time to assort documentation according to quality and evidential importance.

Whereas documentation is assessed at the record group and series level during scheduling, it is assessed at the file level during archival appraisal. Performing the first phase of appraisal at the time of scheduling greatly accelerates and facilitates appraisal during the second phase.

Scheduling is the primary mechanism for conducting an appraisal of active contemporary records. Appraisal-oriented scheduling depends largely on well-informed decision making. Thus, a body of information should be gathered to assist the decision makers. Surveys and inventories should provide a basic resource for informing scheduling decisions. Because of their interactive role, scheduling forms, survey forms, and inventory forms should be designed in conjunction with each other.

Although the data and information needed to complete the scheduling process may be collected and recorded by junior staff members, the final assessment and decision should be made by senior staff members.

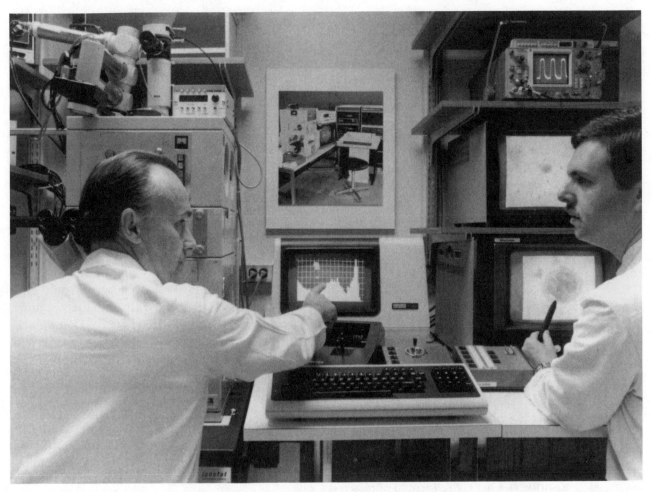

Fig. 10.4 **A scanning transmission optical microscope.** Research practices may employ equipment that produces multimedia documentation. *Source: Alan Mason Chesney Medical Archives, the Johns Hopkins Medical Institutions.*

Setting New Directions for User Services

Managing Access and Use   A system of access to and retrieval of holdings must be designed for the contemporary records component. It may be a manual system or an automated one, or a combination of the two. The major advantage of an automated system is speed. The database may be structured to link data attributes, such as the location of the actual materials, to the key terms used in a search.

There are several features that should be included in either a manual system or an automated one. At a minimum, the system should include concise descriptions of each record group and should identify the office and the employee that released the records and the current storage location of the records. The system may also contain information on retention and disposition, and details concerning the receipt of the records, such as the date received and the individual who accepted the items. It is important to link the access and retrieval system of the contemporary records component with the systems for other collecting components of the archival program.

Policies for access and use should evolve from the overarching policies for the repository. Because of the current nature of contemporary records, more time-related restrictions may apply to these holdings. Thus, a significant portion of the contemporary records component may not be opened for general use. In administering the user service activities of a contemporary records component, a balance must be struck between efficient access for the user and security for the depositor of the records. Permission for access should be granted only to those who have been authorized by the depositor. In practice, this means that in most cases only designated individuals from the records' office of origin will be granted access to the records. The depositor should be consulted whenever an exception is considered, and that individual or office should be involved in negotiating the final decision. Procedures for access should be designed to secure holdings and to facilitate authorized use.

Statistical Databases   The contemporary records component of an archives should function as a clearinghouse for information about the parent institution's current documentation base. This component, as the other components of an archival program, should be highly service oriented. In its service capacity, it should provide a framework of information about the present corporate structure and mandated functions of the parent institution. One viable form of outreach is the development of statistical databases.

In modern institutions where the management of records is decentralized, the location and retrieval of basic institutional statistics (such as the number of faculty members, staff members, patients, or students) may be arduous and time consuming. By compiling summaries of statistical information from annual reports of key departments, the contemporary records unit may be able to create a database of current institutional statistics to be used as a resource for reference queries. In most academic health centers, the development of this type of institutional database would provide a valuable reference service to the institutional community.

Scientific and Clinical Data   For a repository to provide reference service for scientific and clinical data, the holdings must be de-

scribed more thoroughly than is commonly required for regular archival practice. For example, the specific data elements that are contained within each series must be described. These descriptions must account for how each data element was defined in the study and whether there were significant variations in the application of those definitions as the research was carried out; they should assess the accuracy and precision of the data and should be able to provide potential users with enough information to allow them to determine whether the data would be valid for their intended use, and what the limits of such validity are.

There are two options for meeting such requirements. First, the repository could employ staff members with sufficient scientific expertise to handle these issues. This alternative would be difficult in the best of cases and would become more difficult and more costly as the size and the variety of scientific data holdings increased. The other option would be to require, for each data set accessioned, secondary documentation of sufficient quality and comprehensiveness to provide the kind of information described above. This requirement would not be easily met. However, staff should work with the department of origin to assure that such secondary documentation is produced.

Another difficulty stems from the fact that documenting scientific data sets is often very expensive. For one major epidemiological study that had obvious and proven value for a variety of additional research, the National Institutes of Health decided to produce ideal documentation—a comprehensive history of the original project, from research design and execution through data analysis; a bibliography of publications based on the data; a thoroughly detailed description of all the data, including all their forms and formats and an account of significant factors in data collection and processing; and additional documentation that addressed the points summarized above.

The aim of this documentation was to make it possible for the archives to provide adequate reference service for the data with no more staff expertise than is needed to guide a potential user to the first volume of the documentation. The total documentation occupies three feet of shelf space. It is structured so that the first volume is not only an overall introduction to the data but also a guide to the subsequent volumes and individual sections that a user would need to consult.

Obviously, producing this documentation was a major effort: it cost $250,000 (a price, however, that represents less than 1% of the cost of the epidemiological study itself). If a data set is likely to be used, that amount represents a very modest incremental cost. Nevertheless, in absolute dollars it is likely to be a sizeable investment (Thibodeau 1987).

MEETING THE CHALLENGE OF THE ELECTRONIC ENVIRONMENT

Computerization plays a major role in the management of contemporary records. The catalogs of the individual collecting components of an archival program should be standardized and integrated electronically into a joint catalog for the overall repository. Staff of the contemporary records component should also work with the institution's computer personnel to make provisions for the appraisal and transferal of electronic records.

Electronic Records

Records in machine-dependent media, such as magnetic tape or disks, that are not updated as technology changes present special concerns for preservation, access, and retrieval. (See chapter 9 for a more detailed discussion.) Often the institution's computing facility is better equipped than the archives to handle the practical matters of preserving electronic records. Archivists and computer specialists perform very different, yet vital, complementary functions. If the computing facility is chosen as the official repository for electronic data and information, the archives

staff should work with the computing staff to develop policies on retention and preservation for electronic records. In addition, the archives should maintain an inventory of the records retained by the computing facility. The archival program should identify those electronic records that have enduring value, and should act as an important information clearinghouse, directing users to the proper source (Cook 1992).

Micrographics

Although some institutions have successfully employed micrographic applications in their regular records management practices, academic health centers have largely resisted the widespread use of micrographics. Problems experienced in the access and use of micrographic records have led to the unpopularity of these miniaturization processes in the health fields. Some clinicians and scientists even go so far as to say that the micrographic process creates impediments to use.

Accessing and retrieving documentation in micrographic systems is often time consuming and difficult because of inadequacies in indexing and technical processing. Perhaps the greatest problem for personnel in the health fields is that the integrity of content is frequently diminished in micrographic processes. Some parts of the record may be illegible because of inadequate focusing and exposure techniques, or critical parts of a record may not have been photographed because the original was outsized or not turned over to capture the other side of the page. Scientists and clinicians demand that the integrity of content be maintained whenever micrographic processes are employed.

The objections to the use of micrographics in academic health centers usually include concerns about the lack of adequate mechanisms to provide quality control over both the intellectual and the technical aspects of micrographic processes. Users agree that micrographic techniques must be upgraded and carefully adapted to meet the special characteristics and requirements of health care documentation. Better searching and retrieval mechanisms must also be designed so as to ensure more rapid access to micrographic images than is currently available; photographic techniques must be improved to capture extremely subtle and fine details; and stricter procedures for clerical arrangement of original documentation must be imposed.

CONCLUSION

The contemporary records component of an archival program may be started on a limited scale and expanded as resources permit. A small-scale program should begin with coverage of the central administrative offices of the institution and then extend to selected academic and clinical departments. The development of this component is intended to provide a window to the parent institution's contemporary documentation base.

The administration of a contemporary records component should focus on developing and maintaining the following:

- Logs of current institutional records systems
- Profiles of the key research resources that may exist within these systems
- Databases of basic institutional statistics (e.g., important data and information from annual reports)
- Services to help individual departments set up proper technical and intellectual practices for the management of their current records
- An acquisition plan for the selection of contemporary holdings

The underlying objective of a contemporary records component should be to facilitate the use of contemporary documentation for administrative, teaching, research, and patient-care purposes whenever legal and ethical conditions permit.

Archives are having to become increasingly involved in the management of contemporary records at the repository level as well as at the institutional level. The rapid rate at which contemporary documentation is being generated, its accelerated life cycle, and its ephemeral nature require earlier intervention on the part of archivists. The vast expansion of both evidential and informational documentation also presents many new challenges for appraisal and acquisition. The complex issues associated with the generation, use, and maintenance of contemporary documentation in the health fields must be addressed collaboratively by groups that include not only records managers, librarians, and archivists but also computer experts, scientists, and clinicians. Although they may be guided by new forms of topical and technical expertise, archivists still have to shape the processes for appraisal of contemporary documentation. They are ultimately responsible for identifying and preserving a critical core of their institution's contemporary documentation. Archivists must in effect stand guard over the documentation base of their institutions as monks stood guard at the gates of their monasteries in the Middle Ages. In the present era archivists are having to assume greater responsibility for preserving a corpus of contemporary documentation (Taylor 1992).

ACKNOWLEDGMENT

The authors thank Kenneth Thibodeau for his contribution to the content of this chapter.

BIBLIOGRAPHY

ANGEL, H.E. 1984. Archival Janus: The records center. In *A Modern Archives Reader: Basic Readings on Archival Theory and Practice,* ed. M. F. Daniels and T. Walch. Washington, D.C.: National Archives and Records Service.

ASSOCIATION OF ACADEMIC HEALTH CENTERS. 1984. *Executive Management of Computer Resources in the Academic Health Center, a Staff Report.*

ASSOCIATION OF AMERICAN MEDICAL COLLEGES. 1982. *The Management of Information in Academic Medicine.* 2 vols. Washington, D.C.: Association of American Medical Colleges.

———. 1986. Evaluation of medical information science in medical education. *Journal of Medical Education* 61 (suppl.): 487–543.

COOK, T. 1992. Easy to byte, harder to chew: The second generation of electronic records archives. *Archivaria* 33:202–16.

DOJKA, J., AND S. CONNEEN. 1984. Records management as an appraisal tool in college and university archives. In *Archival Choices,* ed. N. E. Peace. Lexington, Mass.: Lexington Books.

ERICSON, T.L. 1992. At the "rim of creative dissatisfaction": Archivists and acquisition development. *Archivaria* 33:66–77.

EVANS, F.B. 1984. Archivists and records managers: Variations on a theme. In *A Modern Archives Reader: Basic Readings on Archival Theory and Practice,* ed. M. F. Daniels and T. Walsh. Washington, D.C.: National Archives and Records Service.

PALMER, R.A., R. ANDERSON, H. BUCHANAN, E. FITZSIMMONS, N. LORENZI, M.K. MAYFIELD, AND J. MESSERLE. 1986. Executive management of information in the academic health center. *Bulletin of the Medical Library Association* 74:45–59.

PEACE, N.E., ED. 1984. *Archival Choices: Managing the Historical Record in an Age of Abundance.* Lexington, Mass.: D. C. Heath and Co.

ROBEK, M.F., G.F. BROWN, AND W.O. MAEDKE. 1987. *Information and Records Management.* 3d ed. Lake Forest, Ill.: Glencoe.

TAYLOR, H.A. 1992. Chip monks at the gate: The impact of technology on archives, libraries, and the user. *Archivaria,* pp. 173–80.

THIBODEAU, K.F. 1987. Consultant's report to the Johns Hopkins Medical Institutions Records Project.

11

Making Provisions for the Management of Historical Records and Personal Papers

Nancy A. Heaton

ARCHIVAL HOLDINGS USUALLY CONTAIN both historical records and personal papers. An institution's historical records are documents that are created and that accrue naturally during the official transaction of business in the institution. For example, the fiscal, administrative, personnel, student, research, and architectural records of a school of public health or a school of nursing constitute collections of historical records. A collection of personal papers comprises documents accumulated by an individual throughout his or her life and may include correspondence; teaching and research notes; manuscripts for lectures, speeches, articles, and books; photographs; diaries; and vital records. Properly speaking, personal papers should be regarded as distinct from the records that an individual generates as an employee. The distinction between the two types of collections is important to maintain in an archives, though the boundaries between the two are often ill-defined. For example, the dean of a medical school will write letters that belong to the historical records group of the office of the dean of the school of medicine. (Such documents written "for hire" are legally owned by the institution for which they are produced.) The dean will also, of course, produce personal correspondence that is appropriately part of a collection of personal papers.

Both historical records collections and personal papers collections are defined functionally, rather than by type of medium. Included along with the traditional paper-based and photographic materials are magnetic tapes, various forms of electronic media, and records produced by various imaging techniques. Generally excluded from the collecting purview of an archives are books and other types of published materials that are regularly collected by libraries. Exceptions are often made for reprint collections that relate to record groups or personal paper collections in the repository's holdings. In addition, the collecting mission of an archives often includes a range of institutional publications (e.g., annual reports, academic catalogs, directories, etc.).

SYSTEMATIZING THE MANAGEMENT OF HISTORICAL RECORDS AND PERSONAL PAPERS

An administrative framework for managing archival holdings serves a number of interrelated functions. It constitutes a means for preserving and enhancing relations with donors and prospective donors, establishes legal ownership of and rights to documentation, protects holdings from deterioration, and helps to determine the priorities for collecting and processing. It also regulates access to documentation, so as to balance the needs of scholars against privacy and literary rights; protects holdings from abuse or theft by users; stimulates research through appropriate organizing and cataloging of documentation; and serves to disseminate information about the intellectual resources of the repository.

The archivist charged with establishing or updating a processing program for archival records may be frustrated by a lack of uniform practice among repositories. Unlike the li-

brarian, who is guided by clearly defined procedures for processing, the archivist will find almost as many approaches to processing as there are archives. Record-keeping schemes vary from repository to repository. Catalogs may take the form of the traditional card catalog, a series of loose-leaf binders, or an elaborate computer database. Furthermore, records are processed and housed differently, and a variety of systems exist to protect confidential records while guaranteeing legitimate scholarly access. To a large extent, variations in management reflect differences in the character and scope of collections; to a lesser extent they result from a continuing struggle within the profession to delineate those practices that ought to be universal, and then to agree on the details of common practice.

Employing a Top-down Strategy

A top-down strategy of processing may be of great value for managing historical records and personal papers. Such a strategy dictates that the actual processing advance from the general to the specific, from the basic to the extensive. That is, an established minimal amount of record keeping and processing (preliminary processing) should be accorded each group of records or papers as it is received. Then, when time and resources allow, or as new staff members are hired or new funding is received, increasingly elaborate levels of processing may be given to collections on the basis of planned priorities. In other words, an overall system should first be planned, and then individual collections will be processed on some fundamental level before more detailed processing or cataloging is undertaken. Minimal preliminary processing

Fig. 11.1 **An entry from the Executive Committee of the Board of Trustees of the Johns Hopkins University (26 December 1892).** Through the records of governance, the evolution of corporate structure may be seen. Founding documents such as executive board minutes provide the basis for corporate policy. *Source: Alan Mason Chesney Medical Archives, the Johns Hopkins Medical Institutions.*

At a meeting of the Executive Committee held at the house of the Chairman, Mr C. J. M. Gwinn, on December 26th 1892 there were present Mr Gwinn, Mr McLane, Mr Stewart, Dr Thomas and Mr White.

The chairman ~~explained~~ said that he thought it was desirable that Miss Garrett should be notified that her offer of the fund ~~referred~~ in aid of the Medical School had been accepted by the Board upon the terms set forth in her offer.

Mr C. Morton Stewart was thereupon requested by the Committee to write to Miss Garrett informing her of the fact of such acceptance and that duly certified copies of her letter and of the resolution of the Board would be forwarded to her.

It was suggested by Mr Gwinn that the letter of Miss Garrett and the resolution of the Board, accepting her offer, should be published in the daily news- papers which had been selected

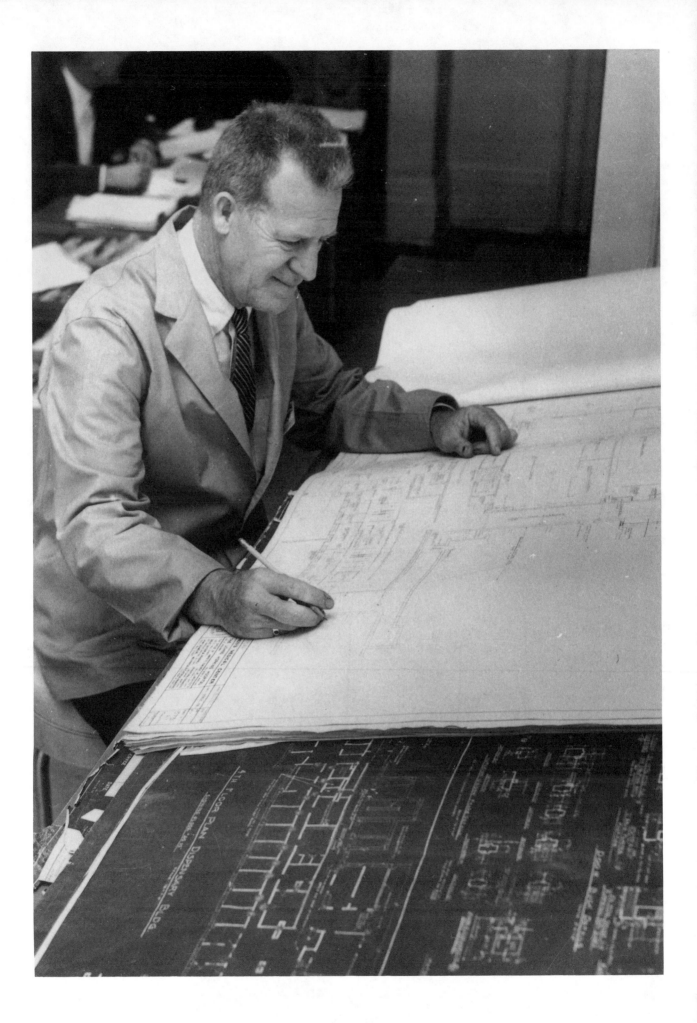

includes the completion of various accessioning and processing forms, prophylactic conservation measures, an initial assessment and general summary of the contents of the collections being processed, and the reboxing of the records or papers in appropriate archival containers. The rationale for preliminary processing of each and every collection may be explained best by examining the consequences of storing unprocessed records.

Uncataloged documents are lost to researchers who do not learn of their existence or know their whereabouts. An archives cannot provide access to such documents because the collection may contain sensitive material, because theft is easy from such an unprocessed and uncataloged collection, and because fragile documents may be compromised by handling. As unprocessed collections multiply, staff members will quickly lose an overview of the holdings, especially when staff turnover leaves gaps in the institutional memory. In this situation, collecting and processing priorities are also extremely difficult to develop. Furthermore, the collecting programs of related repositories will be impaired when the holdings of their sister repositories are not described at least in general terms.

Developing a Framework for Basic Record Keeping

The following record-keeping systems constitute the fundamental units of operation for an archival program: (1) a donor (and, perhaps, a lender) file; (2) accession records; (3) collection files; (4) restricted access files; (5) a shelf list; (6) a catalog of holdings; and (7) user services records. Whereas the form of these records will vary, the substance and purpose generally will not.

At the outset the question will arise as to whether it is wise to computerize the record-

keeping process. Naturally the answer will depend on available resources and staff expertise. For those worried about being left behind in the computer age, it is reassuring to recognize that such a conversion project need not be immediate and total but can, and sometimes should, take place gradually. Furthermore, it may be applied to some but not all of the processing files. For each type of processing file created, the many advantages of going on-line must outweigh the expense, the difficulty of training staff members, and the potential inconvenience caused by the necessity of using computer terminals in fixed locations. In some cases, alternative means of recording data may be easier and more convenient.

Although computerization is optional for most record keeping, the catalog of holdings should be done on-line, preferably using the MARC-AMC (machine-readable cataloging, archives and manuscripts control) format, which is designed specifically for describing historical records and papers. If this option is not practical in the beginning, cataloging should be done in such a way that information may be converted easily when resources are available. Computerized cataloging is desirable because the catalog records can then be uploaded into a public network that allows patrons and other repositories to gain remote access to the catalog. Furthermore, the widespread use of the MARC-AMC cataloging format encourages the adoption of uniform cataloging practices by archival programs. The advantages of computerized cataloging are not limited to increased ease of reference service. Once the contents of collections have been entered into the computer, key-word searching may be used to answer questions pertaining to the management of those collections. A key-word search might be used, for example, to survey collections containing photographs that are in need of conservation. Computerized searching might also be used in a survey to establish patterns of collecting. The possibilities are almost limitless, providing the data have been carefully entered in the first place.

Fig. 11.2 **The ongoing use of architectural records.** Early architectural records may be utilized in historical research as well as in the current facilities design of an institution. *Source: Alan Mason Chesney Medical Archives, the Johns Hopkins Medical Institutions.*

A carefully structured record-keeping system will be enormously helpful in guiding processing procedures. Many archives are likely to create a host of additional record-keeping forms to meet specific needs, such as photocopying, exhibiting documents, or processing special collections of medical artifacts or photographs. The record-keeping system suggested here comprises the core of most systems, and however much it may be adapted or modified in a particular application, its function remains unchanged. An archival program's record keeping should be designed to promote the physical, legal, and intellectual security of its collections and to facilitate relations with donors, donor institutions, and scholars.

ESTABLISHING PHYSICAL AND INTELLECTUAL CONTROLS

The heterogeneity of the holdings in archival repositories in the health fields requires the use of an array of processing techniques. A collection may comprise a single medical diary, or eight hundred linear feet of records of a director of oncology outpatient services. The papers of a medical professor may include, among other items, audiotapes or videotapes of lectures, along with a large collection of 35-mm slides. Records from a department of internal medicine may contain confidential patient records. Records from a department of radiation oncology may take the form of computer disks and printouts, mathematical data, and images produced by various scanning techniques. Records from a pathology department may include specimens, or medical drawings that have both clinical and artistic significance. Records from a research laboratory often contain numerous copies of grant applications. A collection may consist of manuscripts and oral history interviews made in preparation for a biography of a recognized scientist. Almost any collection may harbor correspondence with important literary figures, or valuable memoirs concerning non-medical topics. Personal papers may chronicle the rise and fall of a football team, the leisure

activities of a medical fraternity, the diplomatic and social problems of a missionary nurse. With respect to size, complexity, subject matter, and document format, the boundaries of a collection are remarkably fluid.

Whereas the documentation found in archival holdings ranges from the traditional letter or photograph to a myriad of electronic media, one feature is held in common: seminal information tends to be buried in a daunting volume of records, often without signposts to herald its existence. Also hidden within the collections are the agents of destruction (e.g., microorganisms, acid in paper, thiosulfates in photographs). The dual purpose of processing is to establish intellectual control over the content of the collections and to prepare the collections to resist deterioration. The processing procedures described here include accessioning, arranging, and cataloging. Given the varied character of collections, however, it is possible to address only overarching principles of processing. The novice will need to seek information and training relative to specific types of documentation from the available archival literature and the many programs offered in archival management.

Perhaps one of the most important principles that should govern the management of any collection of historical records or personal papers is a fundamental respect for the original order and provenance of the collection: neither record keeping nor processing should be undertaken without first considering the implications of this principle. Records or papers from one source should not be dispersed but should be kept together as one collection. Even if individual items, or groups of items, such as photographs, need to be *physically* separated from the collection (usually for reasons of storage or conservation) the collection must be kept intact *intellectually* by means of descriptive finding aids. At the very least, separated items need to be marked (e.g., "from the papers of William Welch," or "from the School of Nursing records"). Records or papers from different sources should not be

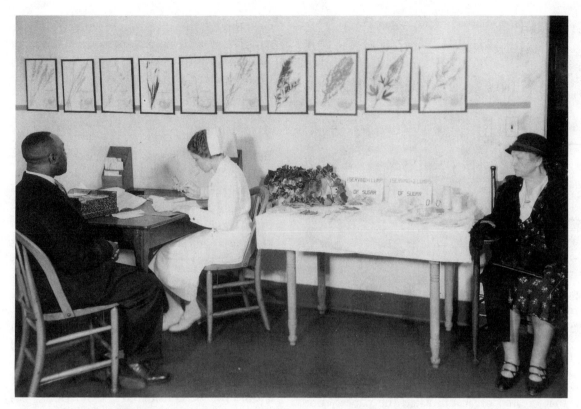

Fig. 11.3 **A student dietician with a patient at the Johns Hopkins Hospital, 1930.** Visual documentation constitutes a major source for studying the activities of teaching, health care, and research. *Source: Alan Mason Chesney Medical Archives, the Johns Hopkins Medical Institutions.*

combined. For example, records or papers pertaining to a particular subject, such as segregation in hospital wards, should not be pulled from various collections and combined in a subject file. (In any case, records or papers rarely deal with only one topic, so selection by one topic often results in the "burying" of other topics covered in the same document.) The original order of the records or papers should be retained (or re-created if possible) unless it is impossible to determine the appropriate order or there are compelling reasons for changing that order.

The principle of respect for provenance and original order is honored by repositories primarily because records are usually more meaningful in their original context, and sometimes are meaningful only in that context. An obvious example is the instance of a photograph that is identified by the surrounding papers. However, the value of the context is often

more subtle. For instance, a research evaluation might be interpreted more accurately when the context in which it was written is clarified by other documents with which it is filed. The internal arrangement of collections may also provide information about the subject of those collections (e.g., by revealing the personal habits and interests of individuals or the functioning of an organization). Therefore, unless the collection has already been disarranged by families, donors, or employees, the original order should generally be retained (at least in its broad outline), though naturally most collections will require a certain amount of "straightening." Experienced historians expect to find records and papers arranged according to the principle of respect for provenance and original order, and such an arrangement will greatly enhance retrieval.

Respect for provenance is reflected in one of the very first processing decisions, that is,

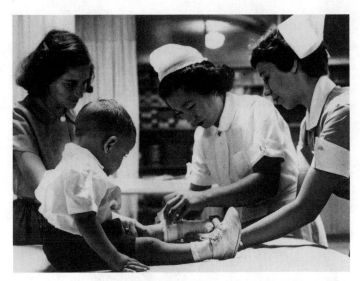

Fig. 11.4   **Nurses dressing the injury of a young patient at the Johns Hopkins Hospital, circa 1955.** *Source: Alan Mason Chesney Medical Archives, the Johns Hopkins Medical Institutions.*

naming the collection. The name of the collection identifies the person or organization that created or accumulated the papers, not the person who later inherited, purchased, or acquired them, and does not necessarily refer to the significance of individuals or topics that may be associated with the collection. The function of cataloging is to highlight information about important people and subjects; the name of the collection should reflect its provenance. For example, if an archives received the personal papers of a little-known physician who had extensive correspondence with William Halsted, the papers should be named for the originating physician, not for William Halsted, even though the papers would contain original letters received from Halsted, and perhaps copies of letters sent by the less well-known physician. (The personal papers of an individual usually contain letters received and copies of letters sent.) Records named after an organization are those produced and acquired by the organization and kept in its working files, even though these records may later be found in the hands of an individual who figured prominently in the organization. For example, the records of the Committee on Problems of Drug Dependence should be named after the committee,

even though they may reside with an individual. When records and personal papers are combined, as they so often are, it is helpful to describe them in such a way as to make that fact known.

Accessioning

Before a record group or a collection of personal papers is transferred to an archives, an investigation of the materials for insect or microorganism infestation is mandatory, unless the archives has a "quarantine" room for incoming materials. Since molds and insects may disperse rapidly throughout the holdings of the entire repository once introduced, it may be necessary to treat the materials before transfer. In the course of this search, the archivist should also note on the accession form any other conservation problems that need immediate or high-priority attention.

Packing archival materials for shipment should not be considered a menial task, because a certain amount of appraisal, arranging, and weeding often needs to be done in the field. Equally important, the packing needs to preserve whatever arrangement or organization may already exist. Packing must be done carefully so that historical evidence is not lost (e.g., by neglecting to transfer label information from file cabinets to boxes). Containers should be carefully numbered in sequence, an effort that will immediately draw attention to any boxes that have been lost in transit and will aid in the reassembly of the collection once it is received at the archives. Packing should be done by, or at least supervised by, archives staff. Although it is convenient to have donors or departments do their own selecting and packing, this practice is undesirable. On the one hand, it is not uncommon for donors to have a penchant for clearing attics and closets and inundate an archives with rooms full of marginal and sometimes irrelevant materials; on the other hand, donors may discard dozens of precious documents because they can't imagine that their personal correspondence or photographs are of any historical interest. In other words, the acquisi-

tion of appropriate materials often requires archives staff members to exercise deft interpersonal skills to persuade donors to release the
documents that the repository needs, and this
process continues during accessioning as the
packers assess documents being acquired or
apparently missing.

Appraisal to assess the intellectual value of
various components of a collection should
precede any selection or weeding of documents. Because appraisal requires a clear understanding of the repository's collecting objectives, a knowledge of the subject matter,
familiarity with research practices and methodologies, and appraisal experience, decisions
about what to select should not be left to inexperienced packers. In the case of small collections, it is practical to accession the collection
as is, deferring appraisal to a later stage of processing when the staff has had time to conduct

sufficient background research to make prudent decisions on retention and disposal.

In the case of collections so large that econ-
omy dictates the need to select only a portion
of the collection for retention before the collection is shipped to and housed in the archives, appraisal must begin in the field and
will then continue throughout processing.
Particularly in repositories in the health fields,
it is likely that the archivist's own experience
and expertise will not always suffice to make
informed decisions. In the case of records kept
by a scientist in the course of his or her research career, a first step in appraisal might be
to seek a consensus of the scientist's peers as to
the value and potential use of various documents. Scientists are not historians, however,
and they will have a different—albeit important
—perspective. Another step would be to survey the records of other repositories to see

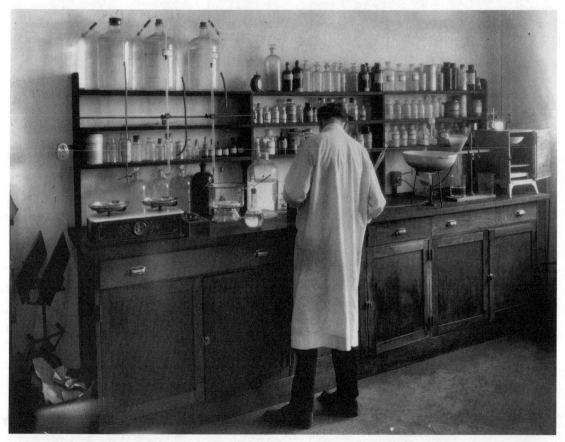

Fig. 11.5   **A laboratory at the Johns Hopkins University School of Medicine, circa 1925.** Photographs
are a major resource for studying the evolution of laboratory practices. *Source: Alan Mason Chesney Medical Archives, the Johns Hopkins Medical Institutions.*

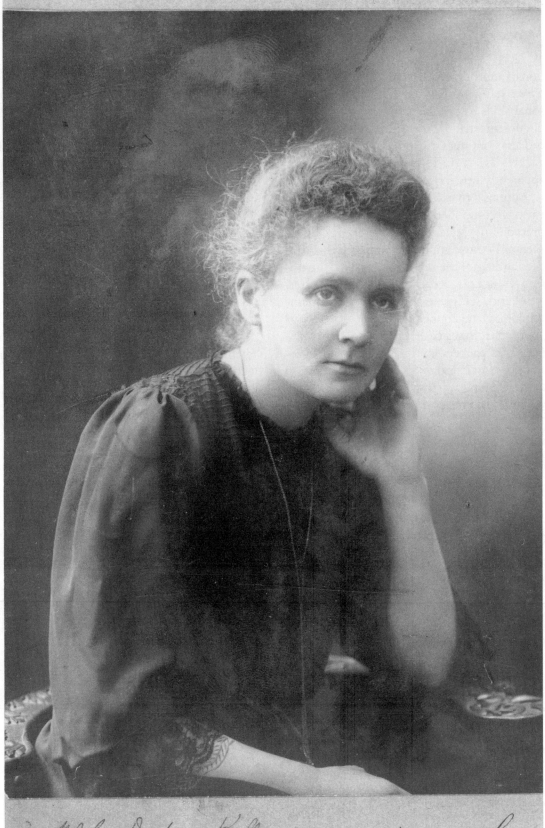

à Mᵉᵉ le Docteur Kelly
M. Curie
Henri Manuel
PARIS

what is already available on the same subject or concerning the same scientist. A third approach would be to query medical historians. Finally, staff members might find it useful to consult experts in the value of certain types of documentation. Such an expert might recognize the hallmarks of a great diary, or high-quality photographs, or valuable artifacts. These approaches will yield differing perspectives and together will assist the archivist in the appraisal. Clearly, such an approach adds considerably to the cost and difficulty of acquiring and processing large, complex collections.

A large collection, or even sometimes a small collection, may require the preparation of an inventory before shipment. Such an inventory is needed for insurance purposes, as a precaution in case there is a loss, or a dispute about what has been transferred. An inventory made on site may also facilitate the interpretation and appraisal of records. For example, the location of a file cabinet may tell the archivist something about the perceived value of the records it contains or its relation to other documents. The way research data are housed may reveal both the methods and the character of a scientist. Preliminary inventories present the pervasive dilemma of processing—the question of balance. How much detail is enough in a preliminary inventory? Should the inventory be a box list, or perhaps a folder list? Is it possible to include too much detail? The answer to the last question is definitely yes. Inventories made before background research and final processing will be provisional and will probably fail to capture the character of either the forest or the outstanding trees. Such inventories should be made for security and as an aid in the later processing and cataloging of collections. Taking an inventory cannot replace cataloging. An inventory is simply a straightforward list, perhaps of folder headings, and as such it is nonevaluative.

Whether or not an inventory is made, the contents of the collection should be summarized in a brief paragraph. This preliminary description should focus on document types and quantities, inclusive dates, and the major subjects and people included. Such a paragraph might read as follows: "Papers (ca. 1900–1980) of W. Horsley Gantt (born 1892, died 1980), behavioral biologist. Approximately 600 Paige boxes of correspondence, posters, photographs, manuscripts, research data, reprints, books, artifacts. Papers relate mainly to his studies with Ivan P. Pavlov in Russia during the early 1920s and to research at his Pavlovian Laboratory at Johns Hopkins."

The précis made during accessioning is most helpful if written in commonsense English without the use of abbreviations, codes, or esoteric conventions of cataloging. It should be as accurate as possible, with names correctly spelled and uncertain dates indicated as approximations. The general nature of the précis should not encourage a lack of attention to accuracy. Rather, it should provide other processors with a sense of the scope and the subject matter of the collection.

The précis, when complete, should be added to the accession form. An accumulation of such summaries is useful when priorities for processing and cataloging are being established. Furthermore, this initial effort to capture the character of a collection may be adapted for on-line entry and used in a temporary preliminary catalog to the holdings of the repository.

A limited amount of arrangement and description necessarily occurs as part of the accessioning procedure. More extensive arranging and descriptive cataloging are often performed concurrently with accessioning, depending on the priorities of the archives, and the time available. If accessions are accumulating, the amount of arranging and de-

Fig. 11.6 **Correspondence with Madame Marie Curie on the early therapeutic uses of radium, from the Howard A. Kelly Papers.** Collections of personal papers provide an important complement to institutional records. They are also a resource for the study of disciplines in the health fields. *Source: Alan Mason Chesney Medical Archives, the Johns Hopkins Medical Institutions.*

scription associated with accessioning should be reduced until it is possible to keep up with minimal accessioning activities for all the collections received.

At this stage of processing, the collection is reasonably physically secure, the provenance and literary rights have been determined, donors have been registered (and probably thanked in writing), the collection has been provisionally evaluated for sensitive documents, major conservation problems have been noted, and a general summary of the contents has been prepared. The accessioning procedure that has now been completed constitutes the bare minimum required, but it affords substantial control over the collection. A reasonable next step is to shelve the collection and move on to another accessioning project. Further processing should be undertaken on the basis of a priority list of all the collections in need of processing.

Even though the collection is now on hold, this is a good time to announce the presence of the collection in the repository by way of a preliminary catalog entry or some other public listing. The announcement may take the form of a simple list of collections by name, or a card catalog or computer file of the collection précis prepared during accessioning. This recommendation of early announcement may seem odd, considering that policy usually precludes scholarly access to unprocessed collections. However, early announcement serves to encourage feedback from scholars and other professionals, and this will assist the archives staff in setting priorities for processing and cataloging. The possibility even exists that inquiries will lead to funding or other assistance. Archivists may be reluctant to "tease" scholars with unavailable collections or to open themselves to pressure that may be brought by users or donors. These concerns have to be weighed against the benefits of sharing information about the archival holdings.

Arranging and Organizing

In a well-managed archives, the arrangement of some record groups and the organization of some holdings will consist of little more than the boxing of documents in the order in which they were received and the application of a general label to the box. That is, arrangement will not proceed much beyond that performed during accessioning. In other cases a record group may be processed and arranged item by item, with individual folders carefully labeled in detail. The correctness or completeness of any method of arrangement depends so much upon the individual record group or personal papers collection that it is impossible to establish firm general rules. An arrangement that works well in one collection may not be practical in another. Completeness may be mandatory in some cases, whereas in others it would be an error in judgment to process the material in any great detail. Experience is the best guide to establishing the relative importance of various collections and various aspects of processing. The extent of processing will depend upon priorities determined in accordance with the mission and documentation plan of the archives.

Many factors influence the extent of processing. One of the more obvious factors is the importance of the institution or person who created the collection, or who may be represented in the collection. A second consideration is the importance of the documents in the collection. Regardless of their intrinsic value, it may not be worthwhile to spend time on documents already available elsewhere. The papers of a prominent scientist are less significant if they contain only information readily available in published sources. Papers may be unique, very early, or very rich in historical information, in which case they are important regardless of whose they are—for example, a medical diary with substantial entries kept by a little-known medical officer in World War I. A collection becomes more important if researchers have expressed an interest in its subject matter. Conservation

K. S. F. S. R.
(Russian Socialistic Federation of Soviet Republics)
N. K. Z.
(Ministry of Public Health)
State Institute of Experimental Medicine
Physiological Laboratory of
Prof. I. P. Pavlov

W. HORSLEY GANTT, Doctor of Medicine, has, for

a period of four and a half years, visited the laboratories

under my direction at the Military Medical Academy, the Academy

of Sciences, and the Institute of Experimental Medicine, and

has become familiar with practically all the works conducted

by those laboratories.   In particular, he has studied

thoroughly and intelligently the surgical operative methods

of the gastro-intestinal tract, and the technique of inves-

tigating the conditioned reflexes.   Besides this, he has cond-

ucted several independent researches relating to the physi-

ology of digestion and the physiology of the cerebral

hemispheres.

     To the whole teaching of conditioned reflexes,

he has devoted especial attention and much time, having famil-

iarized himself with the articles bearing on the subject,

and also he has frequently participated in the laboratory

discussions of the various problems and questions arising

therefrom.   This knowledge is evidenced by his excellent

rendition of my book on conditioned reflexes.

Prof. Dr. I. P. Pavlov

Leningrad,
1 July 1929.

Fig. 11.7   **Correspondence with Ivan Pavlov, from the Horsley Gantt Papers.** *Source: Alan Mason Chesney Medical Archives, the Johns Hopkins Medical Institutions.*

needs may also influence processing priorities: occasionally a collection of mediocre interest will be given priority because of the need for emergency conservation treatment. Space may dictate priority in processing if extensive weeding of a large collection will alleviate a shortage of space. The sensitivities of donors must also be taken into account. Some will be obstreperous in their demand that processing be immediate and thorough; others will be more considerate, but satisfying their expectations may be prudent. Concentrating upon collections that are largely restricted and cannot be made widely available for use is probably not a wise allocation of processing time. If additions to collections are expected, it may be best to postpone processing. Size may also be a factor: a very small collection is easy to process and catalog in depth, even if it is not as important as a larger collection. Any or all of these factors will influence the degree to which a particular collection is processed.

Conducting Background Research The processor making decisions about the arrangement of a collection should, of course, be familiar with the person or organization involved and the subject matter of the collection. It is virtually impossible to find a processor who has expert knowledge of the work of not just one Nobel laureate but a whole host of scientific luminaries, and who is conversant with the functioning of departments, which range from budget offices to neuroscience departments. Fortunately, it is not necessary at the outset to be an authority on the person or organization to process the collection well. Beyond a solid general education in arts and sciences, the skill that is most relevant is knowing what information needs to be gathered and where to find it.

In addition to learning about a specific person or organization, processors need to spend time learning about various types of documentation. For example, a processor who is examining financial records for the early years of a hospital must understand what kinds of data are found in an accounting journal and what kinds of data are found in a statement-of-account logbook.

Preliminary Arrangement Once the processor is comfortable with the subject matter of the collection, he or she should give thought to various arrangement schemes. The process of replacing file folders with acid-free folders to prevent the deterioration of the contents provides a convenient opportunity to review the existing arrangement and consider modifications. It is not uncommon for the processor to thumb through the collection numerous times, first during accessioning and packing, then while making an inventory and while re-

placing the folders holding the collection, and eventually when establishing the final arrangement. This repetitive review is not wasted effort, because an appreciation of the records emerges gradually, and during each review the arrangement and description of the collection's contents can be refined. It is usually a mistake to begin alphabetizing or processing without these preliminary forays into the collection, because they assist the processor in capturing the large picture—an essential element of the top-down processing strategy.

Although the original arrangement of records should have been retained up to this point, a great deal of organizing usually remains to be done. In most cases, a certain tension exists between the original order of the collection and alternate arrangements that might be more suitable for research. If such alternative options can be implemented without disrupting the pattern of the original order and without destroying historical evidence by altering the proper context of documents, then modifications may be acceptable. For processors with little or no experience, the conservative course of action is the recommended approach.

Skillful arrangement is too complicated a subject to be treated in a matter of paragraphs. The questions that arise during the arrangement of correspondence will serve to illustrate the kinds of concern that must be addressed. Similar questions of arrangement arise for most types of documentation.

Correspondence is typically organized alphabetically or chronologically, or by subject. There is no one correct arrangement. Rather, an appropriate choice is made by asking how historians and other relevant researchers will use the records. An alphabetical arrangement is convenient if interest focuses on individuals or groups and works best if there is voluminous correspondence for each correspondent or if the time frame covered by a body of letters is limited. Alphabetizing correspondence destroys historical evidence, however, to the extent that the time sequence is lost. It is difficult to reconstruct the history of someone's research, for example, if the correspondence comprises file folders for several hundred people, each folder spanning a different time period. A chronological arrangement will capture this history, and although it may be inconvenient to retrieve the correspondence of one individual or organization in this arrangement, it is still quite possible, particularly with computerized cataloging. A chronological arrangement might be regarded as the default condition, to be used unless there is a good reason to do otherwise. Hybrid solutions, such as chronologizing almost all of the correspondence but separating correspondence with a particular individual or group, are also common. Subject arrangements may be advisable for major topics, but letters rarely concern only one subject. Subject arrangements are generally selected, however, if the records arrive already arranged by subject.

The preliminary arranging of a collection might be limited to reboxing the collection or perhaps transferring the collection to new folders and organizing large categories of files. For example, one might group scientific manuscripts into one unit, correspondence into another, and so on. In accordance with the principle of top-down processing, the extent to which arranging is continued down to the level of individual items is a matter of priorities and expedience, and arranging can be done either all at once or as time and resources become available. Collections are not arranged in isolation; elaborate processing of one collection is always carried out at the expense of others.

Restricted Access The management of collections that contain restricted documents is a challenge for most archives. Because the ramifications of mistakenly granting access to confidential records are potentially so grave, it is wise not to depend on the memory or the judgment of individual staff members, particularly since temporary, part-time, or nonprofessional assistants are often employed to assist researchers. Collections or portions of collections to which access is restricted should be clearly marked. Finding these markings on

a box of records should lead a reference staff member to consult the relevant access policies for guidance in meeting a request for access.

A termination date for restrictions is particularly important because many sensitive records become less sensitive as time passes; at the same time it also becomes more and more difficult to locate the person(s) empowered to make decisions or provide advice about access. Therefore, decisions about the duration of limited access should be made at the time of accessioning if at all possible, and provisions should be made to review the decision periodically. A termination date may be a particular year, or may be set with reference to a particular event, such as the death of the donor.

Cataloging

Traditionally, archives have met the need to inform with such finding aids as simple checklists of holdings, inventories, card catalogs, entries in the *National Union Catalog of Manuscript Collections* (NUCMC), published brochures and formal guides, and on-line catalogs. All of these descriptive tools have their place, both as end products and as interim measures. A sensible approach today is to direct the energies and resources of archives staff to the immediate or eventual adoption of the MARC-AMC catalog format and MeSH headings. The use of the MARC-AMC format and MeSH headings serve as a means of standardizing intellectual control of a repository's holdings. At the same time, these controls enable wider dissemination of information about the holdings. The MARC-AMC format is the standard format for archival and library data bases such as RLIN and OCLC. MeSH headings constitute the standard descriptive terminology for the health fields.

Cataloging is a time-consuming, demanding skill, requiring good judgment about historical, clinical, and scientific significance; a talent for summarizing both the substance and the essence of voluminous records in a few well-chosen sentences or phrases; the ability to choose the relevant key words for optimal indexing and retrieval; unusually good writing skills; familiarity with archival terms and conventions; a working knowledge of practices in the health fields and the terminology and principles of classification in those fields; an understanding of the administrative structure of the parent institution and similar institutions in the U.S. health care system; and experience. Even the best cataloging software cannot substitute for these skills. In other words, cataloging is best reserved for trained and experienced specialists.

It is in cataloging, more than any other function, that the principle of top-down processing is so useful. Unless there is a compelling reason to withhold information about a collection, all collections should be cataloged, if only in the broadest terms. When resources are strained, an archives should begin (without apology) by providing at least a simple listing of its collections. An advantage of the MARC format, even for neophyte catalogers, is that cataloging data may be corrected and expanded easily when they are recorded on-line, making this computer format a useful tool in the top–down approach. MARC provides the structure in the form of data fields, and catalogers can enter as little or as much data as availability, time, and skill allow. The MARC format protects against the omission of important data by inexperienced catalogers. For partially cataloged archives, conversion to the MARC format may be employed as a tool for standardizing and polishing the cataloging that has already been done. An uncataloged collection presents a challenging opportunity to begin the use of the MARC-AMC format, or at the very least to develop a cataloging convention that is compatible with MARC.

However convenient the computerized format, filling in the blanks or fields does not automatically produce a coherent, balanced description of a collection. For this reason, the experience of writing freehand descriptions before undertaking computerized cataloging is instructive. An excellent way to learn cataloging is to read the descriptions written by accomplished professionals. Every year professional societies of archivists give awards for

outstanding finding aids. A study of such publications, whether they relate to the health fields or not, is a wise practice. A common procedure in archives is to have all cataloging critiqued by the other staff members, not only to correct errors and improve writing style but also to keep the entire staff informed about the repository's holdings.

A good description of a collection captures the overall scope and significance of the collection and places the collection in context while it performs the more obvious function of bringing out important subjects, names, and dates. For the cataloger, skill is involved in writing a description that is objective and free from value judgments, yet informative enough to help a researcher decide whether a certain group of records should be consulted. Given the volume of contemporary records collections and the geographic dispersion of repositories, researchers need help in discovering where *not* to look as well as where *to* look. For example, a researcher may be able to make a simple choice between two equally large bodies of correspondence in the personal papers of two equally important scientists if one set is described as "mostly routine correspondence relating to family vacations," and the other as "lengthy correspondence with John Falk concerning progress and problems in research."

The scope of a collection can be captured in several ways. One is a simple indication of quantity: "records, ca. 800 linear feet." Another is a brief summary that focuses on the relative quantities and quality of various types of record: "multiple drafts of published papers and lectures and of correspondence (73 letters dated 1976–1979) with publishers." In the case of personal papers, the context of the collection is established by providing enough biographical and historical information to

Fig. 11.8 **William Welch with Mayor Jackson of Baltimore at the site of a radio broadcast in 1932.** Aural documentation (e.g. sound recordings) augments the written record with the enlivenment of the spoken word. *Source: Alan Mason Chesney Medical Archives, the Johns Hopkins Medical Institutions.*

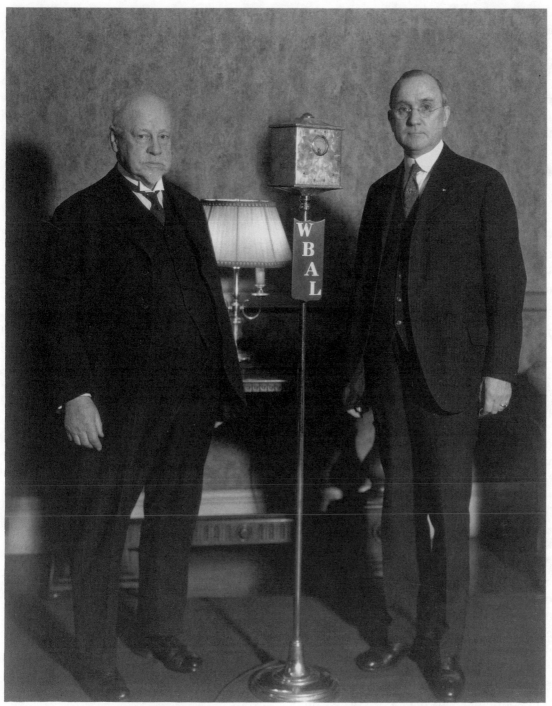

William H. Welch

January 1932

(mayor Howard Jackson

place the papers in time, in place, and in relation to colleagues and others in the field. A description of the records of an institution begins with a brief history of the institution.

Cataloging in an archives with health-related holdings, of course, focuses on descriptions of records that have significance to the health, life, and biological sciences. An accomplished cataloger will not, however, neglect important documents that fall outside the realm of the health fields or the collecting purview of the archives. The unexpected—such as correspondence with an eminent writer such as F. Scott Fitzgerald—is in particular need of cataloging because researchers will not normally search for such correspondence in a repository with clinical and scientific holdings.

A particular problem arises in large collections containing voluminous correspondence. Although it is possible and sometimes advisable to produce computerized listings of the names of hundreds of correspondents, it may be necessary to provide a selective list when cataloging. Indeed, such a selection is usually quite helpful to researchers. Choices will normally be made on the basis of the importance of the person and the importance of the correspondence, but one should not fall into the trap of cataloging only the great names, because such an approach leads to unbalanced research.

Archives often supplement in-house finding aids and computer cataloging with more traditional publications. Published guides vary in size from brochures to multivolume works and range in content from descriptions of individual collections or special collections to comprehensive guides covering the entire holdings of a repository. Since each of these types of finding aids makes special contributions, an archives contemplating publication should survey many different finding aids to determine which type best satisfies its goals. Guides serve the dual purpose of actively facilitating scholarship and stimulating reference and research use of holdings. These goals do not always mesh nicely, since serious scholarship is usually better served by extensive cataloging in humble clothing, whereas stimulants for research and reference demand selective summaries of salient information and reproduction of choice visual materials in attractive presentations. In addition, these enticing sorts of publications are expensive and time-consuming to produce. A compromise is often to be found in desktop publishing, which offers a less expensive way for an archives to list its holdings in various forms of attractive presentations.

CONCLUSION

Consistently good processing is critical to the overall intellectual and physical management of archival holdings. Through intellectual organization and description of contents, processing illuminates the informational value of holdings. Finding guides that are prepared during processing assist the staff in planning its priorities, and provide pathways for access and retrieval by users. Processing also entails a comprehensive system of physical controls, from housing of collections in the stacks to ensuring the well-being of individual items within collections. In a user-oriented archival program, processing plays an especially strategic role. Although the immediate purpose of processing is to protect the physical and intellectual integrity of the materials, the ultimate purpose is to make collections easily accessible for reference and research. Because processing functions to facilitate access and use, the processing staff should work in concert with the user services staff to monitor patrons' needs.

Specific processing goals for individual collections must be in keeping with the ultimate processing goals of the overall archival program. Whereas many small processing steps occur simultaneously or in close sequence, the total effort must always be guided by larger objectives. The ability to judge when to move from one step to another is learned by experience. Processing staff may serve the archives best if they are well versed in general principles and practices of research in the health fields and other related fields and well informed in the subject areas pertinent to the collection. Understanding legal and ethical precedents and regulations concerning the use of archival materials is equally important. An essential duty of processors is to keep abreast of professional standards in the archival field through professional societies like the Society of American Archivists, through professional journals and conferences, and through the Academy of Certified Archivists. Researchers who patronize archives depend on the training and judgment of the processors who organize and safeguard the documents without which history cannot be written.

BIBLIOGRAPHY

Compiled by Robert Sink

GAILLARD, A.J. 1988. Automating intellectual access to archives. *Library Trends* 36:495–623.

HAM, F.G. 1992. *Selecting and Appraising Archives and Manuscripts*. Chicago: Society of American Archivists.

HENSEN, S.L. 1989. *Archives, Personal Papers, and Manuscripts: A Cataloging Manual for Archival Repositories, Historical Societies, and Manuscript Libraries*. Chicago: Society of American Archivists.

HOLMES, O.W. 1964. Archival arrangement: Five different operations at five different levels. *American Archivist* 27:21–41.

LUCAS, L. 1981. Efficient finding aids: Developing a system for control of archives and manuscripts. *American Archivist* 44:21–26.

MICHELSON, A., ED. 1989. *Archives and Authority Control*. Technical Report no. 6. Pittsburgh: Archival and Museum Informatics.

MILLER, F. 1990. *Arranging and Describing Archives and Manuscripts*. Chicago: Society of American Archivists.

NEW YORK STATE ARCHIVES AND RECORDS ADMINISTRATION. 1991. *Guidelines for Arrangement and Description of Archives and Manuscripts*. Albany: New York State Education Department.

PEDERSON, A., ED. 1987. *Keeping Archives*. Sydney, Australia: Society of Archivists.

SMIRAGLIA, R. 1990. *Describing Archival Materials: The Use of the MARC AMC Format*. New York: Haworth Press.

SOCIETY OF AMERICAN ARCHIVISTS, COMMITTEE ON FINDING AIDS. 1976. *Inventories and Registers: A Handbook of Techniques and Examples*. Chicago: Society of American Archivists.

12

Making Provisions for the Management of Material Evidence

Philip D. Spiess II

THREE-DIMENSIONAL OBJECTS and other nontextual materials are often found in archives of the health fields. Such materials are referred to as material culture by anthropologists, cultural historians, and museum professionals, and are viewed by scholars in those fields as primary documentary resources. The term *material evidence* is used in this chapter to refer collectively to three-dimensional objects and other nontextual materials (e.g., specimens and artifacts, which include examples of the fine arts). Artifacts generally divide into decorative arts and technical arts.

In archives with holdings from the health fields, material evidence may include medical instruments and equipment; scientific apparatus;

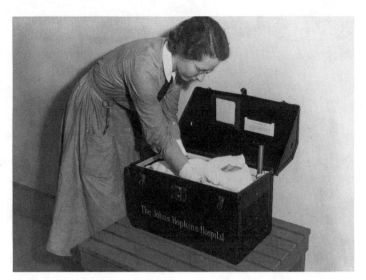

Fig. 12.1   **A carrier used to transport premature infants in 1938.**
Examples of equipment may be selected to demonstrate basic changes
in health care practices. *Source: Alan Mason Chesney Medical Archives,
the Johns Hopkins Medical Institutions.*

human remains and other biological specimens; medicines, drugs, and chemicals; examples of the fine arts, (e.g., paintings,
prints, and sculptures of prominent physicians and scientists and of important events in
the history of medicine, as well as medals,
plaques, and other testimonials and memori-
als); and examples of the decorative arts (e.g.,
furniture and furnishings from the homes, offices, and laboratories of prominent physicians and scientists, and articles of dress such
as uniforms and protective gear).

The classification of material evidence is divided into two broad categories: natural specimens and artifacts. A specimen is any object
found in nature and left in its natural state; it is
usually collected for examination or study. A
specimen may also be a sample that is used for
analysis and diagnosis. It may also be an element or compound used in or produced by
chemistry. An artifact is any object made or
altered by human activity with a view to subsequent use. A historic medical herb garden is
an artifact, even though it contains specimens;
so, too, is a laboratory or hospital room that
an archives may choose to acquire for historical research or exhibition. Thus, a collection
of pathological rarities may be composed of

multiple artifacts (historical specimen jars)
and multiple specimens (the rarities), while
being in itself an artifact.

PLANNING FOR THE DEVELOPMENT OF MATERIAL EVIDENCE HOLDINGS

Archives acquire examples of material evidence in order to augment holdings that are
largely textual. As a result, collections of material evidence present a twofold problem for
archival management: because they complement and supplement other evidence in the
archival holdings, they must be linked, intellectually and administratively, with the holdings of the other program components (e.g.,
historical records, personal papers, and contemporary records); however, because they
vary from the other holdings in terms of com-
pository material, shape, and size, they have to
be managed in accordance with the curatorial
standards of museum practice. Thus, the management of material evidence collections in archival repositories is essentially museum collections management carried out within the
larger framework of archival management.

The material evidence holdings of a museum or an archives comprise both a physical
collection and an intellectual collection. The
physical collection is the sum total of artifacts,
specimens, antiquities, and works of art accumulated by the repository for various com-
memorative and documentary purposes. The
intellectual collection is the body of data, records, publications, copyrights, and other documents and information accumulated by the
repository that relate to the contents of the
physical collection.

Collections of material evidence in archival
holdings are utilized for at least four major
purposes. They may serve as: reference resources for documenting scientific, clinical,
and educational activities; research resources
for in-house study and for visiting scholars to
use; exhibition resources for educational, com-
memorative, or publicity purposes; and educational resources for use in teaching, publications, lectures, and other forms of outreach.

Archives will not be able to put collections of material evidence to effective use until they employ the proper curatorial controls for their development, management, and use. Collections management controls should be applied to all material evidence under the care of an archives, regardless of its status in terms of legal ownership or institution-designated conditions of use (for example, as part of a permanent collection, a study collection, or a teaching collection; or as an exhibit "prop," a sample for conservation analysis, or an asset for sale or trade).

The mission of a material evidence component should be defined at the outset of planning for the archival program. It should flow out of the overall mission for the archival program and correspond with that statement's general provisions; likewise, the collecting plan for the material evidence component needs to be fully compatible with the overarching collecting plan for the repository. Since the collections of material evidence in archives are essentially adjuncts of the textual holdings, the collecting priorities of the former revolve around those of the latter. Whatever the collecting priorities of the repository, the material evidence holdings should relate directly to some aspect of the textual collections; otherwise, a separate museum collection is apt to be started on a de facto basis. The scope of the material evidence holdings, while consistent with the overall collecting scope of the repository, should be spelled out clearly in the collecting plan. Finally, the collections management policy for the material evidence component should correspond with the collections management policies for the program as a whole. It should identify the range of materials to be collected and specify criteria and standards for selection. Specific guidelines for drawing up a collections management policy for material evidence are given in chapter 3 of Marie C. Malaro's *Legal Primer on Managing Museum Collections* (1985).

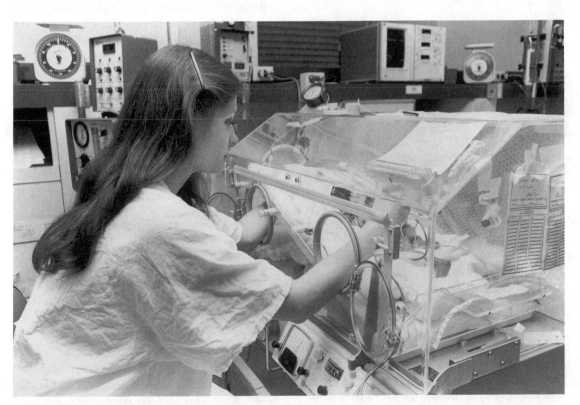

Fig. 12.2   **An incubator used for premature infants in 1981.** *Source: Alan Mason Chesney Medical Archives, the Johns Hopkins Medical Institutions; photograph by Virginia Brown.*

ESTABLISHING INTELLECTUAL AND LEGAL CONTROLS

The first step in defining the scope of the material evidence component in an archival repository is to determine what objects or types of object are needed to fulfill the component's mission. It is then necessary to decide how those objects will relate to the textual materials in the repository's other holdings. The material evidence component should be designed to augment and enhance the repository's acquisition plan. Objects should be appraised according to the criteria and standards outlined in chapter 7 of this volume.

Surveying and Assessing Existing Holdings

Once the question of scope has been addressed, the entire institution should be canvassed to locate artifacts and specimens that relate to the component's collecting plan. Having a prepared mission statement, a definition of collecting scope, and a collecting plan in hand may help the archives to establish a legitimate claim to items that are discovered or protect it

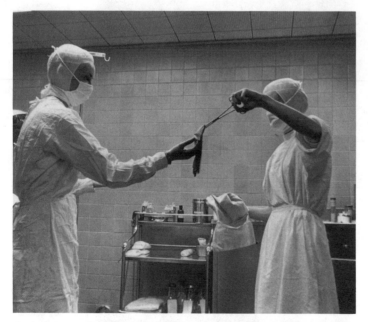

Fig. 12.3 **Examples of operating room apparel.** Apparel represents an important source for documenting change in health care practices. *Source: Alan Mason Chesney Medical Archives, the Johns Hopkins Medical Institutions; photograph by Werner Wolff, Black Star.*

from being forced to accept unwanted and irrelevant materials.

Likewise, the other holdings of the repository should be surveyed for items of material evidence. The items found should then be assessed to determine their relevance to the component's stated mission. At the same time, every object under the administrative jurisdiction of the archives, regardless of collection status, should be registered: the archives should have on file a brief, permanent record that identifies each object and its legal status to distinguish it from every other object. These records form the basis for the collection files, the documentation that physically identifies all the material evidence for which the archives has assumed responsibility, describes the legal status of each object, and traces its use, condition, location, and physical status.

Inventorying the Collection

The most basic procedure for establishing intellectual and legal control over a collection of material evidence is the inventory: the process of creating and maintaining a contemporaneous, reconciled, itemized record that identifies and locates the objects and collections for which an archives has assumed responsibility. The ability of the archives to identify accurately each item in its collection of material evidence and to locate that item has legal ramifications, whether the archives is operated as a private trust or as a public or charitable one.

A thorough inventory serves several purposes. Not only is it a systematic means of verifying that each object is registered and that its location records are accurate but it is also a useful planning tool, for a series of inventories over time will chart the collection's patterns of use, as well as its growth, storage, and security. Furthermore, an inventory serves as a review of whether each object is stored properly, and thus may alert the curator to a need for conservation treatment in a timely manner. Routine spot checks of an inventory may also serve as a deterrent to theft; furthermore, if a theft does occur, the spot checks will detect the loss relatively quickly. Prompt action then can be taken, with inventory records serving as documentation of the loss and indicating the time interval during which the theft most likely occurred.

The development of curatorial controls for the management of the material evidence component should begin with a baseline inventory: an initial, thorough, and standard-setting inventory on which later inventories can be based. This baseline inventory will usually identify a number of objects for which information about provenance or status is lacking, and it may even identify objects that have no documentation whatsoever; these objects should be designated "found in collection." Inventories from other components should also be consulted because they may contain references to objects that cannot be located. Once the baseline inventory is complete, a thorough attempt should be made to match the "unidentified" objects with the missing items' information; such reconciliation is an important follow-up to any major inventory.

Acquisition

Acquisition is the act of gaining possession; the term *acquisition* refers not only to the act itself but also to the object or group of objects to which an archives has acquired legal title. Such rights of ownership may be acquired in a number of different ways: by acceptance of a gift or bequest, by purchase, or by exchange. Archivists should be aware that many circumstances affect the quality of the legal title acquired with an object, and they should consult Malaro's *Legal Primer on Managing Museum Collections* (1985) for a thorough discussion of such factors.

The acquisition of an object by an archives does not automatically imply that it will be accessioned into the repository's collections; instead, it may be reserved for use in a study collection or a teaching collection, as background or supportive material for an exhibit, as a sample for analysis in conservation work (in the process of which it may be destroyed), or as an asset for sale or trade. Before acquiring an object, therefore, archivists should as-

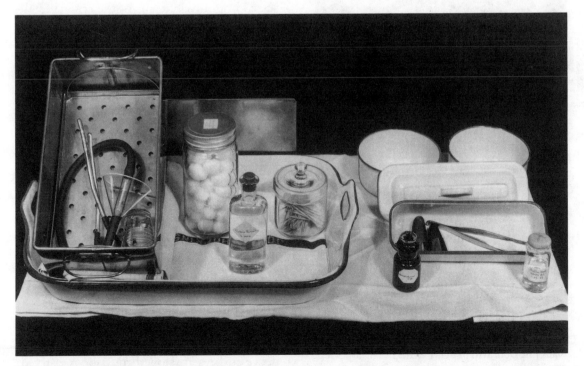

Fig. 12.4   **Clinical supplies.** Samples of material evidence may illuminate and help to interpret the written record. *Source: Alan Mason Chesney Medical Archives, the Johns Hopkins Medical Institutions.*

sess it (1) to ascertain whether its acquisition would be consistent with the mission of the material evidence component; (2) to determine whether it falls within the stated collecting scope for the component; (3) to anticipate how it will be used if acquired; (4) to determine whether it is of sufficient quality, and separate it from lesser-quality items in a large group of objects (such as a gift or bequest); (5) to ensure that the person or institution from whom the archives is acquiring the object currently possesses legal title to that object; and (6) to ensure that the archives has the wherewithal to store and care for the object properly. In short, a careful and thorough assessment of each object at the acquisition stage may prevent legal, ethical, and administrative problems at later stages in the process of collections management.

It is important for an archives to specify who has the authority to accept material evidence for the collection, regardless of whether

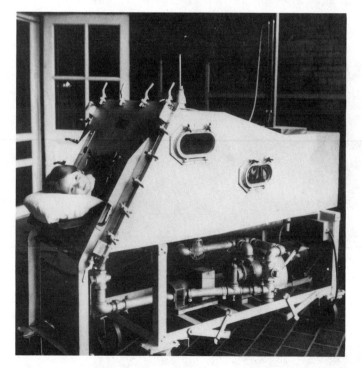

Fig. 12.5 **A Drinker Respirator at the Harriet Lane Home, circa 1931.** When it is impractical to preserve examples of large-scale equipment, photographs may serve as substitute documentation. *Source: Alan Mason Chesney Medical Archives, the Johns Hopkins Medical Institutions.*

that authority resides in an individual staff member or in a committee. Formal delegation of such authority, usually through the collections management policy, is a protection for both the institution and its staff. The policy should be developed by the staff, with the guidance and approval of the advisory committee, and should address the following questions:

- Who has the authority to purchase items of material evidence for the collection?
- Who has the authority to accept gifts of material evidence on behalf of the archives?
- Who has the authority to acknowledge gifts?
- Who is responsible for seeing that all necessary documentation of title has been obtained and promptly recorded?

Donations may serve as an important source for the development of material evidence components; most often artifacts and specimens will arrive as part of a larger donation of textual materials. These items must be assessed not only in terms of the criteria established for the acquisition of textual collections but also in terms of the criteria established for the material evidence collections. When material evidence is donated to an archives (either separately or as part of a textual collection), the archives should use a formal deed of gift as the legal document that establishes and records transfer of title.

Accessioning

Once an object has been acquired by an archives, it must be accessioned if it is destined to become a permanent part of the holdings of the archives. Accessioning is the formal process of recording an addition to the archival holdings; it is not a rote task but a process that requires careful thought and critical judgment about the appropriateness of the material being accessioned. Those items of material evidence to be accessioned must be registered, and all the relevant documentation must be gathered and organized. They must then be numbered and marked, cataloged, and perhaps classified. These procedures are discussed in detail in the following sections.

Numbering and Marking Objects

Each individual object in a collection of material evidence should be given a unique and permanent number, a catalog number, that establishes the object's individuality and links it to the written records that document its creation, its physical form and condition, its technology and/or iconography, its ownership, its use, and its scientific and cultural meaning throughout its existence (that is, all of its history as presently known). The purpose of such a number is simple: it establishes both physical and intellectual control over the material evidence holdings of the archives. Unlike an object name or title, the catalog number refers to one specific object only and

can be easily retrieved from large files of data by automated means.

In the past, museums often created a plethora of numbers and numbering schemes to identify every object transaction and activity. The result was a confusion of registration numbers, accession numbers, catalog numbers, identification numbers, inventory numbers, donor numbers, and classification numbers, with the result that the very purpose of numbering —quick, easy, and unique identification— was defeated. Museums also tried to create and use catalog numbers based on library classification systems (e.g., the Dewey system, the Cutter system), but this approach proved unworkable as well. In recent years, therefore, most museums have reduced their numbering schemes so as to use one main number for identification purposes. This number is usually the catalog number, and it may be formed in several ways. It may be a multidigit

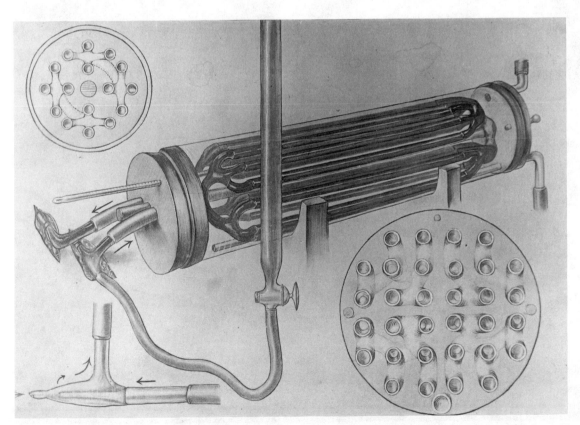

Fig. 12.6 **The vividiffusion apparatus designed by John Jacob Abel, circa 1915.** Design specifications are another source of documentation that may be preserved in lieu of the actual equipment. *Source: Alan Mason Chesney Medical Archives, the Johns Hopkins Medical Institutions; photograph by Nelson Edwards.*

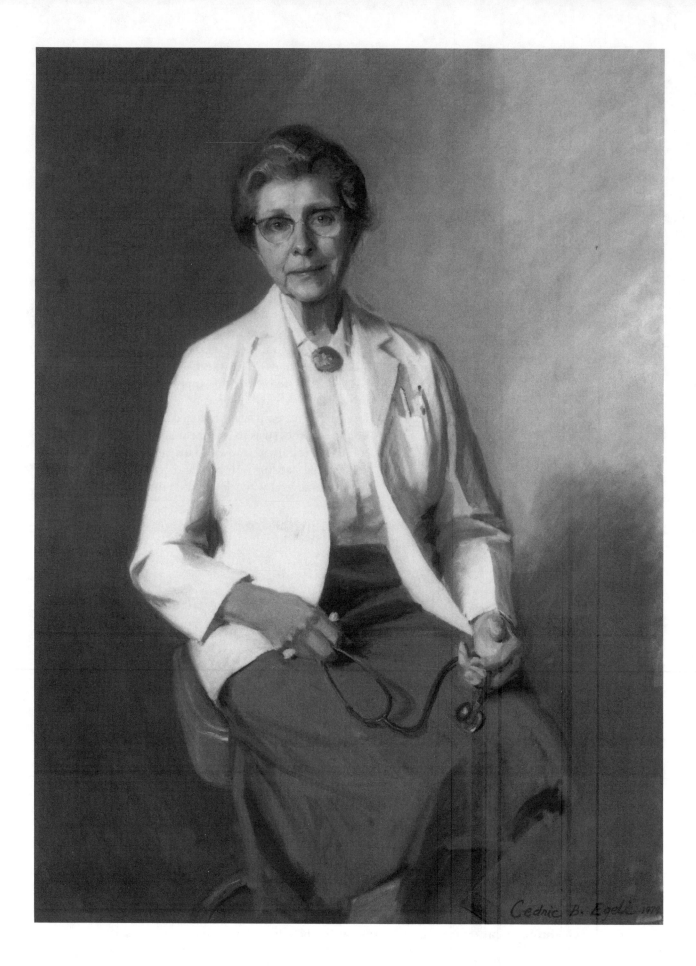

Cedric B. Egeli 1978

number of uniform length that is assigned in sequence. It may be an encoded number, indicating that the object has a particular collection status. Or it may be, as many museum catalog numbers now are, a tripartite number (often with a suffix) based on accessioning data.

Time has proven the usefulness of accession-based catalog numbers composed of multiple parts, particularly when the numbers are to be used in an automated system. For example, such a number could be constructed in four parts (each separated by some form of punctuation) that identify, respectively, the year of acquisition, the transaction number, the specific object, and the specific disjoint part (for example, an accessory) of the object being cataloged. Thus, "92.0012.133.04" would designate the fourth disjoint part of the 133d object in the twelfth transaction of 1992.

Such a numbering system could easily be adapted for archival use. However, as archivists do this, they must remember that in the case of museums the catalog number generally relates to a single, object-oriented acquisition, whereas in archival settings most material evidence is acquired as part of a collection of textual materials, and catalog numbers should reflect that relationship to the textual collections. Thus, the archival catalog number for an object should be composed of at least two segments: it should begin with the archivally assigned number that identifies the overall acquisition, transaction, or accession to which the object belongs; and this number should be followed by a unique suffix that specifically identifies the object itself and any disjoint parts it might have.

Whatever the system used, the number assigned to the object must tie the object to its parent acquisition and to its individual collection file (including registration documents,

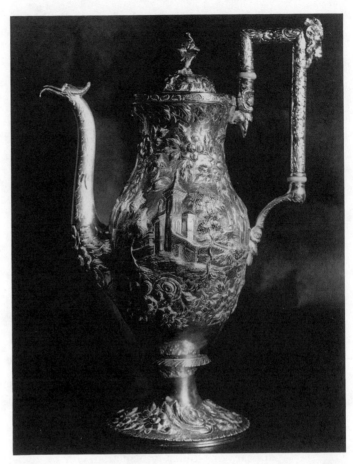

Fig. 12.8 **A silver coffeepot from the estate of Johns Hopkins.** Institutional relics may comprise another major part of material evidence collections. *Source: Alan Mason Chesney Medical Archives, the Johns Hopkins Medical Institutions.*

location records, research files, photographic records, conservation records, and any published accounts or analyses of it or of similar objects). If its number cannot be easily obliterated, the object may be identified quickly and accurately in cases of similarity, misplacement, or theft.

Thus, it is vital to place a mark, usually the catalog number, on the object. Because of the greater variety of types of material involved, the marking of objects differs in some particulars from the marking of manuscripts, records, and other paper- or electronics-based textual materials in archives, yet the principles of marking remain essentially the same. These principles are simple and based on common sense: the mark should be placed on the object

Fig. 12.7 **Portrait of Harriet Guild, M.D. (1899–1992) by Cedric B. Egeli.** Portraits of faculty and staff may constitute a large segment of material evidence collections. *Source: Alan Mason Chesney Medical Archives, the Johns Hopkins Medical Institutions; photograph by Aaron Levin.*

where it may be found relatively easily but will not be obtrusive when the object is displayed; and the mark should be affixed securely enough to prevent its casual removal but should be removable if necessary (for example, when the object is deaccessioned). In every case, care should be taken not to damage the object. If questions arise about the proper way to mark a particular object, a knowledgeable objects conservator should be consulted.

Cataloging

Cataloging, as the term is used in museums and archives, is the recording of all known information relating to an object, whether that information is physical, intellectual, cultural, or scientific. Such information may be a single entry (e.g., an object's spatial measurements) on a cataloging work sheet or many entries in a computer file (as in the case of data from a research project involving the object).

Cataloging is an ongoing, never-ending process. There is always the possibility that some new information about an object will appear, that older information will be reinterpreted in the light of new thinking, or that the object's physical properties will be reexamined using new analytical techniques. The information gleaned, recorded, organized, and stored in the course of cataloging provides the foundation for the preservation and interpretation of the material evidence held by the archives and, indeed, points the way to future collecting, research, and exhibition activity. An object's file is therefore never closed and never complete.

Cataloging is not merely a clerical task; each piece of data that documents a given object or group of objects represents an intellectual decision on the part of the cataloger. The everyday challenges of cataloging include making decisions about what to record, how to record it, how to describe the object(s) being cataloged, how to verify information, where to research, and what to name an unnamed object or a baffling object part. Thus, cataloging requires knowledge, training, and

determination; above all, it requires experience, which comes only from doing the actual work of cataloging.

The cataloging of material evidence, therefore, should be placed in the hands of persons who have studied material culture and are trained in the use of objects as cultural documents, individuals who know intimately the details of the kinds of material evidence being cataloged and who are practiced in "reading" objects, not only as items of science-oriented material culture but also as symbolic reinforcements of the ideas, beliefs, and values of the persons, societies, and institutions that created, owned, and used the objects.

In all cases, the object to be cataloged should be before the cataloger as it is examined and described. Using printed, written, oral, or pictorial information or documentation to catalog an object without having studied the physical details of that object at first hand is the equivalent of relying on hearsay evidence. At best, it may lead to the object's being confused with other, similar objects; at worst, it may foster errors in the cataloging of the object. To verify, clarify, or augment the data obtained from the object itself, the cataloger's own direct knowledge of the object, gained through examination and manipulation as well as through training and experience, should then be supplemented by the other forms of documentation (printed, written, oral, and pictorial) that may exist for the object.

The common procedure for cataloging objects is to devise a simple work sheet (of not more than one page, front and back) on which to record the data being gathered. The work sheet should be compatible with the form that is used for cataloging the other types of documentation in the holdings of the archives. Which data are recorded depends in large part on the individual archives doing the recording, but any archives that is developing a cataloging work sheet should take into account both the mission of the material evidence collection and the likely uses of that collection.[1]

The data being recorded about an object should be broken down into small units of information, rather than being described in long narrative paragraphs. This approach makes it easier to retrieve data and to compare them with similar data on other objects; it also leads to greater standardization in the recording of the data. Furthermore, recording data in small "bites" of standardized information makes it much easier for an archives to prepare the data for automated retrieval.

An excellent technical guide to cataloging is *Common Databases Task Force: Final Report to the Field* (1989).[2] This publication explains the standardization processes for contemporary cataloging in museums of history and/or technology, lists standard data fields for individual objects, and describes these fields in a data dictionary. It also provides sample data cards that may be adapted as cataloging work sheets.

Among the activities involved in cataloging is the process of identifying and describing the disjoint parts of an object. These are items, pieces, or parts of an object that are separate or that can easily be separated (i.e., physically removed) from the core of the object or from other parts of the object. Modular components, accessories, attachments, spare parts, and containers are all considered disjoint parts, as are tools and supplies (such as wrenches, graph paper, ink, oils, or keys) for operating or repairing the associated object when they are being viewed as part of an object group. Some items to be cataloged can be considered aggregate objects (i.e., they may consist of a group, a pair, or a set of items). For example, a balance scale and its weighing pans together make up one aggregate object.

Catalogers also need to research and document the provenance and association of each item being cataloged. The term *provenance* refers to the origins, background, and circumstances (including legal ownership) of an object or collection before it came into the custody of the museum or archives. On the whole, the more that is known and documented about an object's provenance, the greater the research and interpretive potential of that object. The term *association* refers to any relationship between or among objects, persons, institutions, and/or events. In museum work it is most commonly used to indicate a linkage between a given object or group of objects and one or more persons, institutions, or events. Any available data that relate to an object's provenance and associations should be carefully recorded on a cataloging work sheet.

When all of the information currently available about an object has been recorded on a work sheet, some or many of the data fields will still be blank. This is not a cause for concern, because it is highly improbable that any given work sheet will ever be filled out completely. However, these records should be completed as accurately and thoroughly as possible, because they are a central part of the file for a given object.

The cataloging of an object often includes several other activities, including the marking and photographing of the object (if this has not already occurred during accessioning).[3] The catalog number should be "permanently" marked on the object, and one or more black-and-white photographs should

---

1. It is desirable to use the same cataloging form for all archival holdings, both recorded documentation and material evidence. However, there is disagreement in the museum community as to the utility of library-based cataloging practices (such as the MARC format). Many museum professionals find MARC inadequate for cataloging museum objects. Currently, a project is under way to catalog museum objects at seven institutions in Ohio, using MARC format and MeSH headings. Early reports of this project indicate its success in adapting the MARC format to object cataloging (Gerstner 1992).

The goal of cataloging the material evidence in an archives using MARC format (or whatever cataloging format is being used for recorded documentation) is to integrate the intellectual controls for the overall holdings, thus making all documentation in the archives (regardless of format or media) more accessible to users.

2. This guide, which was published jointly by the American Association for State and Local History and the National Museum of American History, represents a major effort in the museum field to bring about greater professional collaboration in dealing with a common agenda of issues and standards.

3. For purposes of clarification, it is important to note that cataloging extends beyond accessioning; also, objects may be cataloged which are not accessioned. Hence, marking and photographing are done either at the time of accessioning or, if the object is not to be accessioned, at the time it is cataloged.

be taken of the object and, perhaps, of its key parts. In addition, legal documents relating to the acquisition of the object by the archives, together with other relevant textual documents (such as operating or instructional manuals, trade catalogs, laboratory notes, transcribed reminiscences, and exhibition catalogs), should be reconciled with the object.

Whereas museums store all the documentation on a particular object in an individual file, archival repositories need to treat most material evidence and its documentation as an integral part of the overall holdings, because in almost every case the material evidence is part of an acquisition and/or accession that is composed primarily of textual materials. For example, an archives might acquire a surgeon's personal papers, together with an instrument that the surgeon had developed and used; the surgeon's notes regarding that object would probably be housed with the rest of the papers. Some items of an archival object's documentation (e.g., operating manuals and/or handwritten memoranda on the object's creation or use) will therefore be filed with the other textual materials of that acquisition. The object's collection file will contain all collections management documentation on that object since its acquisition by the archives: e.g., the deed of gift, the cataloging work sheet, location records, loan records, and condition reports. In addition, the archives should include one or more photographs of the object in its file; such pictorial records will expedite intellectual access to the collections while reducing the need to handle objects or visit storage areas to review material evidence holdings.

No matter how the object and its related documentation are stored, it is most important that the two be linked by catalog number, preferably by the use of a numbering scheme such as that described earlier in this chapter. If the archives acquires new material that happens to relate to a previously acquired object, however, the new material must be treated as a discrete entity, a new and separate accession that cannot be directly linked by catalog num-

ber to the previously acquired object. Instead, the new material and any other items that should be linked to the previously acquired object can be listed by catalog number on that object's cataloging work sheet under the heading "Associations." A fuller description of this practice is given in *Common Databases Task Force: Final Report to the Field* (1989).

Classifying

An archives may want to classify its material evidence, an activity that is part of the cataloging process. Classification is the identification and placement of an object or object group within a systematic arrangement on the basis of its physical characteristics, origin, function, or other noteworthy features. Objects are classified in museums to organize them or to group them by certain distinguishing characteristics for purposes of physical and/or intellectual control. The classification of material evidence, therefore, is similar to the classification of library holdings or of natural specimens; it begins with the broad division of material evidence into two groups: specimens (including chemical elements), and artifacts (including fine and decorative arts).

Most natural specimens in material evidence collections are classified according to systems developed in taxonomy and pathology for such objects. In the case of artifacts, however, the situation is more complex. There are many different ways of categorizing the various physical and cultural aspects of artifacts, because in addition to their properties of material, construction, and form, artifacts carry with them important properties relating to their use, ownership, history, and cultural and symbolic import or meaning. The diverse nature of these properties has prevented the museum profession (and others in the field of material culture) from developing a single satisfactory and universally applicable classification system for manufactured objects, despite many attempts to do so.

Each archives, therefore, must develop for itself a workable classification system for its material evidence, based in part on any classification or subject-indexing scheme it has developed for its collections as a whole (i.e., the textual collections) and in part on the kinds of material evidence being collected and the ways in which they are being used. Elaborate classification systems have been designed for several of the major medical museum collections in the United States, notably the national collections in the Division of Medical Sciences of the National Museum of American History (at the Smithsonian Institution, in Washington, D.C.) and in the Howard Dittrick Museum of Historical Medicine (Cleveland, Ohio). Because of the size and complexity of these collections, their systems probably are not immediately applicable to smaller archival programs, except perhaps as models.

Controlling Access and Use

To conserve, study, and interpret the material evidence in its collections, an archives must ensure that it maintains both physical and intellectual control over those collections. The rules and guidelines that are established regarding the intellectual control of material evidence should correspond with those that determine access to the repository's textual collections. Such regulations, which are to be incorporated into the collections management policy for the material evidence component, should cover who has access to material evidence and to data about particular objects; what staff members are allowed to make decisions about access; and how decisions on such questions are to be made. Archivists should carefully review and apply the appropriate freedom of information and privacy laws, whether their repository is part of a publicly or privately funded institution (see chapter 8).

Patent rights, trademark rights, and copyrights are legal property rights that affect most material evidence in museum and archival collections, and these rights are distinct from the right to possess the object. For example, an archives may have acquired a particular type of patented hypodermic syringe

for its collection, or it may have been given the original artwork for a famous medicine's advertisement (e.g., the advertisement for "Lydia E. Pinkham's Vegetable Compound"), but ownership of the physical object does not automatically carry with it the right to reproduce the object and distribute or sell the reproductions. Likewise, certain company images or logotypes ("logos") may be protected by trademark or copyright, with these rights remaining with the inventor, the manufacturer, or the distributor of the object on which the image appears rather than being transferred to the archives with the other rights of ownership in the object.[4]

This distinction may not, at first glance, seem to be a matter about which an archives need concern itself. However, there will be occasions when patrons request to photograph an object, reproduce or publish a photograph of an object, or even exhibit an object that is protected by patent, trademark, or copyright (or has a particular part or label that is so protected). In responding to these requests, the staff should be careful not to infringe upon patent or trademark regulations or copyrights.

The issue is complicated, particularly because of the copyright law that became effective in January 1978. According to this legislation, copyright owners control five uses of copyrighted material: the right of reproduction; the right of adaptation; the right of distribution; the right of performance; and the right of display. (The last two rights depend on the nature of the material in question.) When an archives is in the process of acquiring an object that appears to be protected by copyright, it is therefore important that the repository establish who holds the copyright and whether any existing copyright interests pass to the archives with the object.

---

4. In some instances an inventor may sell the rights of the invention to a distributor, who in turn licenses a manufacturer to produce the object to be distributed.

Deaccessioning and Disposition

Deaccessioning is the process of permanently removing from the holdings an object that was once accessioned, then formally recording that removal. In deaccessioning an object, both legal and ethical standards must be applied. Because the act of accessioning an object implies that an intellectual judgment was made that the object was worthy of indefinite preservation by the archives, so the act of deaccessioning an object must be carried out thoughtfully, with serious consideration given to the reasons the object is no longer of value to the collection. Two major questions should be asked: should this object be removed from the collection? and if so, what is the appropriate method of disposal for the object? Disposal, the physical removal of an object from the collection (by sale, exchange, transfer, donation to another institution, or actual destruction of the object), may sometimes raise more difficulties than the decision to remove; where and how the object should go must be weighed, therefore, as thoughtfully as whether the object should go.

In all cases of deaccessioning, a repository must be able to justify its decisions concerning the removal and disposal of materials. No difficulty should arise if the decisions were made in accordance with the mission statement and collecting plan for material evidence. To ensure that the component's mission and its holdings continue to correspond with one another, the staff should periodically review the holdings to reevaluate the relevance, condition, and quality of the objects.

ESTABLISHING PHYSICAL CONTROLS

The repair and conservation of material evidence deemed worthy of preservation by a museum or an archives should not be carried out by a nonspecialist. There are, however, many everyday matters of object care that staff members working with material evidence collections should know. A particularly useful reference work on this subject is *The Care of Antiques and Historical Collections,* by Per Guldbeck (1985). Archivists should note, however, that advice concerning conservation is likely to change as previously unknown hazards emerge, as new tools and products are developed, and as ongoing research points to improved conservation methods. For conservation beyond everyday care, the reader is directed to the American Institute for Conservation of Historic and Artistic Works's *Guidelines for Selecting a Conservator* (1985).

CONCLUSION

All repositories of museum objects have two basic functions: to preserve objects, and to ensure the utilization of those objects as stated in the mission. The material evidence component in an archival program fulfills the same broad functions of preservation and utilization that are the functions of the other components of the program. In most respects the policies, precepts, and management procedures that govern the holdings of recorded documentation should be used to govern the material evidence holdings as well. A description of the subject content of the material evidence should be fully integrated with the content descriptions of all other archival holdings, and documentation of the objects' creation and use should be well represented in the textual collections.

Only material evidence that has direct relevance to recorded documentation in the archival program should be collected; to do otherwise surely would be to exceed the archival mandate. Objects should not be collected if they cannot be cared for properly, and incoming objects should be accepted with specific archival uses in mind. A statement of the scope of collecting for the material evidence component should dictate which kinds of objects are to be accepted into the collection and which are not.

Objects worthy of preservation require certain basic but professional treatment in archives; the current management precepts designed to ensure such treatment have been presented in this chapter. The particular user services offered by an archival program will further influence how its collections of material evidence are to be managed, and the use of specific objects by researchers and teachers will create the need for additional attention to be paid to those items. A firm grounding in basic conservation methods, therefore, is of great importance to any member of an archives staff who has responsibility for a collection of material evidence.

ACKNOWLEDGMENTS

The volume editors wish to thank Mary Garofalo for her contribution to the genesis of this chapter.

BIBLIOGRAPHY

AMERICAN INSTITUTE FOR CONSERVATION. 1985. *Guidelines for Selecting a Conservator.* 2d ed. Washington, D.C.: American Institute for Conservation of Historic and Artistic Works.

BACHMANN, K., ED. 1986. *Basic Principles of Storage.* New York State Conservation Consultancy Bulletin no. 1. New York: Cooper-Hewitt Museum (Smithsonian Institution) and New York State Conservation Consultancy.

BOROWSKI, E., WITH R. BURKE. N.D. [ca. 1983]. *On Guard: Protection Is Everybody's Business.* OGV-92. Washington, D.C.: Smithsonian Institution, Office of Museum Programs.

BOROWSKI, E.; WITH D.M. BRETZFELDER, J. CHAMBERS, B. COFFEE, J. DODD, C. LUSH, J.A. MAHONEY, E. MCMILLAN, J. NICHOLSON, R.M. ORGAN, AND E. ROBINSON. 1979. *Protecting Objects on Exhibition.* Series on the Preventive Care of Museum Objects for Non-Conservation Museum Personnel. POS-10. Washington, D.C.: Smithsonian Institution, Office of Museum Programs.

BURKE, R.B., AND S. ADELOYE. 1986. *A Manual of Basic Museum Security.* Leicester, England: International Committee on Museum Security, with the Leicestershire Museums, for the International Council of Museums.

Caduceus: A Museum Journal for the Health Sciences. 1985–. Springfield: Southern Illinois University School of Medicine, Department of Medical Humanities, Pearson Museum.

COMMON AGENDA FOR HISTORY MUSEUMS, COMMON DATABASES TASK FORCE. 1989. *Common Databases Task Force: Final Report to the Field.* Washington, D.C.: American Association for State and Local History and National Museum of American History.

DARIUS, J. 1988. Beware the lab cannibals. *Scientist* 2 (February 8): 11.

DEISS, W.A. 1984. *Museum Archives: An Introduction.* Chicago: Society of American Archivists.

DUDLEY, D.H., I.B. WILKINSON, G. BRUCKNER, ET AL. 1979. *Museum Registration Methods.* 3d ed., rev. Washington, D.C.: American Association of Museums.

FALL, F.K. 1973. *Art Objects: Their Care and Preservation.* La Jolla, Calif.: Laurence McGilvery.

FORCE, R.W. 1975. Museum collections: Access, use, and control. *Curator* 18:249–55.

GERSTNER, P.A. 1992. A stethoscope among the books, a scalpel in the archives: Cataloging artifacts in the historical collection. *Watermark* 16 (1): 1–3.

GULDBECK, P.E. 1985. *The Care of Antiques and Historical Collections.* 2d ed., rev. and exp. by A. B. MacLeish. Nashville, Tenn.: AASLH Press.

International Journal of Museum Management and Curatorship. 1989. Museums and the study of material culture. 8:259–62.

JOHNSON, E.V., AND J.C. HORGAN. 1979. *Museum Collection Storage.* Protection of the Cultural Heritage: Technical Handbooks for Museums and Monuments no. 2. Paris: United Nations Educational, Scientific, and Cultural Organization.

LEE, W., B.M. BELL, AND J.F. SUTTON, EDS. 1982. *Guidelines for Acquisition and Management of Biological Specimens.* Lawrence, Kans.: Association for Systematics Collections.

LESTER, J. 1983. A code of ethics for curators. *Museum News* 61:36–40.

LIGHT, R.B., D.A. ROBERTS, AND J.D. STEWART, EDS. 1986. *Museum Documentation Systems: Developments and Applications.* London: Butterworths.

MCHUGH, A. 1980. Strategic planning for museums. *Museum News* 58:23–29.

MAINE STATE MUSEUM. 1990. *Accessioning and Cataloging Museum Collections.* Augusta, Me.: Maine State Museum.

MALARO, M.C. 1979. Collections management policies. *Museum News* 58:57–61.

———. 1985. *A Legal Primer on Managing Museum*

Collections. Washington, D.C.: Smithsonian Institution Press.

———. 1991. Deaccessioning: The American perspective. *International Journal of Museum Management and Curatorship* 10:273–79.

MUSEUM DOCUMENTATION ASSOCIATION, MUSEUM DOCUMENTATION SYSTEM. 1981. *Practical Museum Documentation.* 2d ed. Duxford, England: Museum Documentation Association.

O'REILLY, P., AND A. LORD. 1988. *Basic Condition Reporting.* Southeastern Registrars Association.

PHILLIMORE, E., COMP. 1976. *A Glossary of Terms Useful in Conservation, with a Supplement on Reporting the Condition of Antiquities.* Ottawa: Canadian Museums Association.

The Prescription: Newsletter of the Medical Museums Association. 1985–. London, Ont.: Medical Museums Association.

REED, P.A., AND J. SLEDGE. 1988. Thinking about museum information. *Library Trends* 37 (Fall): 220–31.

ROBERTS, D.A. 1990. *Planning the Documentation of Museum Collections.* Duxford, England: Museum Documentation Association.

ROTH, E. 1990. Deaccession debate. *Museum News* 68:42–45.

ROWLISON, E.B. 1975. Rules for handling works of art. *Museum News* 53.

SAMUELS, H.W. 1986. Who controls the past? *American Archivist* 49:109–24.

SPIESS, P.D., II, COMP. 1991. *Cataloging Handbook: For the Museum Objects Collection of the DeWitt Stetten, Jr., Museum of Medical Research, National Institutes of Health, Bethesda, Maryland.*

———, COMP. AND ED. 1988. *Museums and Their Operations: A Basic Bibliography.* 5th ed., rev. Washington, D.C.: Smithsonian Institution, Office of Museum Programs.

TAYLOR, L.W., ED. 1987. *A Common Agenda for History Museums: Conference Proceedings, February 19–20, 1987.* Nashville, Tenn.: American Association for State and Local History; and Washington, D.C.: Smithsonian Institution.

U.S. DEPARTMENT OF THE TREASURY, INTERNAL REVENUE SERVICE. *Determining the Value of Donated Property.* Publication no. 561, rev. Washington, D.C.: U.S. Government Printing Office.

WARD, P.R. 1978. *In Support of Difficult Shapes.* Museum Methods Manual no. 6. Victoria, B.C.: British Columbia Provincial Museum.

WEIL, S.E. 1987. Deaccession practices in American museums. *Museum News* 65:44–50.

Conclusion

Nancy McCall and Lisa A. Mix

IN THIS BOOK our overarching goal has been to promote a greater awareness of the archival issues associated with twentieth-century documentation in the health fields. One of our major objectives has been to draw attention to the intellectual potential of this documentation and to suggest ways in which it can be harnessed and better utilized through changes in archival theory and practice. The approaches presented for reconceptualizing archival programs are grounded primarily in principles of use. Our recommendations for the archival selection, organization, and management of documentation have been guided mainly by the evidential and informational usefulness of the documentation for ongoing teaching, research, and health care delivery. Consideration has been given to the teaching and research needs of the health, life, and biological sciences as well as to those of the social sciences and the humanities.

Our main hope is that this book will stimulate wider appreciation of the informational and evidential values of documentation in the health fields. In turn, we encourage archival programs at institutions in the health fields to adopt more focused criteria and higher standards in the selection of their holdings. We urge that these programs broaden the scope of their acquisitions to include scientific as well as clinical documentation and at the same time promote wider research use of their holdings. To facilitate active study and scholarship, they must commit themselves to making the holdings more intellectually accessible through standardized and integrated systems of cataloging. They should design finding aids to enable the widespread sharing of data and information for purposes of research whenever legal and ethical conditions permit.

The strategies for archival administration and management that we present are intended to motivate self-assessment by individual programs and to activate a self-directed course of change. Whereas we suggest that archives in the health fields adopt a core set of curatorial and ethical principles, we recommend also that they adjust the scope and scale of their programs to fit the resources of their particular institutions. Each program must ultimately assume responsibility for charting its own course of development.

ASSUMING A PROACTIVE MODE FOR THE MANAGEMENT OF CONTEMPORARY DOCUMENTATION

The changing intellectual, physical, and technical characteristics of contemporary documentation in the health fields require a proactive mode of archival management. In confronting the scale of contemporary materials, their complexity of content, multiplicity of formats, and fragile media, archival programs must adopt new approaches to collections management. To identify significant documentation and to take the necessary measures for its preservation and utilization, archival intervention must come at an earlier stage in the life cycle of documentation.

Whereas new means of verbal and nonverbal communication have altered many basic clinical, research, and teaching practices, they also hold implications for change in archival practice. Some of these new means of intellectual communication have altered basic ways in which documentation is created, transported, and utilized. As a result, documentation has been transformed in terms of its physical composition and cognitive format, and the technical means by which it is activated and communicated.

Archivists and records managers can no longer rely upon the incubation of time to guide their appraisal and selection decisions. The fragility and ephemeral nature of much of the media of contemporary documentation demands that retention decisions must be made more promptly in the present rather than at a future time when the intrinsic value of the documentation might be better understood. In instances when the documentation cannot be preserved for a long period of time in its original physical state, archivists and records managers have to intervene to preserve its intellectual content. They must act promptly to assure that the content of the documentation may be preserved either by processes of regular refreshment, as in the case of computerized documentation, or by transfer to a more stable and durable medium such as microfilm or paper. Archivists and records managers are thus compelled to shift their focus from the preservation of documentation in its original physical state to preserving the integrity of its original content as it is converted to different formats and media in the passage of time. With some documentation, archivists will have to follow its path of conversion in conjunction with its provenance.

No longer able to rely exclusively on the maturation of time, archivists and records managers are now compelled to appraise the value of content while documentation is relatively new. Compounding this situation is the accelerating life cycle of documentation in the health fields. Some types of documentation pass rapidly from the stages of creation and active use to those of retirement and inactive use in short spans of time. Whereas archival and records management disposition policies have centered around documentation in more durable media with longer cycles of active use, these policies are now having to accommodate the presence of ephemeral media and accelerated cycles of activity. The limited life-span of the media of some contemporary documentation, together with its shortened cycle of active use, is forcing archivists and records managers to alter and expedite their appraisal practices.

The model of knowledge management in the medical library field offers an approach that may be followed for the appraisal of contemporary documentation. Designed to assist the creation and management of scholarly knowledge through computerized applications for storage and representation, the model of knowledge management draws upon the collaboration of a multidisciplinary team. The expertise of the team is pooled to develop and manage bases of knowledge in a particular field. Archivists and records managers should follow the lead of the librarians in the health fields and begin to work more closely with the creators as well as the users of documentation. They need to develop a more informed means of appraisal and a more proactive approach to the management of contemporary documentation.

Ascertaining what documentation is significant requires that each institution establish criteria for the range of documentation that is needed to support its current and long-range mission. The documentation of major institutional functions such as health care delivery, teaching, and research should be given precedence. Whereas the scope of collecting has to be broadened to consider the full spectrum of documentation at each institution, it should also be firmly grounded in a highly specific acquisition plan. The scale of collecting will inevitably be adjusted to fit the availability of institutional resources. Collecting documentation without the means to preserve and utilize it is almost as much a disservice as is the failure to collect. The act of collecting is a responsibility that includes obligations to maintain materials both physically and intellectually and to guarantee their availability for access and use.

ADAPTING CURATORIAL THEORY AND PRACTICE TO MEET THE KNOWLEDGE NEEDS OF THE HEALTH FIELDS

The fact that documentation in the health fields is strongly interrelated in terms of content makes it necessary to integrate the administration and management of these materials at the curatorial level. Although an individual procedure in some aspect of research or health care delivery may generate different formats in various media, it is important to recognize that these manifestations of documentation share an inherent intellectual relationship even though they may be physically diverse. As a result of curatorial conventions, some of these formats may be placed in different types of repositories. However, if they are maintained in separate locations, it is critical that provisions be made for integrating access and retrieval of these materials on the basis of the intellectual content. Theory and practice for archival, records management, manuscript, and museum programs in the health fields should be united in common functional areas. These curatorial practices should adopt a common language and style for description. This will enable them not only to work more effectively with each other in the administration and management of related holdings but also provide cross-cutting access to and use of those holdings.

ACKNOWLEDGING THE PLACE OF COMPUTERIZATION

Of all the new technologies, the advent and growth of computerization has had the greatest impact upon the nature and the use of documentation in the health fields. Computerization has brought about fundamental changes in the format of documentation, the physical composition of media, and the communication of intellectual information. Computer applications present numerous options for the management of documentation in both hard-copy and electronic formats. Finding aids and catalogs to collections in hard copy may be computerized to facilitate more rapid access to and retrieval of documentation in a repository's holdings. Some selections of documentation in hard copy may even be converted to a computerized system so as to enable more rapid access to and retrieval of the elements of content. In the acquisition of documentation that is already computerized, new possibilities exist for streamlining modes of collections management and user services. In some instances, collections of computerized documentation may be processed more quickly than comparable collections in hard copy, and thus be made available in a more timely manner for active reference and research. Computer applications may also be used to assist the administration of collections development, collections management, and user services. In taking advantage of the powerful tools of computerization, archival programs also assume new responsibilities for safeguarding computer software and hardware. Whereas computer applications have enhanced and rapidly accelerated the generation, collection, and transmission of data and information, they have also introduced a new set of preservation issues.

Archivists, however, must embrace the advantages that computerization brings to archival administration and management while also making a concerted effort to deal with the physical and technical fragility of electronic media. The ability to transmute data and information from one medium to another creates exciting new possibilities for the organization and preservation of documentation, as well as its retrieval and use.

DEALING WITH CHANGE

An underlying difficulty for archival theory and practice in the health fields is that these fields exist in a milieu of rapid and constant change. Just as the knowledge base of the health, life, and associated biological sciences is continuously evolving, technologies, laws, and regulations are also in a continuum of change. As a result, archival theory and practice must keep pace with the changing environment of the health fields and be responsive to developments in the intellectual, physical, and technical nature of documentation. As contemporary issues force a reexamination of archival theory and practice, new approaches to the administration and management of archives will be implemented. Dealing with change may arouse uncertainties, but it may also stimulate new ideas and thus energize modes of archival practice.

MAKING PRACTICAL AND CREATIVE CHOICES

In the selection and development of archival holdings at institutions in the health fields, many options exist for practical as well as creative choices. The abundance of documentation presents both opportunity and difficulty for collections development. Individual archival programs must examine the choices that are available to them and define their own acquisition plans. The criteria and standards for selection should consider not only the evidential and informational value of documentation, but also the practical requirements and the costs that would be entailed in maintaining it and making it available to a user population. In determining the scope of its acquisition plan, an archival program should be guided primarily by the mandated functions of the parent institution and their relevance in the larger context of the U.S. health care system. In examining institutional functions, planners should consult Joan Krizack's *Documentation Planning for the U.S. Health Care System*. Krizack and her co-authors describe the types of institutions that make up the U.S. health care system and their mandated functions.

Selection should be guided not only by the scope of the institutional mission and the program's acquisition plan, but also by the level of resources available for the management of the materials under consideration. When the intrinsic value of documentation is significant and yet the resources are not immediately available for its maintenance and use, the archival program should be encouraged to find alternative and supplemental sources of funding. Thus the development of holdings is not a simple linear progression but a dynamic process that entails the constant balancing of priorities and options.

Although archival programs in the health fields are labor-intensive to operate, administrative costs may be defrayed by an intra-institutional job-sharing approach. In this way a core staff of professional archivists run the program in conjunction with support from specially appointed committees and personnel from institutional departments who serve as liaisons to the archives. The departmental liaisons help to coordinate the transferal and processing of materials, while the committees guide the implementation of policy. Although it may be conceded that the administrative and intellectual returns from an archival program help to justify the operating costs of the program, careful financial planning is still an imperative. The philosophic objectives of an archival program must always be offset by the pragmatic requirements of practice.

DESIGNING ARCHIVAL PROGRAMS TO ADVANCE KNOWLEDGE

The ultimate aim of this volume is to stimulate archival programs in the health fields to be more focused and selective in the development of their holdings. We urge that when selecting holdings archival programs consider not only the immediate evidential needs of their institutions but also the larger informational needs of health care delivery, research, and teaching.

In addition to urging the development of coherent and well-focused holdings, we also advocate that efforts be made to promote the use of these primary source materials whenever legal and ethical conditions permit. By facilitating better means of access to and retrieval of these materials through improved processing and user services procedures, archival programs will heighten the usability of their holdings for activities of reference and research. It is our hope that users who are pro-

vided with a rich array of primary source materials and ease of access for study will have greater opportunities to advance new areas of knowledge.

Hospitals That Participated in the National Records Survey of Academic Medical Centers

One hundred and sixteen teaching hospitals (designated academic medical centers by the Council of Teaching Hospitals) were contacted. The seventy-eight respondents to the survey are listed below, arranged according to state.

Arizona
University Medical Center

Arkansas
University Hospital, University of Arkansas for Medical Science

California
Loma Linda University Medical Center
University of California, Los Angeles, Hospitals and Clinics
University of California, Davis, Medical Center
University of California, San Francisco
Los Angeles County–University of Southern California Medical Center
University of California, Irvine, Medical Center
San Francisco General Hospital and Medical Center

Connecticut
Yale–New Haven Hospital
John Dempsey Hospital, University of Connecticut Health Center

District of Columbia
Georgetown University Hospital
George Washington University Hospital

Florida
Jackson Memorial Hospital
Shands Hospital
Tampa General Hospital

Georgia

Crawford W. Long Memorial Hospital
Emory University Hospital
Medical College of Georgia Hospital and Clinic

Illinois

Northwestern Memorial Hospital
Foster G. McGaw Hospital

Indiana

William N. Wishard Memorial Hospital

Kansas

University of Kansas Medical Center

Kentucky

University Hospital, University of Kentucky
Medical Center
Humana Hospital-University

Louisiana

Louisiana State University Hospital

Maryland

Johns Hopkins Hospital

Massachusetts

Beth Israel Hospital
Massachusetts General Hospital
New England Medical Center
University of Massachusetts Medical Center

Michigan

University of Michigan Hospital

Minnesota

Saint Mary's Hospital

Missouri

Truman Medical Center
Barnes Hospital
University of Missouri Hospitals and Clinics
University Hospital

Nebraska

Saint Joseph Hospital
University of Nebraska Hospitals and Clinics

New Hampshire

Mary Hitchcock Memorial Hospital

New Jersey

University of Medicine and Dentistry of New
Jersey, University Hospital

New Mexico

University of New Mexico Hospital

New York

Albany Medical Center Hospital
State University of New York Health Science
Center at Brooklyn
University Hospital
State University Hospital, Upstate Medical
Center

New York Hospital
New York University Medical Center
Strong Memorial Hospital
Mount Sinai Hospital
Westchester County Medical Center

North Carolina

North Carolina Baptist Hospital, Inc.
Duke University Hospital

Ohio

Cleveland Metropolitan General–Highlandview
Hospital
University Hospitals of Cleveland
Ohio State University Hospitals
University of Cincinnati Hospital
Medical College of Ohio Hospital

Oklahoma

Oklahoma Teaching Hospitals
City of Faith Medical and Research Center

Oregon

Oregon Health Sciences University Hospital

Pennsylvania

Hospital of the University of Pennsylvania
Thomas Jefferson University Hospital
Hospital of the Medical College of Pennsylvania
Temple University Hospital
Pennsylvania State University Hospital–Milton
S. Hershey Medical Center

Rhode Island

Rhode Island Hospital

Tennessee

Vanderbilt University Hospital

Texas

Parkland Memorial Hospital
University of Texas Medical Branch
Hermann Hospital
Methodist Hospital

Utah

University of Utah Hospital

Vermont

Medical Center Hospital of Vermont

Virginia

Medical College of Virginia Hospitals

Washington

University of Washington Hospital

West Virginia

West Virginia University Hospitals, Inc.

Wisconsin

University of Wisconsin Hospitals and Clinics

Index

laws: pertaining to archival holdings, 133–36, 141–44; pertaining to copyright, 217
*Legal Primer on Managing Museum
Collections* (Malaro), 207
Lehmann, Harold, 74
Levine, Robert J., 135n
libraries, 88; and collaboration
with archivists, 149; use of
computers in, 80–81
Library of Congress subject headings, 149, 150
"life-cycle" concept, 222–23
Ludmerer, Kenneth M., 28n

machine-readable cataloging. *See*
MARC
MacNeil, Heather, 140, 145
Malaro, Marie C., 207
manuscripts, 88, 92, 93, 185, 213.
See also personal papers
MARC (machine-readable cataloging), 148–49, 150, 158,
189, 199, 200, 215n
Marks, Harry, 20n, 31n, 50, 59n
material evidence, 205–6, 218–
19; accessioning, 210–11; acquisition of, 209–10; assessing, 208; cataloging of, 214–
16; classification of, 206, 216–
17; controlling access and
use of, 217; deaccessioning,
218; development of hold-
ings, 206–7; inventorying,
208–9; numbering of objects,
211–14; physical control of,
218
media: defined, 2; new, 7; range
of, 122
medical libraries. *See* libraries
medical records. *See* patient records
medical records laws, 134–35
medical research. *See* biomedical
research
medical schools. *See* academic
health centers
Medical Subject Headings. *See*
MeSH
Medicare, 35, 36, 37
MEDLINE, 78, 78n, 80
MENTOR, 81
Merton, Robert, 57
MeSH (Medical Subject Headings), 109, 128, 149, 150, 158,
199, 215n
microfilm, 41–42
micrographics, 181–82
museums, 88, 211–13, 214
MYCIN, 81

National Academy of Sciences,
62
National Archives and Records
Administration (NARA), 149
National Institutes of Health, 29,
31, 62, 180–81
National Library of Medicine,
80–81; Medical Subject Headings, 149
National Records Survey of Academic Medical Centers, 40–
41, 73n, 101n, 167, 167n, 227–
28
National Science Foundation, 62
*National Union Catalog of Manu-
scripts Collections* (NUCMC),
199
nondisclosure statements, 144
NREN, 159

OCLC, 159, 199
ONCOCIN, 81
optical disk systems, 161
OVERSEER, 81

patient records, 33–35; administrative functions of, 38; ancillary diagnostic media, 37, 38;
computerization of, 78–80; as
distinguished from scientific
records, 54; evolution of, 35–
37; long-term retention of,
42–49; record-keeping procedures for, 40–42; research value of, 38–40; retention policies
for, 40–42; role of at academic
health centers, 37–40; unit
medical record, 35–37
PDQ (Physicians Data Query),
80
Pernick, Martin, 50
personal papers, 22–23, 88, 92,
131, 132n. *See also* manuscripts
personnel records, 29–30
PIP (Present Illness Program), 81
PLATO, 81
preservation, 103–4, 116–17
Pressman, Jack, 50
Price, Derek de Solla, 59
Privacy Act of 1974, 64
privacy issues, 30, 64, 130–35,
138–40
publishing. *See* scientific publishing

QMR (Quick Medical Refer-
ence), 81

radiology, 26; use of computers
in, 79
record-keeping systems, 40–42,
176–77; computerization of,
189–90
records management programs,
88, 92; at academic health centers, 167–68; computerization
of, 159; redefining concepts
of, 168–74; and regulatory
environment, 172. *See also*
contemporary records;
twentieth-century documentation, archival programs for
records scheduling, 177–78
repository catalog, 148
research. *See* biomedical research;
historical research
Research Libraries Information
Network (RLIN), 149, 158,
199
research protocols, 60n
restricted access file, 148
retroconversion, 161
Richter, Curt, 65, 65n, 67, 68
Robbin, Alice, 140
Rosenberg, Charles, 19n, 25n

sampling: of ancillary diagnostic
media, 47–49; of patient records, 42–47, 116; of scientific
records, 54–55, 116; systematic, 44–47, 49–50
Samuels, Helen, 10n
scheduling. *See* records scheduling
scientific publishing, 59–60, 67
scientific records: alternative research uses for, 64–67; archival issues in acquisition of,
55–58; conversion to
computer formats, 160–61; as
distinguished from patient records, 54; management of,
171–72, 180–82; reanalysis of
for processes of research, 61–
63; retention of, 54–55, 62–
63, 68, 116–17; reuse of,
60–61, 96–97; sampling
approaches, 54–55; sharing of,
57–64, 68–69; types of data,
56–57. *See also* biomedical research
shelf list, 148
Sieber, Joan, 63, 69
Sink, Robert, 203
Society of American Archivists,
139, 140, 203
Sociometrics, 67n
Spiess, Philip D., II, 149